Genetic Mosaics and Chimeras in Mammals

BASIC LIFE SCIENCES
Alexander Hollaender, General Editor
Associated Universities, Inc.
Washington, D.C.

A Continuation Order Plan is available for this series. A continuation order will bring delivery of each new volume immediately upon publication. Volumes are billed only upon actual shipment. For further information please contact the publisher.

Genetic Mosaics and Chimeras in Mammals

Edited by

Liane B. Russell

Oak Ridge National Laboratory
Oak Ridge, Tennessee

PLENUM PRESS · NEW YORK AND LONDON

Library of Congress Cataloging in Publication Data

Main entry under title:

Genetic mosaics and chimeras in mammals.

   (Basic life sciences; v. 12)
   "The chapters . . . are based on talks presented at the Symposium on Genetic Mosaics
and Chimeras held April 3—6, 1978 at Gatlinburg, Tennessee . . . sponsored . . . by
the Biology Division of the Oak Ridge National Laboratory as part of its annual
research conference series."
   Includes bibliographical references and index.
   1. Mammals — Genetics — Congresses. 2. Mosaicism — Congresses. I. Russell, Liane
B. II. Symposium on Genetic Mosaics and Chimeras, Gatlinburg, Tenn., 1978. III.
United States. National Laboratory, Oak Ridge, Tenn. Biology Division. [DNLM:
1. Chimera — Congresses. 2. Mosaicism — Congresses. 3. Mammals — Genetics —
Congresses. W3 BA255 v. 12/QH445.7 S989g 1978]
QL738.5.G46   599'.01'51   78-23172
ISBN 0-306-40065-0

Proceedings of the Symposium on Genetic Mosaics and Chimeras
held at Gatlinburg, Tennessee, April 3—6, 1978

© 1978 Plenum Press, New York
A Division of Plenum Publishing Corporation
227 West 17th Street, New York, N.Y. 10011

All rights reserved

No part of this book may be reproduced, stored in a retrieval system, or transmitted,
in any form or by any means, electronic, mechanical, photocopying, microfilming,
recording, or otherwise, without written permission from the Publisher

Printed in the United States of America

PREFACE AND SUMMARY

Liane B. Russell

Biology Division, Oak Ridge National Laboratory
Oak Ridge, TN 37830

Composite individuals have always excited mankind's imagination. Even the earliest recorded mythologies are full of fanciful
examples of creatures such as centaurs, mermaids, androgynes, and
winged horses. While real, naturally occurring, mosaics might not
appear as spectacular to the popular mind, their study -- particularly in *Drosophila* and plants -- has made important contributions
to genetics, starting relatively early in this century. In mammals,
too, examples of mosaics resulting from early or late somatic mutations and from abnormal egg maturation and/or fertilization events
have been known since the 1930's and exploited for the information
they could provide on such subjects as the origin of the germline
and the extent of cell mixing (see Russell 1964).

Two major, and unrelated, advances, both published 17 years
ago, suddenly provided a wealth of material for the study of mammalian mosaicism. One was the successful manipulation of early
embryos to make viable aggregation chimeras (Tarkowski 1961; Mintz
1962) -- a feat made possible by earlier advances in embryo culture
and transfer. The other was the hypothesis that only one X chromosome of a mammal is active (Lyon 1961; Russell 1961) and that, by
virtue of the fact that the choice of the active X is made at random early in development, the normal mammalian female is a mosaic
for any X-linked genetic heterozygosity.

The ensuing activity in these areas of research has formed one
of the most fruitful interfaces between scientific disciplines --
in this case genetics, embryology, cell biology, and reproductive
biology, to name a few. The coexistence in the same individual of
two different types of cells, recognizable by genetic markers, has

facilitated studies on cell lineage and clonal growth, totipotency
versus determination, autonomy versus inductive influences, cell
interactions, surface phenomena, cell selection, and the action of
hormones and antigens. Thus genetics has been used as a tool in
the study of development and physiology. On the other side, the
developmental studies on mosaics and chimeras have served to shed
light on such genetic problems as the turning off (and on) of
genes, spreading effects, the relation between sex-chromosome constitution and gametic sex, and the nature and time of occurrence
of spontaneous gene mutation, nondisjunction, and X inactivation.
Several of these problem areas were summarized in McLaren's stimu-
lating book "Mammalian Chimeras" (1976), which covers publications
through 1974.

In the four years since, the field has seen new explosive
growth as a result of recent advances in a number of areas. Among
these are the great sophistications in embryological microsurgery,
including immunosurgery, that have made possible the study of
minute cell groups and the transfer of single cells to recipient
embryos; the increased capacity for cytological identification of
chromosomes that has come from advances in banding and labeling
techniques; the more widespread use of cell hybridization; and the
healthy growth in mouse and human genetics that has led to the discovery and characterization of useful biochemical markers, sex-
reversal genes, and valuable chromosome translocations. One of the
most exciting components of the new chimera work is the utilization
of the teratocarcinoma system developed by Leroy Stevens (1975,
review) both *in vivo* and *in vitro*.

The chapters in this volume are by investigators who are ac-
tively engaged in contributing to the exciting areas of knowledge
that have been opened up by the new opportunities in mosaic research. Their findings will be briefly summarized.

Use of teratocarcinomas

Teratocarcinoma cells of various different derivations have
been shown to be totipotent when combined with normal cells in chimeras, indicating that the ordinarily malignant phenotype results
from a reversible change in gene expression rather than from a
permanent genetic change; and, in the case of LT cells, that the
block to parthenogenetic development is not a cell-lethal defect
(see chapters by Illmensee, Stevens *et al.*, Eppig *et al.*). The
establishment of cell lines from various teratocarcinomas has opened
opportunities for *in vitro* selection for specific mutations, and
for subsequent analysis of the developmental potential of the
mutant cells following blastocyst injection (Illmensee). The value
of teratocarcinoma stem cells for the study of X inactivation in an

in vitro system (Martin *et al.*)[*] and possibly for investigating X derepression (Kahan) has also been demonstrated.

X-chromosome differentiation

The problem of X chromosome differentiation has recently been readdressed in novel ways by a number of laboratories. By dosage measurements on individual embryos of products coded for by X-linked genes, several investigators (Monk; Chapman *et al.*; Kratzer and Gartler) have shown the early existence of bimodal distributions and a subsequent transition to unimodality. The cytological sexing of embryos in which dosage measurements were made (Epstein *et al.*) has confirmed that the high and low mode (which are related by a factor of about 2) are, as assumed, due to XX and XY embryos, respectively. These results show that X differentiation is due to inactivation of one of two previously active X's, rather than activation of one of two previously inactive ones. They also provide clues as to the stages when this event occurs.

There is increasing evidence that X differentiation occurs in the trophectoderm of the blastocyst before it occurs in the inner cell mass, the precursor of the embryo proper (Monk; Kratzer and Gartler). The suggestion has been made that X inactivation is associated with the departure of cells from the undifferentiated "stemline" (Monk); and there is evidence that the earliest inactivation that occurs is nonrandom. The preponderance of a presumed inactive X^P demonstrated by Takagi in yolk sac and chorion (descendants of the earliest tissues to differentiate) has been confirmed by West *et al.* with biochemical markers. Both laboratories have ruled out selection by the maternal environment, indicating that the parental origins of the X's have, in fact, "marked" them. Attempts to demonstrate nonrandom inactivation in extraembryonic membranes of humans were unsuccessful (Migeon and Do), possibly because no material earlier than newborn has to date been examined.

The rodent yolk sac and chorion, so far, provide the best demonstration of the existence of primary nonrandomness in placental mammals. Other examples of nonrandomness could be shown to be secondary, presumably resulting from cell selection (Russell and Cacheiro; Migeon). The appearance of nonrandomness may also be obtained as a result of transfer of gene product between cells (Migeon).

The inactive X of a female presumably becomes reactivated in her oocytes (although it is equally possible that the germline is

---

[*] All citations without dates refer to chapters in this book.

set aside from cells in which inactivation has not taken place).
Attempts to derepress the inactive X in somatic cells have made
various ingenious uses of human-mouse cell hybrids, translocation
markers, and *in vitro* selection for a specific gene product (Kahan;
Migeon, Sprenkle, and Do). In the very rare cases when derepression was achieved, this was a localized event not extending into
flanking regions of the chromosome. There is evidence (Kahan) that
the influences that maintain X repression are not trans-acting ones.
The likelihood that there is a single inactivation center in the
mouse X chromosome has been deduced from the inactivation pattern
in an assortment of X-autosome translocations (Russell and Cacheiro).

Gamete differentiation, sexual development, origin of the germline

Inactive-X mosaicism (with the added tool of "sex-reversal"
genes), nondisjunctional mosaicism (XO///XY and/or XYY), and chimeras
have all been used to study certain aspects of gamete differentiation and sexual development. While XX↔XY chimeras most often
develop into males, occasionally females, and only rarely hermaphrodites, the nondisjunctional mosaics in the BALB/c mouse appear
to be a particularly fruitful source of hermaphrodites possessing
ovotestes (Beamer *et al.*); and hermaphrodites are also found
in XX↔XX;*Sxr* chimeras, indicating that *Sxr* is not as strongly male-
determining as Y. There is considerable speculation about the
role of a testis-organizing antigen; and about which of the gonadal
cells possess or lack antigen receptors (Ohno; Gordon). Morphogenetic processes in the entire male genital tract are influenced
partially by autonomous cellular responses to testosterone and partially by cellular interactions (Drews; Ohno). With regard to the
gametes themselves, the evidence of several investigators (discussed by Tarkowski) indicates that XX cells cannot undergo functional sex-reversal, whereas it is possible that XY rarely can
become an oocyte, and XO is known to undergo spermatogenesis when
Sxr is present. The influence of the gonad's somatic cells on
gamete characteristics other than functional sex can be studied
in various ingenious ways by the use of chimeras (McLaren).

That the germline is set aside as a small number of cells has
been deduced from independent lines of evidence. One is the very
wide distribution of progeny ratios produced by mosaics resulting
from early somatic mutation either of mutable genes (Searle) or
at ordinary loci (Russell 1978). The other is a similar finding
for chimeras, which often have only one component represented in
the germline (McLaren).

Developmental problems addressed by the use of chimeras

Chimeras are being used in ever more sophisticated ways to approach a variety of developmental problems. For example, to answer the question of whether certain general, overt phenotypes are controlled by specific tissues, as many tissues as possible are analysed with respect to their chimeric composition. In the case of body weight, it appears that the overall phenotype may depend on cellular genotype throughout the body (Falconer *et al.*). In the case of behavior traits, on the other hand, some behaviors were found to co-vary with the cellular composition of specific brain portions, while others were found not to be correlated with the central nervous system (Nesbitt). Chimeras are also being used to analyse the action of certain lethal genes. An electron-microscope study of *t* alleles found one to be not strictly autonomous with regard to cellular phenotype, while the apparent autonomy of another may result from failure of cell surface association (Spiegelman). The importance of cell-surface interactions in relation to biochemical differentiation in one cell type has also been explored in cell-culture aggregates (Kozak).

Chimeras have lately been employed to determine the origin of carcinogen-induced tumors (Iannaccone), following the general type of analysis used by other investigators on spontaneous tumors arising in women heterozygous for X-linked markers. The induced tumors appear to be clonal growths.

Mathematical approaches to mosaicism

Studies of mosaics and chimeras entail interpretations of complex patterns and conclusions concerning precursor cell population sizes. Valuable mathematical and statistical models are found in three of the chapters. West, who has contributed much-needed definitions of spots formed in various ways, has concerned himself with analysing variegation patterns to tell something about their developmental history in terms of cell mingling and clonal growth. Whitten has produced a classical computer analysis of random mosaics in one, two, or three dimensions. Kane's statistical treatment of various data sets aims at estimating cellpool size at the time of X inactivation and organ-precursor selection. Future analysis of patterns will be aided by the development of useful cell markers (Gearhart and Oster-Granite).

———————

All of the chapters included in this volume are based on talks presented at the Symposium on "Genetic Mosaics and Chimeras" held April 3-6, 1978 at Gatlinburg, Tennessee.* The symposium was sponsored and supported by the Biology Division of the Oak Ridge Na-

tional Laboratory as part of its Annual Research Conference series.
Travel support for some of the overseas speakers was generously
provided by the National Science Foundation (Agreement No. PCM77-
26622). In planning the program and making arrangements for the
conference, I was assisted by an organizing committee (Drs. E. G.
Bernstine, J. Papaconstantinou, R. J. Preston, and R. W. Wallace)
and by the superb administrative talents of Mrs. Mary Jane Loop.
My very special thanks go to Mrs. Janet Varnadore for her unfailing
efficiency in the typing of this book.

---

* Only two of the scheduled symposium talks, those by C. E. Ford and
  by R. J. Mullen, are not included here. One of these was based on
  a paper printed elsewhere (Mullen and Herrup 1978).

REFERENCES

McLaren, A. 1976. Mammalian Chimeras. Cambridge University
Press, Cambridge, London, New York, Melbourne.

Mintz, B. 1962. Formation of genotypically mosaic mouse embryos.
Amer. Zool. 2: 432.

Mullen, R. J. and K. Herrup. 1978. Chimeric analysis of mouse
cerebellar mutants. In, Topics in Neurogenetics, X. O. Breakefield,
Ed. Elsevier North-Holland, New York.

Lyon, M. F. 1961. Gene action in the X-chromosome of the mouse
(Mus musculus L.). Nature, Lond. 190: 372-373.

Russell, Liane Brauch. 1961. Genetics of mammalian sex chromosomes. Science 133: 1795-1803.

Russell, Liane B. 1964. Genetic and functional mosaicism in the
mouse. In, The Role of Chromosomes in Development, Michael Locke,
Ed. Academic Press, New York, pp. 153-181.

Russell, L. B. 1979. Analysis of the albino-locus region of the
mouse. II. Mosaic mutants. Genetics, in press.

Stevens, L. C. 1975. Comparative development of normal and parthenogenetic mouse embryos, early testicular and ovarian teratomas,
and embryoid bodies. In, Roche Symposium on Teratomas and Differentiation, M. Sherman and D. Solder, Eds. Academic Press, New York,
pp. 17-32.

Tarkowski, A. K. 1961. Mouse chimeras developed from fused eggs.
Nature, Lond. 190: 857-860.

CONTENTS

USE OF CHIMERAS AND CELL AGGREGATIONS TO STUDY DEVELOPMENTAL POTENCY, GENE EXPRESSION, CONTROL OF PHENOTYPE, AND TUMOR ORIGIN

MATHEMATICAL AND STATISTICAL ANALYSES OF MOSAIC PATTERNS

Use of Chimeras and Cell Aggregations to Study Developmental Potency, Gene Expression, Control of Phenotype, and Tumor Origin

REVERSION OF MALIGNANCY AND NORMALIZED DIFFERENTIATION OF

TERATOCARCINOMA CELLS IN CHIMERIC MICE

Karl Illmensee

Department of Biology, University of Geneva, Switzerland

In this review, I should like briefly to summarize some new
approaches in experimental research on mouse teratocarcinomas.
During the past few years, these tumors have been tested for their
developmental potential, genetic constitution, and state of neoplastic transformation in the living organism, using microsurgery to
introduce the malignant stem cells into early mouse embryos. What
exactly are teratocarcinomas, and why are they becoming such a useful tool in analyzing gene expression during mammalian differentiation?

Mouse teratocarcinomas are tumors that either develop spontaneously in the gonads or can be produced experimentally from
embryos and primordial germ cells (see reviews by Damjanov and
Solter 1974; Graham 1977). Unlike most other tumors, they normally
contain a number of well-differentiated tissues, derived from all
three germ layers, such as brain and skin (ectoderm), gut and glandular epithelium (endoderm), muscle, cartilage, and bone (mesoderm).
The chaotic arrangement of the various tissue elements gives this
kind of tumor a monstrous appearance, as the ethymological root
(Gk: teraton) implies. Teratocarcinomas also contain a rapidly
dividing undifferentiated stem-cell population of embryonal carcinoma cells that is responsible for the malignant properties of
these transplantable tumors. By contrast, teratomas are composed
only of differentiated tissues and lack embryonal carcinoma cells;
they are therefore benign (Sherman and Solter 1975).

4

KARL ILLMENSEE

ORIGIN AND CHARACTERISTICS OF TERATOCARCINOMAS

Teratocarcinomas in the ovaries and testes of mammals have been known for some time, and their morphology and developmental behavior had been analyzed to some extent (see review by Askanazy 1907). However, little progress in understanding the ontogeny of this tumor was made until the first teratocarcinoma was found in the mouse (Stevens and Little 1954). Since then, considerable advances in teratoma research (Pierce 1967; Stevens 1967a) have established the mouse as an experimental system for a better understanding of the related human cancer (Dixon and Moore 1953; Norris, Zirkin, and Benson 1976).

Teratocarcinomas are relatively rare in humans, and it is usually not possible to trace the origin of individual tumors (Simpson and Photopulos 1976). On the other hand, there are two strains of mice that have high incidences of gonadal tumor formation. In the 129/Sv strain, about 10 to 30% of the males, depending on their genetic background, will spontaneously develop testicular teratomas (Stevens 1970a). In another strain, the LT/Sv, about 50% of the females spontaneously develop ovarian teratomas (Stevens and Varnum 1974).

FIGURE 1. Mouse teratocarcinoma OTT6050 derived from a 129-*Sl*/+ male embryo that had been grafted to the testis of a syngeneic adult host. In the ectopic site, the day-6 embryo transformed into a malignant tumor which could be propagated subcutaneously as a transplantable teratocarcinoma (Stevens 1970).

A. The pluripotent tumor is composed of various kinds of differentiated tissue of which only a few are represented here, e.g., cartilage (c), glandular epithelium (g), muscle (m), and primitive neuroepithelium (n). It also contains embryonal carcinoma cells (ec) as the undifferentiated stem-cell population.

B. After intraperitoneal injection into syngeneic mice, the solid teratocarcinoma has been converted into an ascitic form of "embryoid bodies." These round structures, the size of a preimplantation embryo (about 100 μm in diameter), consist of embryonal carcinoma cells (ec) surrounded by a layer of endoderm cells (e) that secrete Reichert's membrane (arrow).

C. After mild proteolytic treatment of small embryoid bodies (eb), the rind of endodermal epithelium (e) can be removed mechanically in order to collect the core of embryonal carcinoma cells (ec) for microinjection. ⟶

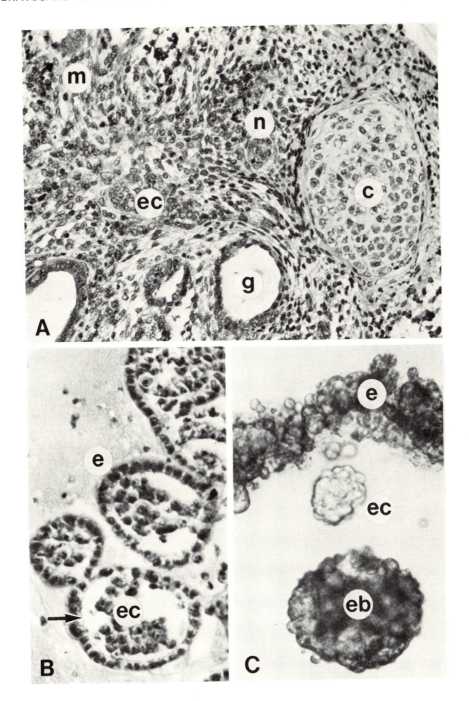

Figure 1

Testicular teratomas start developing within the seminiferous tubules of 129/Sv mice as early as the 15th day of gestation and are derived from primordial germ cells (Stevens 1967b) which, for unknown reasons, become neoplastic and escape the regular growth control during testicular ontogeny. Ovarian teratomas in LT/Sv mice also originate from germ cells, inasmuch as they arise from parthenogenetically activated eggs that grow quite normally into early embryos but then become disorganized, invade the ovary, and differentiate into various kinds of tissues without orderly *in situ* topography (Stevens 1974).

Teratocarcinomas may be experimentally produced by grafting genital ridges of day-12 embryos, or whole day-6 embryos, under the testis capsule of syngeneic hosts (Stevens 1967b, 1970b). In this ectopic site, they soon grow and proliferate progressively, leading to transplantable tumors that are morphologically and developmentally indistinguishable from spontaneous testicular or ovarian tumors. Some of those pluripotent teratocarcinomas (Fig. 1A) have been successfully converted into a modified ascites form dubbed "embryoid bodies" (Fig. 1B) because of their close resemblance to normal embryos (Stevens 1960). Presumed similarities between embryonal carcinoma cells and undifferentiated embryonic cells have further been revealed at the ultrastructural (Pierce and Beals 1964), biochemical (Bernstine et al. 1973), immunological (Edidin and Gooding 1975; Babinet et al. 1975), and developmental levels (Stevens 1974; Pierce 1974a).

Of the two presently available *in vivo* sources of teratocarcinoma cells, the solid tumors are deemed unfavorable because the malignant, multipotential stem cells are erratically intermingled with their benign, differentiated cellular progeny. The intraperitoneally propagated embryoid bodies, on the other hand, seem to be quite promising, since the location of their embryonal carcinoma cells has been revealed: the latter comprise a "core" surrounded by an endodermal epithelial "rind" of yolk-sac-like cells (Fig. 1C).

POTENTIAL OF *IN VIVO* PROPAGATED TERATOCARCINOMAS

Pluripotency of the embryonal carcinoma was conclusively demonstrated when single cells from completely dissociated embryoid bodies gave rise to solid tumors of varied tissue composition after subcutaneous transfer to syngeneic graft hosts (Kleinsmith and Pierce 1964; Jami and Ritz 1974). However, the apparent stability of the malignant phenotype, the consistent absence in teratocarcinomas of certain tissues, such as kidney, thymus, lung, and liver, and the immaturity and abnormal differentiation of other tissues has until recently left open the question whether embryonal carcinoma cells are, in fact, totipotent and therefore comparable to

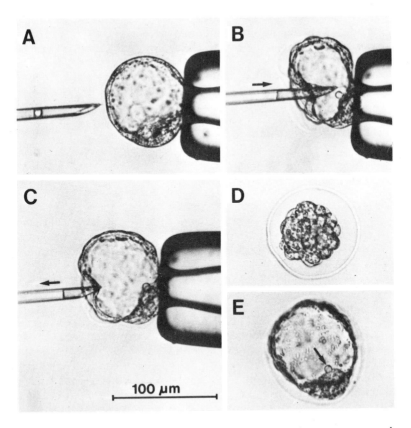

FIGURE 2. Procedure for microinjection of single teratocarcinoma
cells into mouse blastocysts.

A. With the aid of a blunt holding pipette, a well-expanded
blastocyst (4 days p.c.) is kept in the appropriate position.

B. The sharpened injection pipette, into which a cell has been
previously sucked, is gently pushed through the zona pellucida
and trophoblast into the blastocoel. The cell is then injected
and subsequently attached to the inner cell mass, the presumptive embryonic region.

C. The injection pipette is withdrawn slowly from the blastocyst in order to prevent detachment of the implanted cell.

D. Shortly after manipulation, the blastocyst collapses and
entraps the injected cell.

E. About 1 hr later, the blastocyst expands again to its normal size. The injected teratocarcinoma cell can still be seen
near the inner cell mass (arrow). After a brief *in vitro* incubation, the experimental blastocyst is surgically introduced
into the uterus of a pseudopregnant foster mother to allow further development.

normal early embryonic cells as far as their developmental capacity
is concerned. The absence of certain tissues in the many solid
tumors examined was consistent with the possibility that the stem
cells might not be comparable to totipotent cells of the preimplantation embryo but rather to some cells from later stages during
which they had become somewhat restricted in their developmental
capacity. Moreover, it was conceivable that during the process of
malignant transformation, the embryonal carcinoma cells eventually
lost their "genetic normalcy."

Male teratocarcinoma

     The similarities between embryonal carcinoma cells and early
embryonic cells pose the crucial question of whether the tumor
cells can, in fact, participate in normal development after being
brought into close association with cells of early embryos so that
the latter can provide an environment suitable for *in situ* differentiation. The most promising recipient is probably the blastocyst into which embryonal carcinoma cells can be injected microsurgically so as to entrap them near the inner cell mass, the presumptive embryonic region (Fig. 2). Here, during development, the
tumor cells eventually become integrated into the embryo after it
is subsequently transferred to a pseudopregnant foster mother.
Recent microinjection experiments have shown that teratocarcinoma
cells contribute to the coat (Brinster 1974, 1975). Unfortunately,
the recipient had not been otherwise marked genetically, so that
it was impossible to distinguish between any *internal* tissue contributions derived from the injected tumor cells and the random-
bred recipient.

     While this observation of coat chimerism was certainly encou-
raging, a more extensive genetic labeling seemed necessary to demonstrate normal tissue differentiation (Mintz and Illmensee 1975).
Orderly functioning of these tissues was attested to by the production of tumor strain-specific adult type of hemoglobin in erythrocytes, immunoglobulins in plasma cells, liver proteins in hepato-
cytes, glucose phosphate isomerase (GPI) heterodimers in muscle
cells, black eumelanin in melanoblasts, and phaeomelanin in follicle cells (Fig. 3). According to conventional classifications,
all germ layers were included in these differentiations. However,
since the old germ-layer concept probably undervalues flexibility
in development (Oppenheimer 1940), it is perhaps more relevant to
emphasize that the results show normal contributions of teratocarcinoma cells to many developmentally unrelated tissues, including
those tissue elements never seen in the solid tumors.

     While a haphazard integration of the injected tumor cells into
a limited number of tissues was occasionally observed, the terato-

carcinoma-derived chimeric mice did not significantly differ in
their mosaic tissue composition from normal embryo-derived chimeras
(reviews by Mintz 1974; McLaren 1976). Additionally, in two instances, tumor cells also formed reproductively functional sperm (Fig.
4). Thus, after almost eight years as a highly malignant tumor,
the male carcinoma stem cells appeared to be developmentally pluripotent and able to express their genetic repertoire in an orderly
sequence of differentiation of somatic and germ-line tissues.
Moreover, singly injected teratocarcinoma cells proved to be capable of contributing to virtually all tissues of an adult mouse,
thereby demonstrating their developmental totipotency (Illmensee
and Mintz 1976, and unpublished data).

    In a few instances, however, only tumors appeared postnatally,
and there was no participation in normal tissue formation, as
judged from biochemical and histological analysis. These transplantable tumors proved to be well-differentiated teratocarcinomas,
similar to the original OTT6050 tumor (Table 1). Of course, one
could argue that the embryonal stem-cell population is still
heterogeneous with respect to the malignant phenotype and that,
for example, one cell was able to become normalized whereas another
cell formed a tumor. The alternative explanation is that the embryonal carcinoma cell can either differentiate normally or give
rise to a tumor, depending upon the microenvironment into which the
injected cell happens to have been placed during ontogeny. In order
to distinguish between these two possibilities, a single teratocarcinoma cell was cloned *in vitro*; one daughter cell was then injected
into a blastocyst and another implanted subcutaneously into a syngeneic adult host. In some cases, the cell injected into a blastocyst
participated in normal tissue differentiation, whereas the subcutaneously implanted daughter cell produced a tumor, indicating once
again that the embryonic environment seems to be important in
bringing about reversion of the malignant phenotype.

    Additional evidence to support this interpretation comes from
another kind of experiment in which the inner cell mass of the blastocyst (i.e. the presumptive embryo) has been replaced microsurgically
by a core of about 20 embryonal carcinoma cells (Illmensee and Mintz,
unpublished data). While the remaining trophoblast of the recipient
predominantly served as implantation vehicle, the introduced malignant stem cells should have then exhibited their potential to normally
progress in differentiation without any participation by the embryo.
However, although implantation did occur in several instances, the
embryonal carcinoma cells were unable to develop into embryos but
rather formed teratomas after subcutaneous transplantation of the implantation sites to syngeneic hosts. It therefore appears as if the
malignant stem cells retain their neoplastic properties if left by
themselves and revert to normality only in close association with
normal embryonic cells.

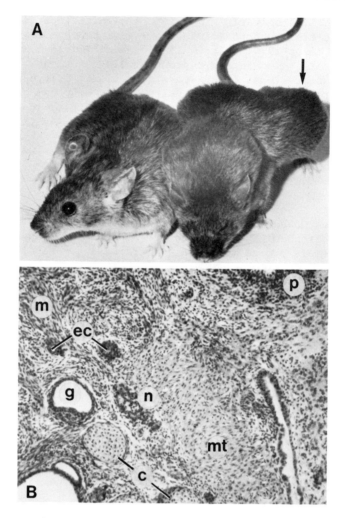

FIGURE 3. The *in vivo* potential of OTT6050 teratocarcinoma under
different environmental conditions.

A. Following microinjection into a C57BL/6-*b*/*b* blastocyst,
the teratocarcinoma cells become integrated and are capable
of contributing normally to the coat as well as to internal
tissues. A one-year-old healthy male chimera (left mouse)
shows teratocarcinoma-derived *agouti* hair-follicle clones
(darker areas) among the *brown* melanoblast clones (lighter
areas) derived from the recipient *b*/*b* genotype. Mosaicism
can be noted on the patchy tail as well. Additionally the
chimeric male had tumor-derived sperm in its testes, as demonstrated in matings with C57BL/6-*b*/*b* females. All the offspring exhibited the diluted *agouti* 129 teratocarcinoma phenotype and segregated in a Mendelian ratio for *Sl*/+ and +/+.

Female teratocarcinoma

As mentioned above, ovarian tumors develop spontaneously in adult females of the LT/Sv strain. The ovaries of some of these females contain embryos in various pre- and early postimplantation stages that result from parthenogenetic activation of mature oocytes (Stevens and Varnum 1974). Here, in the ectopic site of the ovary, the early embryo cannot develop properly but soon becomes disorganized and forms a tumor which is usually benign, but occasionally classifiable as a malignant teratocarcinoma (Fig. 5A). Only the latter form may be established as a transplantable solid tumor containing well-differentiated tissues as well as embryonal carcinoma cells -- similar to the testicular tumor. In order to test their developmental potential, we transplanted single LT72484 ovarian teratocarcinoma tumor cells into genetically different blastocysts (Table 1). Some of the resulting chimeric mice showed tumor-derived contributions (Fig. 5B) and internal organ mosaicism, as verified by GPI analysis (Illmensee and Mintz, unpublished data).

Totipotency of the ovarian teratocarcinoma cells, and their reversal to normalcy, were demonstrated by substantial contributions in all major tissues. Additionally, in one case, the tumor cells populated the germ line and developed into functional eggs, giving rise to healthy offspring. Limited tissue participation irrespective of conventional germ-layer theories was also observed (Table 2). Such a sporadic distribution could result either from late integration of injected tumor cells during embryogenesis, or from their restricted developmental potential. Because of the contributions of LT cells to functional, adult tissues of the chimeras, it is very unlikely that the early developmental standstill of parthenotes and their subsequent neoplastic transformation into ovarian teratomas result from an incomplete or altered "genetic make-up." Recent findings that parthenotes can be "rescued" by combination with normal embryos (Stevens, Varnum, and Eicher 1977; Surani, Barton, and Kaufman 1977) also favor the notion that developmental aberrations during parthenogenesis and teratocarcinogenesis are causally related to changes at the organismic rather than the genetic level.

By contrast with the normal development that follows injection into blastocysts, subcutaneous injection of a teratocarcinoma cell into a syngeneic adult host (right mouse) leads to the formation of a large tumor (arrow) after about four weeks.

B. This malignant tumor contains various tissues, similar to those seen in the original OTT6050 teratocarcinoma, e.g., cartilage (c), glandular epithelium (g), muscle (m), mesenchymal tissue (mt), pigmented epithelium (p), immature neuroepithelium (n), and embryonal carcinoma cells (ec).

TABLE 1. Microinjection of mouse teratocarcinoma cells into genetically different embryos at the preimplantation stage

Type of tumor utilized	Cells injected into blastocysts	Blastocysts transferred to foster mothers	Mice developed normally			Mice with tumors		References
			Total	Mosaic	(%)	Total	(%)	
OTT6050 ascites	3—5	280	93	13[†]	(13.9)	1	(1.1)	Mintz and Illmensee (1975)
OTT6050 ascites	1	161	71	18[†]	(25.3)	5	(7.0)	Illmensee and Mintz (1976)
LT72484 solid	1	158	74	8[†]	(10.8)	3	(4.0)	unpublished data
OTT6050 TK⁻ line	3—5	85	31	3	(9.6)	—	—	unpublished data
HxM hybrid cell line*	1	103	49[‡]	3	(7.0)	—	—	Illmensee et al. (1978)

* Clonally propagated cell hybrids derived from Sendai-virus-mediated cell fusion between mouse teratocarcinoma, deficient in thymidine kinase (TK⁻), and human fibrosarcoma, deficient in hypoxanthine phosphoribosyltransferase (HPRT⁻).

[†] Including one germline chimera each.

[‡] To date, biochemical and histological analyses have been carried out on 42 adult mice, of which three were chimeras. No tumors were observed in the experimental mice that developed from hybrid cell-injected blastocysts.

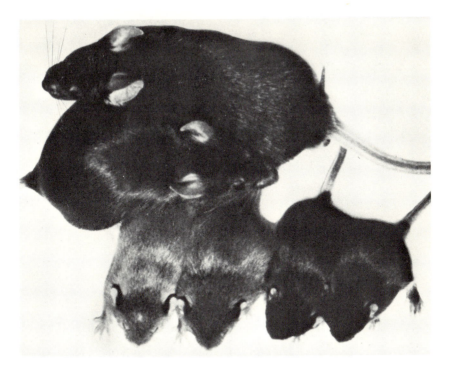

FIGURE 4. Germ-line chimera derived from an OTT6050 teratocarcinoma cell-injected blastocyst. The WH chimeric male, when mated
with a WH female, produced not only offspring with the expected
black WH phenotype but also some that had the diluted agouti
coat color of the 129 tumor-strain type. The tumor cell-
derived progeny segregated for *Sl/+* and *+/+* (first and second
baby from the left, respectively).

POTENTIAL OF *IN VITRO* CULTURED TERATOCARCINOMAS

     During the past few years, quite a number of different terato-
carcinoma cell lines have been produced under *in vitro* culture conditions and shown to be capable of differentiating into various
tissue structures as well as of producing tumors following subcutaneous implantation into adult hosts (Evans 1975; Nicolas, Avner,
Gaillard, Guenet, Jakob, and Jacob 1976; Chung, Estes, Shinozuka,
Braginski, Lorz, and Chung 1977). However, since the *in vitro*
assay systems are generally limited with respect to normal growth
and differentiation (Hsu and Baskar 1974), a more favorable environment is provided when cells are introduced into the living organism
in order to reveal their full potential.

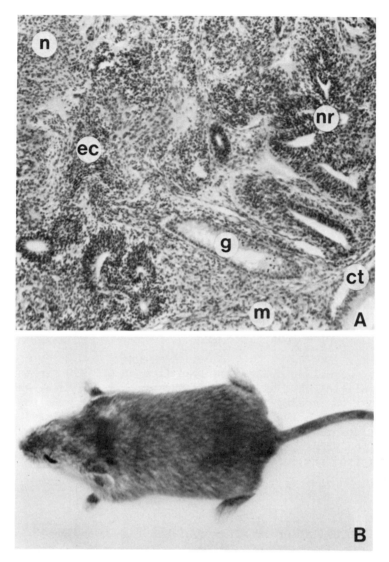

FIGURE 5. Pluripotent teratocarcinoma LT72484, which occurred spontaneously in the ovary of an LT/Sv female. The tumor has been
established as a malignant teratocarcinoma for many transplant
generations (Stevens and Varnum 1974).

A. In subcutaneous sites of syngeneic adult hosts, the tumor
cells differentiate into derivatives of all three germ layers,
e.g., neuroepithelial rosettes (nr), mature neural tissue (n),
glandular epithelium (g), muscle (m), and ciliated tissue (ct).
Among these well-differentiated tissues, there are clusters of

In a bioassay similar to that used for *in vivo* propagated teratocarcinomas, *in vitro* cultured embryonal carcinoma cells from other tumor sources proved competent in contributing to the coat and to several internal somatic tissues, although most of the chimeric mice additionally developed tumors in various anatomical sites (Papaioannou, McBurney, Gardner, and Evans 1975; Papaioannou, Gardner, McBurney, and Babinet 1978). This frequent tumor formation may have resulted from a large number of injected cells, unable to become properly integrated during early development, and/or from accumulated intrinsic changes that occurred during *in vitro* culture. It need not necessarily be pertinent to the original properties of teratocarcinomas.

Recent advances in clonally propagating various cell lines derived from teratocarcinomas (Evans 1972; Martin and Evans 1975; McBurney 1976) opened new ways of selecting somatic mutations (Boon, Kellermann, Mathy, and Gaillard 1975). It has been proposed previously (Mintz, Illmensee, and Gearhart 1975) that teratocarcinomas may provide a unique kind of cell which can be selected *in vitro* for a given mutation and then cycled through mice via blastocyst injection for further *in vivo* analysis (Fig. 6). Following such an experimental scheme, different sources of cultured teratocarcinoma cells that were selected either for hypoxanthine phosphoribosyltransferase (HPRT) deficiency (Dewey, Martin, Martin, and Mintz 1978) or for thymidine kinase (TK) deficiency (Table 1) seemed to retain their *in situ* developmental potential to a remarkable extent. However, the frequency of tissue mosaicism in adult chimeric mice was reduced compared with the rate of integration obtained from embryonal carcinoma cells of the original tumor (see Table 1). Nevertheless, these results indicated that teratocarcinoma cells selected *in vitro* for TK deficiency were still able to

---

embryonal carcinoma cells (ec) which represent the multipotential stem-cell population. Single cells of this ovarian teratocarcinoma were microinjected into CBA-T6/T6 blastocysts in order to assess their developmental capacity and state of malignancy during *in situ* differentiation.

B. Chimeric female with LT72484 teratocarcinoma-derived coat contributions (darker patches) in the head region and over the hindquarters (note also the patchy tail). The remaining agouti coat (lighter areas) originated from the CBA-T6/T6 genotype of the recipient blastocyst. In addition, this female turned out to be a germ-line chimera, with functional eggs derived from the injected tumor cell giving rise to healthy offspring.

TABLE 2. Limited tissue contributions* in postnatal chimeric mice derived from single teratocarcinoma cells after injection into genetically different blastocysts (data from Table 1).

Type of tumor cell injected	Blood	Brain	Spleen	Heart	Kidney	Reprod. tract	Muscle	Liver	Gut and stomach	Pancreas	Thymus	Lung
OTT6050 ascites	—	—	—	40	—	—	—	—	—	—	—	50
	—	—	—	—	—	—	60	—	—	—	—	40
	—	—	—	5	—	—	—	—	5	—	10	—
	—	—	—	—	—	—	—	—	—	—	—	75
	—	—	—	—	—	—	—	—	5	—	—	—
	—	—	—	—	—	—	—	60	—	—	—	—
	—	—	—	40	—	—	—	—	—	—	—	—
LT72484 solid	—	—	—	—	—	—	—	30	25	—	—	—
	—	—	—	—	—	—	33	—	—	—	—	—
	—	—	—	—	—	—	—	—	—	—	—	40
	—	—	—	—	—	60	—	—	—	—	—	—

*
Teratocarcinoma-derived tissue contributions are calculated in percent (i.e., 40 equals 40% in a given tissue) and are estimated from electrophoretic analyses of strain-specific allelic enzyme variants of glucosephosphate isomerase (GPI) in blood-cell lysates and tissue homogenates. The reduced number of mosaic tissues and their sporadic distribution in chimeric mice suggest late integration of cellular progeny of the injected tumor cell into the various organ primordia. In some instances, genetic mosaicism was found in developmentally unrelated tissues (e.g., in the heart and lung, or in skeletal muscle and lung), irrespective of conventional germ-layer theories.

differentiate into a variety of tissues -- e.g., liver, lung, heart, brain, and skeletal muscle -- and therefore could be used as carriers for introducing and analyzing foreign genetic material in vivo.

    In collaboration with Dr. Croce (Wistar Institute), mouse teratocarcinoma cells deficient in TK were fused with human fibrosarcoma cells deficient in HPRT, according to established proce-

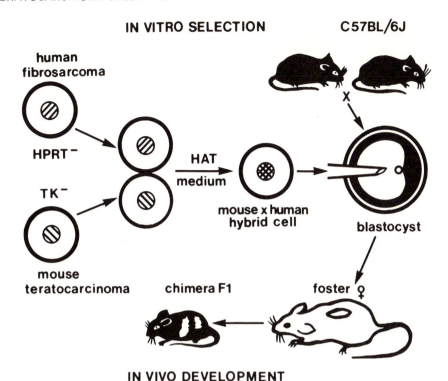

IN VITRO SELECTION   **C57BL/6J**

human fibrosarcoma

HPRT⁻

TK⁻

HAT medium

mouse x human hybrid cell

blastocyst

mouse teratocarcinoma   chimera F1   foster ♀

IN VIVO DEVELOPMENT

FIGURE 6. Experimental scheme of cycling human x mouse hybrid
    cells through mice via microinjection into blastocysts. Hybrid
    cells between human fibrosarcoma, deficient in hypoxanthine
    phosphoribosyltransferase (HPRT⁻), and mouse teratocarcinoma,
    deficient in thymidine kinase (TK⁻), were cultured in HAT
    medium. Single hybrid cells were then injected into C57BL/6
    blastocysts, bearing many genetic markers, in order to detect
    any *in situ* tissue differentiation derived from the injected
    cell. Shortly after micromanipulation, the blastocysts had to
    be surgically introduced into the uterus of a pseudopregnant
    foster mother to allow development to term. The live-born
    experimental offspring were analyzed for hybrid-cell contribu-
    tions in the coat, the various internal organs, and the germ
    line.

dures (Croce, Koprowski, and Eagle 1972). Only the interspecific
hybrid cells can grow in hypoxanthine/aminopterin/thymidine (HAT)
selective medium (Littlefield 1964). By contrast, TK- and HPRT-
deficient parental cells, which lack the enzymes required for the
incorporation of thymidine and hypoxanthine,, respectively, do not
survive in this medium. Under these selective conditions, the

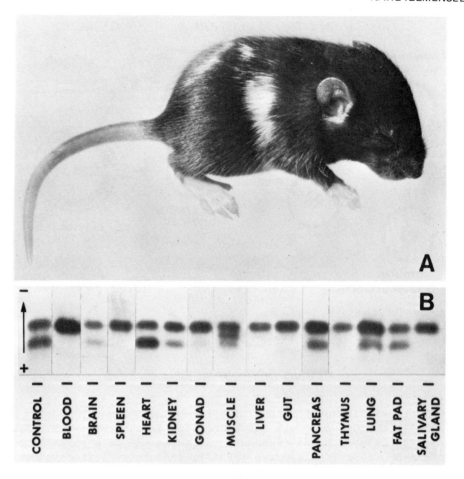

FIGURE 7. Adult normal tissue differentiation from human x mouse
   hybrid cells after injection into C57BL/6 blastocysts.

   A. Chimeric male showing substantial coat mosaicism. Amongst
   the black hairs of the C57BL/6 recipient, there are white
   patches on the hindquarters, tail, and feet, and a large white
   clone extending from the mid-lateral to the ventral side. All
   of these originated from the hybrid cell.

   B. Cellulose-acetate electrophoresis of glucosephosphate isomerase (GPI) obtained from tissue homogenates of a chimeric
   male (shown above). CONTROL represents a 50:50 GPI mixture
   of slow-migrating hybrid-cell type and fast-migrating C57BL/6
   type. Clonal descendants of the injected human x mouse hybrid
   contributed significantly to 7 of the 14 internal organs
   analyzed. They also fused normally with myoblasts of the
   C57BL/6 recipient, as judged from heterodimeric enzyme expression in skeletal muscle (Illmensee *et al.* 1978).

viable hybrid cells, which quickly lose human but not mouse chromosomes, retain at least human chromosome 17 that carries the locus
for TK (Matsuya, Green, and Basilico 1968). This particular
chromosome also carries a second known gene that is closely linked
to TK and codes for galactokinase (GLK) (Elsevier, Kucherlapati,
Nichols, Creagan, Giles, Ruddle, Willecke, and McDougall 1974).
The latter enzyme, with its characteristic electrophoretic mobility
quite different from the equivalent mouse enzyme, serves as another
useful biochemical marker for detecting the presence and normal
expression of the human gene product in the hybrid cells. Although
this experimental series has not yet been completely analyzed, we
have already obtained three chimeric mice, two of them with coat
mosaicism (Fig. 7A), and all three with substantial internal organ
contributions. The presence of heterodimeric GPI activity in
skeletal muscle attested to regular fusion of myoblasts between
host and hybrid cells (Fig. 7B). None of the mosaic tissues examined histologically in serial sections revealed any morphological
abnormalities or teratoma formation. By contrast, the subcutaneous
injection of human x mouse cell hybrids into athymic *nude* mice resulted in tumors, but not in teratoma-derived 129 hosts (Illmensee,
Hoppe, and Croce 1978).

It thus appears that the malignant hybrid cells become functionally integrated during mouse ontogeny and participate in
orderly *in situ* differentiation. But what happens to the human
gene products? At the moment, the answer is not so clear-cut,
since human enzymes have not yet been unequivocally detected in
the mosaic tissues; weak human-specific GLK activity could be
recovered only from the heart of one chimera and from the kidneys
of another. It is therefore obvious that the problems related to
the retention and recovery of human genes must first be solved
before we can effectively utilize our *in vivo* system for cycling
human genetic material through mice.

REVERSIBLE VERSUS STABLE ACQUISITION OF MALIGNANCY

Overwhelming data in cancer research accumulated over the
years have led to the simplistic, and yet quite appealing, notion
"once a cancer cell, always a cancer cell" (discussed by Pierce
1974b). Recently, however, there has been contradictory evidence
in plants (reviewed by Braun 1970, 1972) as well as animals (reviewed by Gardner 1977), suggesting that this kind of dogmatic concept no longer applies -- at least to certain tumors.

Transplantations of malignant cells into early mouse embryos
(the subject of this review) and of nuclei from tumor cells into
amphibian eggs (McKinnell, Steven, and Labat 1976) have shown that
neoplastic transformation can be reversed under appropriate environ-

mental conditions. A further example of presumed reversion is the
normal differentiation of initially malignant erythroleukemia cells
when injected into the spleens of irradiated normal mice (Matioli
1973). It therefore seems conceivable that the malignant state
does not always result from stable alterations in gene structure,
but rather from reversible non-mutational changes in gene expression, thereby leading to particular abnormalities during differentiation (Pierce 1967; Markert 1968).

At present, nothing is known about the "normalizing signals"
that enable an originally malignant cell to take part in normal
development, nor do we have any insight as to the mode of action
of these signals during cellular reprogramming.

CONCLUSIONS AND PERSPECTIVES

In recent years, it has been observed that mouse teratocarcinoma cells share some common developmental features with normal
embryonic cells and might therefore help us better to understand
some of the events occurring during normal cell differentiation
(reviewed by Martin 1975; Jacob 1975,1977). When utilizing the teratocarcinoma as an experimental model for the study of mammalian embryogenesis, one must always bear in mind the malignant properties
of these tumor cells. It is therefore crucial that one resolves
whether or not neoplastic transformation persists as a cell-heri-
table phenotype.

The most rigorous test for reversion to normalcy is to determine whether teratocarcinoma cells can make significant contributions to the normal differentiation in a mouse rather than in a
tumor. For this to occur, the initially malignant cells presumably
have to be brought into close association with cells of early embryos so that the latter can provide an organizational framework
appropriate for normal development. When this was done, it was
indeed found that the teratocarcinoma cells apparently lost their
malignancy and participated normally in organogenesis. With this
necessary prerequisite of a presumably intact genome, it should now
be feasible, at least for this particular tumor, to trace the origin and causes of malignant transformation and to further investigate the mechanisms underlying cell-to-cell interaction during the
process of neoplastic reversion.

Are teratomas unique as far as reversion to normality is concerned, or do other tumors with a similar capability exist? The
in vivo assay of introducing tumor cells into mice may enable us
to reveal whether more specialized neoplastic cells have already
undergone stable genetic changes that prevent reversion to normalcy,
or whether they are still developmentally flexible and, therefore,
might become integrated to some extent during organogenesis.

Considerable progress in establishing *in vitro* cell lines from various teratocarcinomas has opened new opportunities to clonally propagate certain cellular phenotypes, to select for somatic mutations, and to introduce xenogeneic chromosomal material via somatic cell hybridization. It is therefore not presumptous to envisage that our bioassay of cycling teratocarcinoma cells through mice, in conjunction with *in vitro* mutagenesis or selective introduction of foreign genes into these tumor cells, may provide a useful tool for developmental, biochemical, and genetic analyses of mammalian differentiation and diseases *in vivo*.

REFERENCES

Askanazy, M. 1907. Die Teratome nach ihrem Bau, ihrem Verlauf, ihrer Genese und im Vergleich zum experimentellen Teratoid. Verhandl. Deutsch. Gesellsch. Pathol. 11: 39–82.

Babinet, C., Condamine, H., Fellous, M., Gachelin, G., Kemler, R. and Jacob, F. 1975. Expression of a cell surface antigen common to primitive mouse teratocarcinoma cells and cleavage embryos during embryogenesis. In, Teratomas and Differentiation, M. I. Sherman and D. Solter, Eds.

Bernstine, E. G., M. L. Hooper, S. Grandchamp, and B. Ephrussi. 1973. Alkaline phosphatase activity in mouse teratoma. Proc. Nat. Acad. Sci. USA 70: 3899–3902.

Boon, T., O. Kellermann, E. Mathy, and J. A. Gaillard. 1975. Mutagenized clones of a pluripotent teratoma cell line: variants with decreased differentiation or tumor-formation ability. In, Teratomas and Differentiation, M. I. Sherman and D. Solter, Eds. Academic Press, New York, pp. 161–166.

Braun, A. C. 1970. On the origin of the cancer cells. American Scientist 58: 307–320.

Braun, A. C. 1972. The relevance of plant tumor systems to an understanding of the basic cellular mechanisms underlying tumorigenesis. Progr. Exp. Tumor Res. 15: 165–187.

Brinster, R. L. 1975. The effect of cells transferred into the mouse blastocyst on subsequent development. J. Exp. Med. 140: 1049–1056.

Brinster, R. L. 1975. Can teratocarcinoma cells colonize the mouse embryo? In, Teratomas and Differentiation, M. I. Sherman and D. Solter, Eds. Academic Press, New York, pp. 51–58.

Chung, A. E., L. E. Estes, H. Shinozuka, J. Braginski, C. Lorz, and C. A. Chung. 1977. Morphological and biochemical observations on cells derived from the *in vitro* differentiation of the embryonal carcinoma cell line PCC4-F. Cancer Res. 37: 2072–2081.

Croce, C. M., H. Koprowski, and H. Eagle. 1972. Effect of
environmental ph on the efficiency of cellular hybridization.
Proc. Nat. Acad. Sci. USA 69: 1952-1956.

Damjanov, I. and D. Solter. 1974. Experimental teratoma. Current
Topics Path. 59: 69-130.

Dewey, M. J., D. W. Martin, G. R. Martin, and B. Mintz. 1977.
Mosaic mice with teratocarcinoma-derived mutant cells deficient in
hypoxanthine phosphoribosyltransferase. Proc. Nat. Acad. Sci. USA
74: 12, 5564-5568.

Dixon, F. J., Jr. and R. A. Moore. 1953. Testicular tumors —
A clinico-pathologic study. Cancer 6: 427-454.

Edidin, M. and L. R. Gooding. 1975. Teratoma-defined and trans-
plantation antigens in early mouse embryos. In, Teratomas and
Differentiation, M. I. Sherman and D. Solter, Eds. Academic Press,
New York, pp. 109-121.

Elsevier, S. M., R. S. Kucherlapati, E. A. Nichols, R. P. Creagan,
R. E. Giles, F. H. Ruddle, K. Willecke, and J. K. McDougall. 1974.
Assignment of the gene for galactokinase to human chromosome 17 and
its regional localization to band q 21-22. Nature 251: 633-636.

Evans, M. J. 1972. The isolation and properties of a clonal tissue culture strain of pluripotent mouse teratoma cells. J. Embryol.
Exp. Morph. 28: 163-176.

Evans, M. J. 1975. Studies with teratoma cells *in vitro*. In, The
Early Development of Mammals, M. Balls and A. E. Wild, Eds.
Cambridge University Press, London, pp. 265-284.

Gardner, R. L. 1977. Cellular susceptibility to neoplasia and
its reversibility. In, Neoplastic Transformation: Mechanisms and
Consequences, H. Koprowski, Ed. Dahlem Konferenzen, Berlin, pp.
111-124.

Graham, C. F. 1977. Teratocarcinoma cells and normal mouse embryogenesis. In, Concepts in Mammalian Embryogenesis, M. I. Sherman
and C. F. Graham, Eds. MIT Press, Cambridge, pp. 315-394.

Hsu, Y-C. and J. Baskar. 1974. Differentiation *in vitro* of
normal mouse embryos and mouse embryonal carcinoma. J. Nat.
Cancer Inst. 53: 1, 177-185.

Illmensee, K., P. C. Hoppe, and C. M. Croce. 1978. Chimeric mice
derived from human-mouse hybrid cells. Proc. Nat. Acad. Sci. USA
75: 1914-1918.

Illmensee, K. and B. Mintz. 1976. Totipotency and normal differentiation of single teratocarcinoma cells cloned by injection into blastocysts. Proc. Nat. Acad. Sci. USA 73: 549-553.

Jacob, F. 1975. Mouse teratocarcinomas as a tool for the study of the mouse embryo. In, The Early Development of Mammals, M. Balls and A. E. Wild, Eds. Cambridge University Press, London, pp. 233-241.

Jacob, F. 1977. Mouse teratocarcinoma and embryonic antigens. Immunol. Rev. 33: 3-32.

Jami, J. and E. Ritz. 1974. Multipotentiality of single cells of transplantable teratocarcinomas derived from mouse embryo grafts. J. Nat. Cancer Inst. 52: 1547-1552.

Kleinsmith, L. J. and G. B. Pierce. 1964. Multipotentiality of single embryonal carcinoma cells. Cancer Res. 24: 1544-1552.

Littlefield, J. W. 1964. Selection of hybrids from matings of fibroblasts in vitro and their presumed recombinants. Science 145: 709-710.

Markert, C. L. 1968. Neoplasia: a disease of cell differentiation. Cancer Res. 24: 1544-1551.

Martin, G. R. 1975. Teratocarcinomas as a model system for the study of embryogenesis and neoplasia. Cell 5: 229-243.

Martin, G. R. and M. J. Evans. 1975. Multiple differentiation of teratocarcinoma stem cells following embryoid body formation in vitro. Cell 6: 467-474.

Matioli, G. 1973. Friend leukemia mouse stem cell reversion to normal growth in irradiated hosts. J. Reticuloendothel. Soc. 14: 380-386.

Matsuya, Y., H. Green and C. Basilico. 1968. Properties and uses of human-mouse hybrid cell lines. Nature 220: 1199-1202.

McBurney, M. W. 1976. Clonal lines of teratocarcinoma cells in vitro: differentiation and cytogenetic characteristics. J. Cell. Physiol. 89: 441-456.

McKinnell, R. G., L. M. Steven, and D. D. Labat. 1976. Frog renal tumors are composed of stroma, vascular elements and epithelial cells: what type nucleus programs for tadpoles with the cloning procedure? In, Progress in Differentiation Research, N. Muller-Berat et al. Eds. North Holland, Amsterdam, pp. 319-330.

McLaren, A. 1976. Mammalian chimeras. In, Developmental and Cell Biology Series, M. Abercrombie, D. R. Newth and J. G. Torrey, Eds. University Press, Cambridge.

Mintz, B. 1974. Gene control of mammalian differentiation.
Annual Review of Genetics 8: 411-470.

Mintz, B. and Baker, W. W. 1967. Normal mammalian muscle differentiation and gene control of isocitrate dehydrogenase synthesis.
Proc. Nat. Acad. Sci. USA 58: 592-598.

Mintz, B. and K. Illmensee. 1975. Normal genetically mosaic mice
produced from malignant teratocarcinoma cells. Proc. Nat. Acad.
Sci. USA 72: 3585-3589.

Mintz, B., K. Illmensee and J. D. Gearhart. 1975. Developmental
and experimental potentialities of mouse teratocarcinoma cells
from embryoid body cores. In, Teratomas and Differentiation, M. I.
Sherman and D. Solter, Eds. Academic Press, New York, pp. 59-82.

Nicolas, J. F., P. Avner, J. Gaillard, J. L. Guenet, H. Jakob, and
F. Jacob. 1976. Cell lines derived from teratocarcinomas. Cancer
Res. 36: 4224-4231.

Norris, H. J., H. J. Zirkin, and W. L. Benson. 1976. Immature
(malignant) teratoma of the ovary. Cancer 37: 2359-2372.

Oppenheimer, J. M. 1940. The non-specificity of the germ layers.
Quart. Rev. Biol. 15: 1-27.

Papaioannou, V. E., R. L. Gardner, M. W. McBurney, C. Babinet, and
M. J. Evans. 1978. Participation of cultured teratocarcinoma
cells in mouse embryogenesis. J. Embryol. exp. Morph. 44: 93-104.

Papaioannou, V. E., M. W. McBurney, R. L. Gardner, and M. J. Evans.
1975. Fate of teratocarcinoma cells injected into early mouse
embryos. Nature 258: 70-73.

Pierce, G. B., Jr. 1967. Teratocarcinoma: Model for a developmental concept of cancer. In, Current Topics in Developmental
Biology 2, A. Moscona and A. Monroy, Eds. Academic Press, New York,
pp. 223-246.

Pierce, G. B. 1974a. The benign cells of malignant tumors. In,
Developmental Aspects of Carcinogenesis and Immunity, 32nd Symp.
Soc. Dev. Biol., T. J. King, Ed. Academic Press, New York, pp.
3-22.

Pierce, G. B. 1974b. Neoplasms, differentiations and mutations.
American Journal of Pathology 77: 103-118.

Pierce, G. B. and T. F. Beals. 1964. The ultrastructure of primordial germinal cells of the foetal testis and of embryonal carcinoma cells in mice. Cancer Res. 24: 1553-1567.

Sherman, M. I. and D. Solter, Eds. 1975. Teratomas and Differentiation. Academic Press, New York.

Simpson, J. L. and G. Photopulos. 1976. The relationship of neo-
plasia to disorders of abnormal sexual differentiation. In, Birth
Defects: Original Article Series, XII, 1, 15-50. (The National
Foundation.)

Stevens, L. C. 1960. Embryonic potency of embryoid bodies derived
from a transplantable testicular teratoma of the mouse. Dev. Biol.
2: 285-297.

Stevens, L. C. 1967a. The biology of teratomas. Advan. Morphogenesis 6: 1-81.

Stevens, L. C. 1976b. Origin of testicular teratomas from primordial germ cells in mice. J. Nat. Cancer Inst. 38: 549-552.

Stevens, L. C. 1970a. A new inbred subline of mice (129/terSv)
with a high incidence of spontaneous congenital testicular teratoma. J. Nat. Cancer Inst. 50: 236-242.

Stevens, L. C. 1970b. The development of transplantable teratocarcinomas from intertesticular grafts of pre- and postimplantation
mouse embryos. Dev. Biol. 21: 364-382.

Stevens, L. C. 1974. Teratocarcinogenesis and spontaneous parthe-
nogenesis in mice. In, The Developmental Biology of Reproduction,
C. L. Markert and J. Papaconstantinou, Eds. Academic Press, New
York, pp. 93-106.

Stevens, L. C. and C. C. Little. 1954. Spontaneous testicular
teratomas in an inbred strain of mice. Proc. Nat. Acad. Sci. USA
40: 1080-1087.

Stevens, L. C. and D. S. Varnum. 1974. The development of teratomas from parthenogenetically activated ovarian mouse eggs. Dev.
Biol. 37: 369-380.

Stevens, L. C., D. S. Varnum and E. M. Eicher. 1977. Viable chimeras produced from normal and parthenogenetic mouse embryos.
Nature 269: 515-517.

Surani, M.A.H., S. C. Barton and M. H. Kaufman. 1977. Development
to term of chimeras between diploid parthenogenetic and fertilized
embryos. Nature 270: 601-603.

VIABLE CHIMAERAS PRODUCED FROM NORMAL AND PARTHENOGENETIC MOUSE

EMBRYOS*

Leroy C. Stevens, Don S. Varnum, and Eva M. Eicher

The Jackson Laboratory, Bar Harbor, Maine 04609

Parthenogenesis occurs spontaneously in about 10% of ovulated eggs of inbred strain LT/Sv mice (Stevens and Varnum 1974; Stevens 1975) and is experimentally inducible in other strains by various physical and chemical agents (see Tarkowski 1975 for review). The development of most parthenotes seems normal up to the expanded blastocyst stage (Van Blerkom and Runner 1976). They implant in the uterus, but, for reasons unknown, are resorbed within a few days. Although they rarely survive to 8 days of gestation when they develop somites, heart muscle, amnion, and neuroepithelium, Kaufman, Barton, and Suram (1977) obtained two embryos with 25 somites by transferring parthenogenetic blastocysts to the uteri of ovariectomised females treated with exogenous hormones. Even though parthenogenetic embryos do not survive to birth, their cells contain genetic information that permits prolonged survival. If two-cell parthenotes are cultured to the blastocyst stage and then grafted to extrauterine sites such as the testis or kidney, they may survive as teratomas composed of several types of tissues and undifferentiated embryonal cells (Stevens 1974; Ilse *et al.* 1975; and L.C.S. and D.S.V., unpublished). Furthermore, strain LT/Sv spontaneous ovarian teratomas contain numerous differentiated tissues composed of parthenogenetically derived cells. The question remains — why do parthenotes not survive at the organismic level *in utero*? Eicher and Hoppe (1973) used experimental chimeras composed of normal and abnormal embryos to transmit a recessive

*This paper and the succeeding one represent the substance of a short communication presented by L. P. Kozak at the Symposium. They are reprinted, by permission, from NATURE 269(5628): 515-518 (1977).

X-linked lethal mutation, and we considered the possibility that parthenogenetic embryonic cells might also be rescued if combined with normal embryonic cells. Here we present evidence of production of at least two viable chimaeras between normal and parthenogenetic embryos.

Parthenogenetic eight-cell embryos were obtained from F_1 hybrid females produced by mating females of the LT/Sv strain to males of the incipient recombinant inbred strain LTXBJ (L.C.S. and D.S.V., unpublished). (The progenitors of LTXBJ were strains LT/Sv and C57BL/6J. Strain LTXBJ had been inbred for 11 generations of brother x sister matings when the experiments were initiated.) Nearly all of the females of the LTXBJ recombinant strain have bilateral ovarian teratomas at 3 months of age. These teratomas are derived from parthenogenetically activated ovarian eggs. About 30% of their ovulated eggs undergo spontaneous parthenogenetic development. (LT/Sv x LTXBJ)F_1 hybrid females have the same high incidence of spontaneous parthenogenesis as LTXBJ females.

Inbred strain LT/Sv is homozygous for the alleles a, B^{lt}, C, and $Gpi-1^a$ at the agouti, brown, albino, and glucose-phosphate-isomerase-1 loci, respectively. LTXBJ is homozygous for the alleles a, B, C, and $Gpi-1^b$. Although parthenogenetic embryos of the LT/Sv strain are diploid (P. C. Hoppe, personal communication), it is not known whether they result from initiation of mitosis in primary oocytes or secondary oocytes (lack of the second meiotic division), or diploidisation of haploid ootids. Regardless of their origin the parthenogenetic embryos from the (LT/Sv x LTXBJ)F_1 females would appear a/a C/C. Depending on the nature of their origin, however, their genotypes for the brown and glucose-phosphate-isomerase-1 loci could be homozygous (for either allele) or heterozygous. Interpreting the origin of parthenogenetic cells in chimaeras was further complicated because we combined two parthenogenetic embryos per single normal embryo to form each chimaera. The two parthenotes could have different genotypes.

The normal eight-cell embryos were derived from eggs of albino 129/Sv (homozygous A^w, B, c, $Gpi-1^a$ females fertilised by sperm from A/HeJ (homozygous a, b, c, $Gpi-1^a$) males. Thus, these F_1 embryos were genotypically A^w/a, B/b, c/c, $Gpi-1^a/Gpi-1^a$.

Experimental chimaeras were produced by aggregating eight-cell embryos *in vitro* (Mintz 1971). After removal of the zona pellucida with Pronase, one normal and two parthenogenetic morulae were combined in Whitten's medium (Whitten 1971) and cultured overnight. The aggregated 'triplets' were then introduced into the uteri of (SJL x C57BL/10)F_1 pseudopregnant females. To date, 55 'triplet' embryos have been transferred into six pseudopregnant females and two litters have been delivered.

On 30 January 1977 a litter of five mice was delivered by a female that had received eight 'triple' embryos. Of the four live young, one was a male about half the size of his three female littermates. This male was white with small patches of pigmented hair on the back and head that could only have been derived from the parthenogenetic embryos. Some of the pigmented hair was agouti and some nonagouti indicating that the mouse was chimaeric with respect to hair follicle cells. Both irises had pigmented and non-pigmented areas (Fig. 1). No nipples were evident. At 26 days old the chimaeric male weighed 13 g, and his littermates weighed 16 g each.

At 36 days old, blood samples were collected from the male and his four littermates and analysed for GPI (Fig. 2). All of the nonchimaeric females showed only the GPI-1A form of glucose phosphate isomerase. The red blood cells of the chimaeric male apparently included cells derived from the parthenogenetic embryos as shown by a GPI-1B band (Fig. 2) that could only result if cells of parthenogenetic origin were present. In addition, a GPI-1AB band was evident. Its intensity seemed greater than the GPI-1B, as is the normal case of $Gpi-1^a/Gpi-1^b$ cells, suggesting that at least one of the parthenogenetic embryos was of the $Gpi-1^a/Gpi-1^b$ genotype. The presence of a GPI-1AB band would imply that at least one of the parthenogenetic embryos resulted from mitosis of a

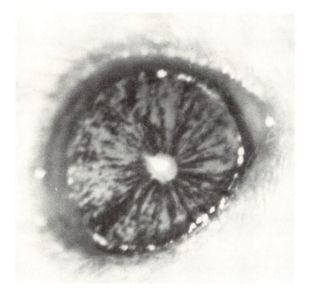

FIGURE 1. Eye of chimaera mouse. The non-pigmented areas were derived from a normally fertilised egg, the pigmented areas from one or two parthenogenetically activated eggs.

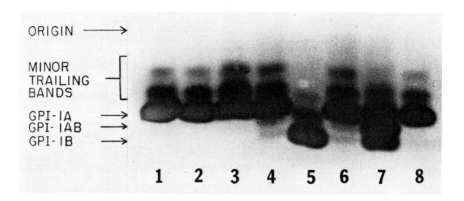

ORIGIN ⟶

MINOR
TRAILING
BANDS

GPI-IA ⟶
GPI-IAB ⟶
GPI-IB ⟶

1   2   3   4   5   6   7   8

FIGURE 2.   Electrophoresis of red blood cell lysates on cellulose
acetate gels stained for glucose phosphate isomerase using
method of Eicher and Washburn (1978). In slots 1—3 and 8 are
lysates from the four normal female sibs (GPI-1A) of the chimaeric male. Slot 5 includes lysate from a C57BL/6J male
(GPI-1B) and slot 7 from a (C57BL/6J x DBA/2J)F_1 male (GPI-
1AB). Slot 4 (repeated in slot 6) contains lysate from the
chimaeric male. Of interest are the two bands present in
slots 4 and 6 that have migrated at a faster rate than the
major band in the position of GPI-1A. These two minor bands
line up such that one is in the same position as the GPI-1AB
(hybrid) band and the other in the position of the GPI-1B
band. It seemed that the slower of the two bands (position
of GPI-1AB hybrid band) stained more intensely than the faster
band (position of GPI-1B), as is the case in lysates from a
$Gpi-1^a/Gpi-1^b$ individual, suggesting that at least one parthe-
nogenetically-derived embryo in the chimaeric male mouse was
of the $Gpi-1^a/Gpi-1^b$ genotype.

primary oocyte or lack of a second meiotic division in a secondary
oocyte (with crossing over between the centromere and the $Gpi-1$
locus), but not diploidisation of haploid ootids. It is also
possible that a polar body nucleus fused with its egg nucleus.

     At 38 days of age the male gonads were examined through an
incision in the abdominal skin and musculature. Both seemed to
be normal testes. The right testis was removed and prepared for
histological examination. There was no histological evidence that
cells of parthenogenetic origin were present in the testis. To
date the chimaeric male has sired 27 albino offspring, none of
which shows evidence of parthenogenetic cells.

On 27 March 1977, a second litter of three mice was delivered. This litter was obtained by transferring 9 'triple' embryos each composed of two LT/Sv parthenotes with one albino 129 embryo. The female of this litter was much smaller than its two male litter-mates. Both her irises were pigmented showing the presence of parthenogenetic cells.

The evidence presented here shows that cells of parthenogenetic origin can survive and participate in normal organ formation. Since both parents of the normal embryo were albino, all of the pigment cells in the coat and irises of both chimaeras must have been derived from parthenogenetic embryos. Since the agouti pattern is determined by the genotype of the hair follicle cells, the presence of agouti hairs in the male chimaera indicates that some of these cells originated from the parthenogenetic member. Finally, the presence in the male chimaera of LT/Sv strain-specific GPI shows that red blood cells were derived from parthenogenetic embryos of the chimaera.

Although our preliminary results indicate that parthenogenetic cells are capable of differentiating normally in combination with normal cells, it is still not clear why parthenotes cannot survive to term *in utero* in strain LT/Sv mice.

It has recently been found that ovarian teratomas in mice are derived from oocytes that have completed the first meiotic division (Eppig *et al.* 1977).

Four male and two female pigmented parthenote ↔ normal albino chimaeras have been produced (Stevens 1978). All were mated to albinos. One of the female chimaeras produced five litters of 29 albino young. Her sixth litter contained three albino and two pigmented young. The pigmented young could only have been derived from ova of parthenogenetic origin. This demonstrates that parthenogenetic embryonic cells are totipotent.[†]

We thank W. K. Whitten and S. Carter for useful discussions and for demonstrating the method of making chimaeras. We thank S. Reynolds and D. Dorr for technical asistance. This research was supported by grant CA 02662 from the USNIH, and GM 20919 from the National Institute of General Medical Sciences.

[†] This paragraph is an addition to the paper originally published in NATURE.

REFERENCES

Eicher, E. M. and P. C. Hoppe. 1973. J. exp. Zool. 183: 181-184.

Eicher, E. M. and L. W. Washburn. 1978. Proc. Natl. Acad. Sci. USA 75: 946-950.

Eppig, J. J., L. P. Kozak, E. M. Eicher and L. C. Stevens. 1977. Nature 269: 517-518.

Ilse, S. A., M. W. McBurney, S. R. Bramwell, Z. A. Deussen and C. F. Graham. 1975. J. Embryol. exp. Morph. 34: 387-406.

Kaufman, M. T., S. C. Barton and M. A. Surani. 1977. Nature 265: 53-55.

Mintz, B. 1971. In, Methods in Mammalian Embryology, J. C. Daniel, Ed. W. H. Freeman, San Francisco, pp. 186-214.

Stevens, L. C. 1975. In, The Developmental Biology of Reproduction, C. L. Markert and J. Papaconstantinou, Eds. Academic Press, New York, pp. 93-106.

Stevens, L. C. 1978. Nature, in press.

Stevens, L. C. and D. S. Varnum. 1974. Develop. Biol. 21: 364-382.

Tarkowski, A. K. 1975. In, The Developmental Biology of Reproduction, C. L. Markert and J. Papaconstantinou, Eds. Academic Press, New York, pp. 107-129.

Van Blerkom, J. and M. N. Runner. 1976. J. Exp. Zool. 196: 113-123.

Whitten, W. K. 1971. Adv. Biosci. 6: 129-139.

OVARIAN TERATOMAS IN MICE ARE DERIVED FROM OOCYTES THAT HAVE

COMPLETED THE FIRST MEIOTIC DIVISION[*]

John J. Eppig, Leslie P. Kozak, Eva M. Eicher, and
Leroy C. Stevens

The Jackson Laboratory, Bar Harbor, Maine 04609

Spontaneous ovarian teratomas are found in about 50% of strain
LT/Sv mice by the time they are 90 days old (Stevens and Varnum
1974). These teratomas result from parthenogenetic cleavage of
ovarian oocytes. Some parthenotes reach a developmental stage
equivalent to 7 d embryo before they become disorganised and further develop into a teratoma. Since some cleaved ovarian oocytes
are accompanied by polar bodies, but others seem to lack them, it
was uncertain whether the teratomas derive from oocytes that complete the first meiotic division or from oocytes that cleave mitotically without previous meiotic division.

A strain of mice having an even higher frequency of ovarian
teratomas than LT/Sv was produced by making a recombinant inbred
line from strains LT/Sv and C57BL/6J (L.C.S. and D. S. Varnum,
unpublished). Nearly all of the females of this recombinant line,
called LTXBJ, have bilateral ovarian teratomas by 90 days of age.
Fortuitously, among the C57BL/6J genes retained in the recombinant
strain is the $Gpi-1^b$ allele at the glucosephosphate isomerase
($Gpi-1$) locus on chromosome 7. Since strain LT/Sv is homozygous
for the $Gpi-1^a$ allele at this locus, (LT/Sv x LTXBJ)F_1 hybrids are
heterozygous at $Gpi-1$ and express the A, hybrid AB and B allozymes
in a ratio of 1 : 2 : 1 (Fig. 1a).

Electrophoresis of 23 teratomas from F_1 female mice revealed
a homozygous A or B allozyme banding pattern in 21 cases (Fig. 1b).
The other two teratomas showed the 1 : 2 : 1 heterozygous banding
pattern, indicating that they were heterozygous $Gpi-1^a/Gpi-1^b$.

---

* See footnote for preceding paper

We concluded from these results that the teratomas found in the (LT/Sv x LTXBJ)F$_1$ female mice originated from parthenogenetically cleaved oocytes which had completed the first meiotic division (Fig. 2). In 21 of 23 cases, this division segregated the Gpi-1^a and Gpi-1^b alleles so that the parthenogenetic embryo and subsequently the teratomas were homozygous for either of those alleles at the Gpi-1 locus. In the other two cases, where the heterozygous banding pattern was found, the most probable conclusion is that crossing-over has occurred between the centromere and the Gpi-1 locus, so that the Gpi-1^a and Gpi-1^b alleles were located on two chromatids attached to the same centromere.

Other studies on the origin of ovarian teratomas in women who were heterozygous for alleles producing allozymes of glucose-6-phosphate dehydrogenase and phosphoglucomutase, have shown that these teratomas were homozygous for the alleles in most cases, and thus that they arose from oocytes that had completed the first division of meiosis (Linder 1969).

Preliminary chromosomal analysis of LT teratoma has indicated that most of the cells are diploid and a small number are polyploid (L.C.S. and D. S. Varnum, unpublished). Also, the parthenotes recovered from the oviduct of superovulated LT/Sv mice are also diploid, although at least one polar body was usually found (P. C. Hoppe, personal communication). Therefore, diploidisation of the egg karyotype must have occurred after the first division. The mechanism of this diploidisation is unknown but it is possible, in principle, that karyokinesis of the second meiotic division occurs without cytokinesis, thus suppressing the formation of polar body II; or that there is a fusion of the second polar body with the ovum. Our preliminary results do not allow us to distinguish between these possible alternatives.

--->

FIGURE 1a. Electrophoresis of supernatants prepared from ovaries
            (slots 1—6, and 8) and spleen (slot 7) from (LT/Sv x LTXBJ)F$_1$
            mice. Male LTXBJ mice were mated with female LT/Sv to produce
            the hybrids. At 8—10 weeks of age, the F$_1$ females were autop-
            sied and teratomas were removed while taking care to contami-
            nate the tumour with as little ovarian tissue as possible.
            Excessively bloody tumours were not used. Pieces of tissue

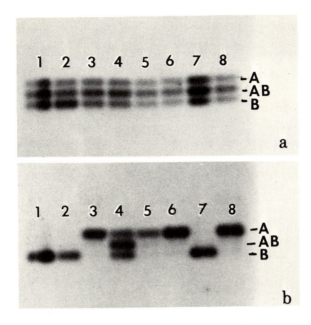

were homogenised with ground glass microhomogenisers in 0.05 ml 50 mM Tris-HCl buffer, pH 7.5, containing 1 mM EDTA and 1 mM β-mercaptoethanol. The homogenate was centrifuged for 20 min at 16,000 g and the supernatant solution used as the enzyme source. Electrophoresis was carried out on Titan-III Zip Zone cellulose acetate plates (Helena Laboratories, Beaumont, Texas) with 0.043 M Tris, 0.046 M glycine buffer, pH 8.6, for 1.75 h at 180 V. Glucose phosphate isomerase (EC 5.3.1.9.) was detected with a 1% agar overlay containing 50 mM Tris-HCl, pH 8.0, 2.5 mM $MgCl_2$, 2.5 mM fructose-6-phosphate, 1 mM NADP, 0.1 mg ml^{-1} nitroblue tetrazolium and 5 IU ml^{-1} glucose-6-phosphate dehydrogenase. The GPI-1B form in slot 2 appears darker than the GPI-1AB, suggesting that this piece of ovary was contaminated with some teratoma tissue which was not obvious when the sample was taken. A piece of F_1 tissue was tested from each animal from which a teratoma was assayed to assure heterozygosity.

b, Electrophoresis of supernatants prepared from teratomas from (LT/Sv x LTXBJ)F_1 female mice. Samples 1–3 and 5–8 show either the GPI-1A or GPI-1B allozyme pattern. Sample 4 is one of the two teratomas that showed a hybrid allozyme pattern. Samples 7 and 8 were taken from contralateral ovaries of the same animal (slot 7, Fig. 1a) and are homozygous for alternative allozymes. In some teratomas, the hybrid AB allozyme and the other homozygous allelic product were detected, but in these cases the amount of the AB form greatly exceeded the minor homozygous form, indicating that the tumour was probably contaminated with normal ovarian tissue.

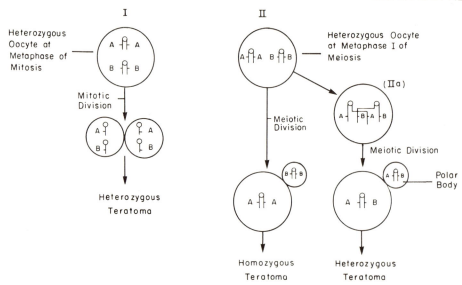

FIGURE 2. Diagramatic representation of alternatives for the dis-
    tribution of alleles at the *Gpi-1* locus (A and B refer to the
    Gpi-1ᵃ and *Gpi-1ᵇ* alleles, respectively). The GPI enzyme
    consists of two subunits which associate randomly. Conse-
    quently, homozygous *Gpi-1ᵃ* or *Gpi-1ᵇ* cells contain enzyme
    with two A or B subunits, respectively. Heterozygous *Gpi-1ᵃᵇ*
    cells contain three forms of the enzyme: one with two A sub-
    units, one with an A and a B subunit, and one with two B sub-
    units in a 1 : 2 : 1 ratio. If teratomas originate from
    oocytes which cleave mitotically without previous meiotic
    division (alternative I), then all teratomas would show the
    heterozygous banding pattern for GPI. If, however, the first
    meiotic division occurs before parthenogenetic cleavage, then
    (as the data presented here indicate) most teratomas would be
    homozygous for either the GPI-1A or GPI-1B allozymes (alterna-
    tive II). In a minority of cases, heterozygous teratomas
    would be found resulting from a chromatid exchange between
    the *Gpi-1* locus and the centromere (IIA).

     This research was supported by NSF (grant PCM 7603047 to
J.J.E.) and the NIH (grant HD 08431 to L.P.K., GM 20919 to E.M.E.
and CA 02662 to L.C.S.). The Jackson Laboratory is fully accredited
by the American Association for accreditation of Laboratory Animal
Care.

REFERENCES

Linder, D. 1969. Proc. Natl. Acad. Sci. USA 63: 699-704.

Stevens, L. C. and D. S. Varnum. 1974. Devel. Biol. 21: 364-382.

GROWTH CONTROL IN CHIMAERAS

D. S. Falconer, I. K. Gauld and R. C. Roberts

Agricultural Research Council, Unit of Animal Genetics,
West Mains Road, Edinburgh EH9 3JN, Scotland

How do chimaeras of large and small strains grow? Is their
growth rate related to the cellular proportions in the body as a
whole, or in any particular organ? Do the cells from the faster
growing component tend to outgrow those from the slower growing?
These are the main questions that we have been trying to answer,
and this paper is a preliminary account of the results.

The strains of mice from which aggregation chimaeras were made
were the Q-strains (Falconer, 1973), selected over 23 generations
for large (L) and for small (S) body size, with unselected controls
(C). There were six replicates each of L, C and S lines. Weight
at 6 weeks of age was the criterion of body size. The Large lines
were about twice the weight of the Small lines at this age. Luckily
some of the replicates in each size group (L, C, and S) were polymorphic for the enzyme GPI-1 and for albino. In each size-group
two stocks were constructed which were homozygous for complementary
alleles at each of these two loci. Thus one stock was $Gpi\text{-}1^a$ and
albino to be referred to as (a), the other $Gpi\text{-}1^b$ and coloured, to
be referred to as (b). For this report we have data from 16 chimaeras of C(a) ↔ L(b) and 15 chimaeras of either S(a) ↔ L(b) or
S(b) ↔ L(a). In addition to these overt chimaeras, there are a
few single-colour animals in both the C ↔ L and S ↔ L groups, and
a few chimaeras of types L ↔ L, C ↔ C and S ↔ S, to be used for
some comparisons. The relation of body-size to the composition of
the coat alone in the C ↔ L chimaeras and in a different set of
S ↔ L chimaeras (not enzyme marked) was described by Roberts, Falconer, Bowman and Gauld (1976).

The chimaeras were scored for percent albino in the coat, and
for the percent of allozyme $Gpi\text{-}1^a$ in various tissues. The results

throughout are expressed as the percent of the Large component. The enzyme was scored by electrophoresis of serial dilutions, as described by Klebe (1975). The proportion of one or other allozyme can be derived from the number of dilution steps separating the last visible bands of the two. This method proved to be highly repeatable, nearly always giving the same reading on repeated runs. Nine organs or tissues were studied: they are listed in Table 1.

The C ↔ L chimaeras were killed for the enzyme assays when they were 10—12 months old, but their body weights analysed were those at 6 weeks of age. The enzyme content of the blood was

TABLE 1. Mean cell proportions (% L) in organs studied, ± standard errors

	C ↔ L	S ↔ L
Coat	49 ± 8	45 ± 5
Brain	46 ± 4	47 ± 4
Spinal cord	41 ± 6	46 ± 5
Pituitary	36 ± 8	50 ± 7
Liver	43 ± 7	58 ± 6
Lung	39 ± 7	53 ± 5
Kidney	45 ± 8	53 ± 5
Spleen	36 ± 6	55 ± 5
Blood	27 ± 7	53 ± 7
Mean*	$40.6 \pm 2.2^{\dagger}$	50.9 ± 1.4
p[‡]	< 0.001	< 0.05

* Unweighted mean of organs.

[†] Significantly different from 50%, $P < 0.01$.

[‡] Significance of variation between organs, from 2-way analysis of variance.

assayed at 6 weeks and at killing: there were no consistent changes. The S ↔ L chimaeras were all killed at 6 weeks of age, so that the weights and cell proportions refer to the same age. In both sets of chimaeras the 6-week weights of females were converted to male-equivalents by multiplying them by 1.2, a conversion factor found to apply equally to all three size-groups (Falconer, 1973). After conversion the sexes were pooled. All body weights were adjusted by regression to a standard litter size of 2 at birth.

We consider first the question of cell selection during development. Table 1 gives the mean cell proportions in each of the organs. In the C ↔ L chimaeras there were less than 50% of cells derived from the Large component in all organs, the overall mean of 41% Large being significantly different from 50%. The organs of the S ↔ L chimaeras varied round 50% with an overall mean of 51%. In both sets of chimaeras the organs were significantly heterogeneous with respect to cell proportions. These results answer one question clearly: there was no tendency for the cells from the larger component to outgrow those from the smaller; indeed the reverse was true in the C ↔ L chimaeras. There is, however, clear evidence of cell selection taking place to different degrees in different organs.

Fig. 1 gives a general impression of the relationship between weight and cell proportions. It plots body weight against the mean cell proportions in all the organs studied, which is the nearest we can get to the cell proportions in the body as a whole. It is very clear from both groups of chimaeras that body weight is influenced by the cell proportions. Both of the linear regressions shown on the graphs are significantly different from zero (P < 0.001). Estimates of the weights of the constituent strains are shown by arrows at the margins of the graphs. The C ↔ L chimaeras seem to show chimaeric heterosis to a marked degree. There are, however, difficulties in getting strictly comparable weights of the constituent strains, so the heterosis may be spurious. The S ↔ L chimaeras show no heterosis, and we think the evidence for chimaeric heterosis is not convincing.

The question now is: can we identify any organ as being more important than the others in influencing body weight? First consider the simple correlations between body weight and cell proportions in each organ. These are given in Table 2, arranged in descending order. The correlations are all high, ranging from 0.85 down to 0.65. The simple correlations, however, tell us very little, partly because the organs do not differ much, but mainly because the organs themselves are all highly correlated one with another in respect of cell proportions. This is illustrated in Table 3, which gives the distribution of correlations in each set of chimaeras. The high inter-organ correlations make it difficult

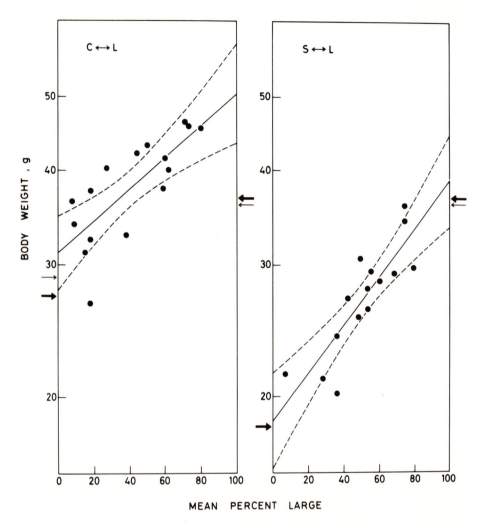

FIGURE 1. Relation of body weight at 6 weeks to cell proportions
    in nine organs or tissues. Weight is plotted on a logarith-
    mic scale. The cell proportions are the means, unweighted,
    of all the organs. Each point is an individual chimaera.
    The straight lines are the fitted linear regressions. The
    broken lines are the 95% confidence limits of predicted mean
    weights. The arrows at the margins are estimated weights of
    the constituent strains as given by Roberts et al. (1976)
    (thick arrows), or from single colour chimaeras and L ↔ L or
    C ↔ C chimaeras (thin arrows).

TABLE 2.   Simple correlations of body weight with % large cells in
    each organ, in order of magnitude of the correlation.   *n* is
    the number of chimaeras.

C ↔ L (n = 16)		S ↔ L (n = 15)	
Coat	0.79	Pituitary	0.85
Pituitary	0.79	Spinal cord	0.84
Lung	0.77	Blood	0.79
Spinal cord	0.76	Kidney	0.78
Kidney	0.74	Lung	0.78
Blood	0.72	Brain	0.75
Liver	0.69	Spleen	0.72
Spleen	0.68	Coat	0.68
Brain	0.65	Liver	0.66
Mean	0.732 ± 0.051	Mean	0.761 ± 0.064

to separate their effects on weight. They also raise another
question, which must be dealt with first. This is: are there
real differences in cell proportions between the organs of the
same mouse? Perhaps each mouse has its overall cell proportions
from which its organs deviate only by errors of estimation. If
there were no real differences between organs the question of
whether any organ is more important than the others in determining
weight could not be pursued further. The differences between
organs within mice were, however, undoubtedly real. First, the
differences were often very much greater than any found in repeat
runs. Second, the error variance was calculated from the differences between left and right kidneys and between two samples of
blood. Tested against this error variance, the mean square between
organs within mice was highly significant ($P < 0.001$).

TABLE 3. Distributions of simple correlations between pairs of
organs in respect of % large cells. The organs are the 9
listed in Table 1, giving 36 pairs.

| | number of organ-pairs | |
correlation	C ↔ L	S ↔ L
.90 - .95	12	4
.85 - .90	6	7
.80 - .85	7	10
.75 - .80	10	7
.70 - .75	1	3
.65 - .70	0	2
.60 - .65	0	2
.55 - .60	0	0
.50 - .55	0	1
Mean	0.852	0.800
s.e.	± 0.066	± 0.092

        To assess the effects on weight of each organ separately one
would like, ideally, to calculate partial correlations. Unfortunately the number of animals is not much greater than the number
of variables and so this approach is inpracticable. The alternative approach adopted is as follows. The organs (i.e. their cell
proportions) are regarded as predictors of weight. When knowledge
of all the organs is utilized, a certain proportion of the variance
of weight is accounted for. The remainder, the residual variance,
is attributable to environmental variance in the usual sense, together with any effects of other organs not studied. We first calculate the multiple correlation, R, of weight with all the organs.
The residual variance of weight, as a proportion of the total, is
$1 - R^2$. We then calculate the residual variance again with one
organ omitted, and ask: is the residual variance now significantly

greater? In other words, does this omitted organ tell us anything
more about weight beyond what all the other organs together tell
us? This was repeated with each organ omitted in turn. Table 4
gives the results. The organs are arranged in order of importance

TABLE 4. Residual variance of weight, as percent of total, when
one organ is omitted from the multiple correlation of weight
with cell proportions in organs.

C ↔ L			S ↔ L	
Omitted	$1-R^2$ %		Omitted	$1-R^2$ %
None	16		None	8
Coat	30		Pituitary	25
Brain	29		Blood	20
Blood	25		Kidney	20
Spleen	18		Spinal cord	18
Lung	18		Liver	16
Liver	17		Spleen	14
Spinal cord	17		Brain	11
Pituitary	16		Lung	11
Kidney	16		Coat	8

	C ↔ L	S ↔ L
Minimum values for significance at P = 0.02 :	43	27
P = 0.05 :	32	19
P = 0.10 :	26	15

as judged by the increase of the residual variance that their omis-
sion causes. In the C ↔ L chimaeras no organ has a significant
effect. In the S ↔ L chimaeras three organs, pituitary, blood and
kidney, have effects significant at $P < 0.05$. The two series of
chimaeras, however, are not at all consistent in the order of importance of the organs. For example pituitary, which has the biggest
effect in the S ↔ L chimaeras, has no effect at all in the others.
The results of this analysis therefore cannot be accepted as revealing any real differences between the organs in their effects on
the control of growth. The proportion of the two cell types undoubtedly does affect weight, but we cannot localize the effect.
There may of course be a localized effect in some other organ or
tissue not studied. We ought therefore to ask whether the residual
variance of weight contains any variance due to cell proportions
that is not accounted for by the nine organs studied.

The variance of weight of chimaeras has three components:
(1) that due to the differing cell proportions, which might be
called 'chimaeric variance', arising from the genetic differences
between the constituent strains, (2) that due to genetic differences
between individuals within the constituent strains, and (3) that
due to environmental differences affecting the chimaeras. There is
no need here to separate (2) from (3) and they will be referred to
jointly as environmental variance. The square of the multiple
correlation, R^2, estimates the chimaeric variance that is accounted
for by the nine organs, as a proportion of the total. The residual
variance, $1 - R^2$, is the environmental variance together with any
chimaeric variance that is not accounted for. The expected amount
of environmental variance (components 2 + 3) can be estimated from
the constituent strains or, better, from chimaeras made from strains
of similar weight, and from single-component chimaeras. Comparison
with the residual variance of the C ↔ L and S ↔ L chimaeras will
then show whether there is any indication of chimaeric variance due
to the cell proportions in any organ not studied. Table 5 gives
the data for this comparison. The environmental variance is shown
separately for the three genotypes (L, C, and S), each genotype
being represented by different types of chimaera as shown at the
foot of the table. The weighted mean of the environmental variance
is 10.8 g^2, whereas the weighted mean of the residual variance is
9.5 g^2. The conclusion is that the cell proportions in the nine
organs account for all the chimaeric variance. There is therefore
no evidence of any other organ or tissue that controls growth.
This does not mean that the existence of such an organ is excluded
by the evidence. Suppose, for example, that connective tissue were
the only controlling tissue, no other organ having any effect on
growth. Being widely dispersed and probably with a large number of
progenitor cells, connective tissue would be highly correlated in
respect of cell proportions with most other organs. The meaning of
the above result would thus be that the nine organs together give

TABLE 5.   Environmental variance of weight (g^2) for comparison
       with residual variance.

Environmental*	d.f.	Variance
L genotype	9	21.2
C genotype	40	9.2
S genotype	3	0.7
Weighted mean	52	10.8
Residual		
C ↔ L	6	13.5
S ↔ L	5	4.6
Weighted mean	11	9.5

* Chimaera types in genotypes, with numbers of animals:

 L genotype: L ↔ L (4 overt, 4 single colour);

              S ↔ L (3 single).

 C genotype: C ↔ C (24 overt, 14 single);

              C ↔ L (5 single).

 S genotype: S ↔ S (4 overt).

 Variance calculated within groups in parentheses and then
 pooled.

 Some of these chimaeras are from earlier series that were
 not enzyme-marked.

us a very accurate estimate of the cell proportions in connective
tissue. Suppose, in contrast, that there was one growth-controlling
tissue derived from very few progenitor cells. In that case, its

cell proportions would not be highly correlated with other organs, and the nine organs would give only a poor estimate of its cell proportions. The evidence rules out this possibility and we can conclude that growth is not controlled by any tissue derived from a very small number of progenitor cells.

Finally, are the sizes of any organs influenced by their own cell proportions? Organ weights are, of course, closely correlated with body weight. If an organ has a higher proportion of 'Large cells' than the rest of the body will it be disproportionately large? To answer this question we calculated the partial regression of organ weight on cell proportions in the organ, with body weight held constant, body weight being the weight at killing without adjustment for litter size. This was done for the brain, kidney, liver, lung, pituitary, spleen, and testis in both sets of chimaeras. There were three significant regressions (spleen, pituitary, testis) out of a total of fourteen, but the two sets of chimaeras were not consistent and we do not think that this is convincing evidence that cell proportions influence organ weights. Since the sizes of most organs are generally thought to be regulated by functional needs it seems unlikely that they would be influenced by their own cell proportions.

From all these results it looks as if growth and body weight are determined by the cellular genotype throughout the whole body, though not by localized effects on the growth of each organ individually.

SUMMARY AND CONCLUSIONS

Aggregation chimaeras were made from strains of mice differing in body size and marked by albino and an enzyme variant (GPI-1). The cell proportions — percent of cells from the larger of the two component strains — in each of nine organs or tissues were estimated by electrophoresis of serial dilutions or by visual scoring of the coat. The object was to look for relationships between body weight and cell proportions.

Body weight was very clearly correlated with the mean cell proportions in all the organs. The organs were all highly correlated with each other in respect of cell proportions, but there were real differences between organs within mice. There was no clear evidence that any one organ by itself had a significant effect on body weight. The nine organs jointly accounted for all the chimaeric variance, leaving no more than would be expected for environmental variance. There was no convincing evidence that the cell proportions in any organ had a localized effect on the weight of the organ itself.

The conclusions about the control of growth are: (1) The cells of the larger component do not proliferate faster than those of the smaller component during development. (2) None of the nine organs studied is predominant in controlling growth. (3) There may be some other organ or tissue that itself controls growth; but, if so, it cannot be one with a small number of progenitor cells. (4) Growth is correlated with the cellular genotype of each of the nine organs studied, either because each contributes something to the control of growth, or because each is correlated, in cellular genotype, with some other controlling organ. (5) If there is no other growth controlling organ, then it seems that growth depends on the cellular genotype throughout the whole body.

REFERENCES

Falconer, D. S. 1973. Replicated selection for body weight in mice. Genet. Res. 22: 291-321.

Klebe, R. J. 1975. A simple method for the quantitation of isozyme patterns. Biochem. Genetics 13: 805-812.

Roberts, R. C., D. S. Falconer, P. Bowman and I. K. Gauld. 1976. Growth regulation in chimaeras between large and small mice. Nature, Lond. 260: 244-245.

ATTEMPTS AT LOCATING THE SITE OF ACTION OF GENES AFFECTING BEHAVIOR

Muriel N. Nesbitt

University of California San Diego, La Jolla,
California 92093

INTRODUCTION

Among the many differences between the C57BL/6J and A/J inbred mouse strains are several differences in behavior. In an effort to understand aspects of the mechanisms underlying these behavioral differences, we have constructed a series of A ↔ C57 chimeras. Study of the chimeras should allow us to find out (i) whether any of the behaviors are governed by single cells or single clones, (ii) how many distinct, independently controlled differences underlie the behaviors we measure, and (iii) which tissues control the behaviors.

THE TESTS OF BEHAVIOR

We chose four behavioral categories to study, on the bases of ease of testing and the magnitude of the difference between our two strains: open-field activity (McClearn 1959, 1960); alcohol preference (McClearn and Rodgers 1959; McClearn 1972); cricket attacking (Butler 1973) and rope climbing.

The test for open-field activity involves placing the mouse to be tested in the center of the floor of a meter-square box, which is marked off in a 64-square gridwork. The test lasts five minutes. During that time, the number of squares the mouse enters while moving around the box is counted, as is the number of times the mouse defecates. In our hands A/J mice run across 62 ± 21 squares and defecate 5 ± 1 times, while C57BL/6J mice enter 206 ± 69 squares and do not defecate.

The test for alcohol preference involves housing the mice
individually in cages equipped with two graduated drinking bottles,
one containing water and the other a 10% V/V solution of ethanol
in water. The amount of fluid drunk from each bottle is recorded
daily. Every four days, the two bottles are switched left to
right, and the entire test lasts sixteen days. The alcohol preference score for a given mouse is the ratio of the volume of
ethanol solution consumed during the test period to the total
volume of fluid consumed. Under our conditions, the C57 mice
score 0.79 ± .11 (they prefer alcohol), while the A score 0.21 ±
0.09 (they avoid alcohol).

Testing for cricket-attacking behavior involves introducing
a cricket into the home cage of a mouse housed alone, and giving
the mouse 20 minutes in which to attack the cricket. Mice appear
to learn from their first exposure to a cricket, so they attack
subsequent crickets more quickly. We therefore tested each mouse
for cricket attacking on two consecutive days. Cricket-attacking
scores are calculated as "latency to attack," that is, time elapsed
before the attack is made. Naive C57 males have a median latency
to attack of 4 minutes, while naive females have a latency of 9
minutes. In the second test, C57 males and females both score
1.4 minutes. A-strain mice usually fail to attack at all in
either test.

Rope-climbing behavior is tested on an apparatus consisting
of a clothesline rope about 18 inches long, stretched vertically
between two platforms. There is a knot in the rope equidistant
from the two platforms. The mouse to be tested is placed on the
knot at time 0. The time it takes the mouse to move off the knot
and begin climbing is called rope latency. This is 16 ± 9 seconds
for C57 mice, and 1.7 ± 0.7 minutes for A. After having moved off
the knot, the mouse can climb up the knot and get off onto the top
platform, or climb down the rope to the lower platform. Rope time
is the time spent by the mouse after getting off the knot, before
reaching one of the platforms. This averages 1.7 ± 0.2 minutes
for C57 and 8.7 ± 0.45 minutes for A mice. The two strains do not
differ in the frequency with which individuals climb up as opposed
to down the rope.

THE CHIMERAS

We used the technique of morula aggregation (Tarkowski 1961;
Mintz 1962) to produce chimeras. We obtained 36 chimeras in all.
Sixteen of them were from a group provided to us by Dr. W. Whitten
of the Jackson Laboratory. These included 10 chimeras of the type
A ↔ B10·D2. The rest of Whitten's chimeras, and all of the ones
produced by us, were of the A ↔ C57BL/6 type. B10·D2 mice are

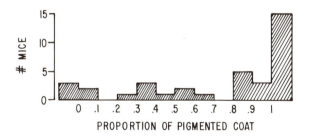

FIGURE 1. Distribution of coat color among chimeras. The column
    to the left of 0 represents totally albino mice. The next
    column contains those mice which had some pigment, but in
    which less than 10% of the coat was pigmented. Similarly
    the right-most column represents completely pigmented mice.

C57BL/10J with the H-2 region of DBA/2J. C57BL/10J has behaved
like C57BL/6J when the two have been compared (e.g., Thompson
1953). Figure 1 shows the distribution of coat color in our chimeras. The three individuals with entirely white coats proved not
to contain a detectable C57 component in any tissue when analysis
of the glucose-phosphate isomerase (GPI) isoenzyme pattern was
done. All other chimeras contained both cell types in at least
some tissues.

BEHAVIOR OF THE CHIMERAS

    If a single clone or single cell controls a particular behav-
ior, the chimeras must behave either like C57 mice or like A mice,
because the cell or clone will be of C57 origin or A origin, and
not mixed. On the other hand, if a multiclonal constellation of
cells controls a behavior, chimeras will be able to behave in
ways other than those characteristic of the parent strains. For
example, the behavior of chimeras could be intermediate between A
and C57. Figure 2 shows the distribution of scores of our seven
behavior tests in the chimeras. In all cases, except latency to
attack cricket 2, some of the chimeras show scores clearly intermediate between those of the parent strains, so that we conclude
those behaviors are not controlled by a clonal cell population.
Although cricket-2 scores show the distribution appropriate to a
clonally-controlled behavior, there are reasons to believe that
the cell population controlling this behavior is multiclonal.
This will be discussed further below.

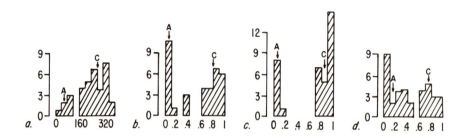

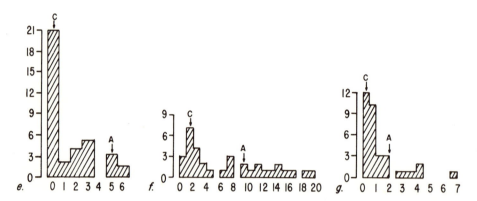

FIGURE 2.   Distribution of behaviors among chimeras. In each distribution the arrow marked "A" designates the mean score of
A/J mice, while the arrow marked "C" designates the mean of
C57BL/6J mice.
   a) Distribution of number of squares traversed in the open-
       field test.
   b) Distribution of scores for latency to attack first crick-
       et. A score of 0 means no attack. A score of 1 would
       mean instantaneous attack.
   c) Distribution of scores of latency to attack second crick-
       et. Scores are as in part b.
   d) Distribution of alcohol preference.
   e) Distribution of number of fecal boli deposited during the
       open-field test.
   f) Distribution of rope climbing time scores. Scores are in
       terms of the fraction of the total available time (5 min)
       that were used in climbing.
   g) Distribution of rope-latency scores. Scores are in terms
       of the fraction of the total available time (5 min) that
       elapsed before the mouse began to climb the rope.

If two behaviors share a common controlling cell population, they should covary in a group of chimeras. The reason is that the composition of the cell population in question will determine both of the behaviors in any chimera. We looked for covariation among our behaviors by means of a technique called factor analysis (Dixon 1975). This technique is designed to identify clusters of highly correlated variables. Our assumption is that traits that are highly correlated share a common cause, or factor. A standard computer program, BMDP4M (Dixon 1975), was used for the factor analysis, specifying options for the method of principal components and varimax rotation. Factors are generated so as to explain all variance of all traits, and so that correlations are maximized within, and minimized between the clusters being defined. The degree to which a factor determines each of the behaviors is given by the factor loading. In other words, the factor loading is the regression coefficient for predicting the behaviors from the factor.

Three factors were described in our analysis. Each of the factors and the factor loadings are given in Table 1. Factor loadings of less than 0.250 represent nonsignificant correlations between factors and traits, and so are designated NS in the table.

The fact that only three factors are required to describe our data suggests that only three mechanisms underlie our seven behaviors, at least at the tissue level. Cricket attacking and rope climbing, though both could be seen as involving activity, are distinct, independently controlled behaviors. A matrix of this size would be expected to contain one or two values spuriously significant at the 5% level. We think the −0.591 loading of open field activity with cricket killing is such a value. The negative

TABLE 1. Factor loadings

	Factor 1	Factor 2	Factor 3
First cricket	0.937	NS	NS
Second cricket	0.902	NS	NS
Defecation	NS	0.366	−0.765
Open field activity	−0.591	NS	0.584
Alcohol preference	NS	NS	0.871
Rope latency	NS	0.901	NS
Rope time	NS	0.822	NS

sign of the loading indicates a negative correlation between
activity and factor 1, and also between activity and cricket
attacking. If activity and cricket attacking shared a common
mechanism they should be positively correlated, because C57 mice
score high both in activity and cricket attacking, while A mice
score low in both. We think the 0.366 loading of defecation with
factor 2 is also likely to be spurious. If defecation and rope
climbing had a common mechanism, they should be negatively correlated in chimeras, since C57 mice score high in climbing and low
in defecation, while A mice are the opposite.

The factor analysis suggests that attacking of first cricket
and attacking of second cricket share a common mechanism. The
cellular control of attacking the first cricket appeared not to be
clonal (see above). Thus, control of attacking the second cricket
must not be clonal. We attribute the sharp bimodality of the distribution for cricket 2 (Figure 2c) to the learning that occurs
after exposure to the first cricket. Mice having long latencies
during the first test nevertheless learn about crickets and attack
quickly during the second test.

It is interesting to us that our results indicate that alcohol preference, open-field activity and open-field defecation have
a common mechanism at the tissue level. The albino locus has been
shown to influence both open-field activity (DeFries and Hegmann
1970) and alcohol preference (Henry and Schlesinger 1967); and
Whitney (1972) found a correlation between open-field activity and
alcohol preference among the F2 of a cross between a high-activity,
alcohol-preferring strain, and a low-activity, alcohol-avoiding
strain. Taken together, these results suggest that alcohol preference, defecation, and open-field activity may share a common
genetic mechanism.

CELLULAR COMPOSITION OF CHIMERAS

A and C57 mice have different alleles at the *Gpi-1* locus, and,
thus, different electrophoretically distinguishable forms of the
enzyme glucose phosphate isomerase (GPI, E.C. 5.3.1.9). We
assayed the cellular composition of the tissues of our chimeras
by comparison of the bands produced upon starch gel electrophoresis of extracts of the chimeric tissues to bands produced by hemo-
lysates of mixtures of A and C57 erythrocytes in various proportions. Chimeras were perfused with heparinized saline prior to
dissection, because GPI activity derived from erythrocytes would
otherwise have contributed to the GPI scores of our chimeric tissues. The major shortcoming of this method is that it does not
allow tissues that cannot be physically dissected apart to be
assayed separately. Thus, our values for liver, for example, are

a mixture of the GPI values for parenchymal cells and those for
connective tissue.

TISSUE CONTROL OF BEHAVIORS

In a series of chimeras, a behavior should covary with the
composition of the constellation of cells by which it is controlled. Having collected data on the composition of our chimeric
tissues, we are now attempting to evaluate covariation between our
three factors and the chimeric tissues. This is a difficult statistical problem, given a sample size as small as ours. Thus far,
we have simply calculated the pairwise correlation coefficients
relating our tissues to our factors. We have observed several significant correlations; but, unfortunately, many spuriously significant correlations are expected in a matrix as large as this. Thus,
because of the preliminary nature of this part of the work, we
will say at this time only that (i) factor 3 (defecation, activity,
alcohol preference) is not significantly correlated with any central nervous system (CNS) part or nerve, (ii) factor 3 is highly
correlated with coat color ($r = 0.74$, significant at 0.0001 level),
(iii) factor 1 (cricket attacking) is correlated with CNS structures (olfactory lobes, brainstem). Our efforts are now being
directed toward finding a suitable method for analysis of our data.

SUMMARY

None of the seven behaviors appears to be controlled by a
clone or single cell. The seven behaviors reflect three separate
mechanisms. One mechanism underlies cricket attacking. A separate
mechanism underlies rope-climbing latency and climbing time. A
third mechanism is common to alcohol preference, open-field activity, and defecation in the open field. Preliminary data suggest
that the mechanism mediating the strain difference in alcohol preference, open field activity, and defecation lies outside the CNS.

REFERENCES

Butler, K. 1973. Predatory behavior in laboratory mice: strain
on sex comparisons. J. Comp. Phys. Psych. 85: 243.

DeFries, J. C. and J. P. Hegmann. 1970. Genetic analysis of open-
field behavior. In Contributions to Behavior-Genetic Analysis:
The Mouse as a Prototype. G. Lindzey and D. Thiessen, Eds. New
York: Appleton-Century-Crofts.

Dixon, W. J. 1975. BMPD Biomedical Computer Programs. University
of California Press.

Henry, K. R. and K. Schlesinger. 1967. Effects of the albino and dilute loci on mouse behavior. J. Comp. Phys. Psych. 63: 320-323.

McClearn, G. E. 1959. The genetics of mouse behavior in novel situations. J. Comp. Phys. Psych. 52: 62-67.

McClearn, G. E. 1960. Strain differences in activity of mice: influence of illumination. J. Comp. Phys. Psych. 53: 142-143.

McClearn, G. E. 1972. Genetics as a tool in alcohol research. Ann. N. Y. Acad. Sci. 197: 26-31.

McClearn, G. E. and D. A. Rodgers. 1959. Differences in alcohol preference among inbred strains of mice. Quart. J. Stud. Alc. 20: 691-695.

Mintz, B. 1962. Formation of genotypically mosaic mouse embryos. Am. Zool. 2: 432.

Tarkowski, A. K. 1961. Mouse chimeras developed from fused eggs. Nature 190: 857-860.

Thompson, W. R. 1953. The inheritance of behavior: behavioral differences in fifteen mouse strains. Can. J. Psychol. 7: 145-155.

Whitney, G. 1972. Relationships between alcohol preference and other behaviors in laboratory mice. Finn. Found. Alc. Stud. 20: 151-162.

FINE STRUCTURE OF CELLS IN EMBRYOS CHIMERIC FOR MUTANT GENES AT THE T/t LOCUS

Martha Spiegelman

Sloan-Kettering Institute for Cancer Research
New York, New York 10021

Since it has been proposed that at least some of the abnormalities in mouse embryos that are homozygous for lethal mutations at the T/t locus are interpretable as due to derangements of cell recognition and response (Bennett 1975), we thought that we might be able to look directly at the affected cells in embryos chimeric for the mutant and wild-type genotypes during the appropriate developmental stages in order to see what kinds of cellular associations occur when cells of the defective type are in proximity to their normal counterparts. Such observations might give a clue to the kind of deficiency, in a mechanical sense perhaps, that is involved in the mutant embryo. In short, do cells of the mutant phenotype remain unchanged, or do they react to the new environment and participate in normal development? With respect to the T/t locus, this question has been approached once before, in 1964 by Mintz for the $t12$ gene.

THE t^{w18} MUTATION*

The mutant embryo that appeared especially promising for analysis via chimeras is the t^{w18} homozygote, which is recognizably abnormal at late 7 to early 8 days of gestation. During this

---

*The gene maintained in this laboratory is t^{w18}, which is in the same complementation group with t^4 and t^9 (Bennett 1975), but not necessarily identical to either one; t^9/t^9 and t^4/t^4 embryos (Moser and Gluecksohn-Waelsch 1967) are less developmentally retarded than those of t^{w18}/t^{w18} genotype.

period, in normal embryos, mesoderm segregates from the primitive
streak, and the neural tube, notochord, and somites organize as
discrete entities. The t^{w18}/t^{w18} embryos are retarded, appearing
like advanced egg cylinders; relatively few mesodermal cells seg-
regate from the primitive streak, which remains disproportionately
large; somites rarely form (Bennett and Dunn 1960).

From electron-microscopic observations it is known that normal
mesodermal cells are typically stellate, with long tapering cytoplasmic processes that contain a finely filamentous network and
frequently terminate in small focal junctions or gap junctions
where they abut on one another. Mesodermal cells in the t^{w18}/t^{w18}
embryo, on the other hand, are rounded in outline and are often
clumped together, with much of their apposed surfaces closely
aligned over large distances. Fine filopodia containing a filamentous lattice as well as gap junctions are infrequently seen (Spiegelman and Bennett 1974).

The striking difference in appearance between the stellate
reticular associations of normal mesodermal cells, and the aggregated groups of rounded mesodermal cells in the t^{w18} mutant led us
to think that we might be able to distinguish two populations of
cells in embryos chimeric for wild-type and mutant genotypes, if
these cells were to retain their typical phenotypes. If, however,
mutant cells in the chimera were to achieve some degree of normal
morphology, identification of the t^{w18}/t^{w18} mesodermal cells would
be less sure, but the nature of the defect might become clearer.
For example, if all of the mesodermal cells in a chimeric embryo
appeared to be normal stellate cells, it would suggest that the
affected cells from the mutant can recognize and respond to associations with normal cells. If, however, distinct clusters of
normal stellate cells and of aggregated rounded cells were present
in the mesoderm of chimeric embryos, then it would seem that the
defective cells lack the necessary recognition and response machin-
ery. The fact that the gross morphology of the t^{w18} homozygote is
so clearly different from that of the normal embryo also encouraged
us to undertake these experiments, since we hoped that some deviations in the primitive streak, neural epithelium, or somites might
persist and permit the identification of presumed mutant↔normal
chimeras.

With these aims in mind, aggregation chimeras were constructed,
transferred to foster mothers, recovered at 8 days of gestation,
and fixed for light and electron microscopy.*

---

*Embryos were fixed in 2% glutaraldehyde, phosphate-buffered, post-
fixed in 1.5% osmium tetroxide, phosphate-buffered, dehydrated
through ethanol and propylene oxide, and embedded in Epon. Sections cut at 1 μm thickness were stained with toluidine blue for
light microscopy. Ultra-thin sections were stained with uranyl
acetate and lead citrate for electron microscopy.

Observations on embryos chimeric for the t^{w18}/t^{w18} *genotype*

Embryos at the 8-cell stage from matings between $+/t^{w18}$ parents were aggregated with known $+/+$ embryos (series I) from wild-type parents, or were paired *inter se* (series II), according to the method of Mintz (1964b) but with modifications by V. Papaioannou. In series I, 20% of the chimeras can be expected to be mutant↔normal and in series II, 32% can be expected to be mutant↔normal and 4% can be expected to be mutant↔mutant. Control chimeras were produced in the same way from $+/+$ embryos obtained from matings of wild-type parents.

In series I, of 58 embryos recovered from foster mothers on the eighth gestational day, 15 (26%) showed some of the abnormalities typically associated with the t^{w18}/t^{w18} genotype, namely, retardation, abnormal primitive streak, and distorted neural tube and mesoderm. Of 44 embryos retrieved in series II, 19 (43%) had some of the mutant features. On the basis of these frequencies, the 34 embryos from the two series were therefore classified as mutant↔normal chimeras. The remaining 68 embryos appeared entirely normal, like the group of 18 control chimeras; stages of development varied from headfold to 16 somites.

By gross morphological criteria, 14 of the 34 presumed mutant↔normal chimeras achieved considerably greater differentiation, including the formation of several pairs of somites, than we had ever seen in several hundred ordinary t^{w18} homozygotes; this result suggested that perhaps normalization of the affected cells can occur. The putative mutant↔normal chimeras were divided into two groups: 20 "t^{w18}-type", which closely resemble the typical monozygotic mutant, and 14 "new abnormals". In general, the new abnormals had more resemblance to normal embryos, at both the gross and microscopic levels, than to the standard t^{w18} mutant; nevertheless, all 14 embryos showed some of the abnormalities typical of the mutant phenotype, such as prominent excess tissue bulging dorsally from the primitive streak or neural epithelium, or showed marked thickenings of the primitive streak, neural epithelium, or somites (Fig. 1).

In sections viewed in the light microscope, the new abnormals invariably show regions of superabundant neural epithelium and mesoderm; no regions of excess tissue were ever seen in littermate normal chimeras or in control chimeras (Fig. 2, 3). The basic body organization of the new abnormal chimera is the same as that of the normal or control chimeras with both types having neural tube or folds, notochord, somites, endoderm, and coelomic mesoderm of regular form. It is evident in those regions of excess tissue in the new abnormal chimeras that mesodermal cells have a more smoothly rounded profile and are often more densely packed than those of the normal chimeras.

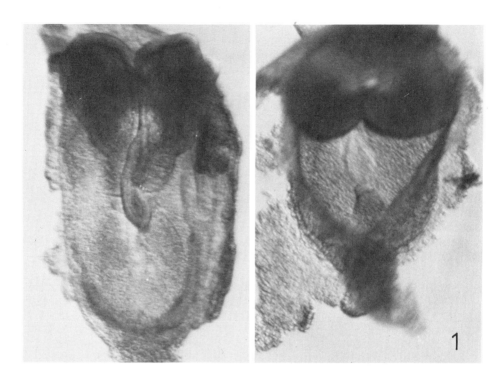

FIGURE 1. Two "new abnormal" chimeras, both having head folds and
somites. The embryo on the left has a large growth extending dorsad and caudad from the posterior border of the head fold. The
embryo on the right has a large cone of tissue projecting dorsad
from the posterior trunk region. (Embryo was not flat and head
folds stand up vertically out of focus.)

        In the electron microscope, mesodermal cells of both the con-
trol and the littermate normal chimeras appear like those of the
normal monozygotic embryo; in all three, the cells are stellate
with tapering cytoplasmic processes frequently joined to neighboring cells by gap junctions as well as small focal junctions (Fig.
4). The broad areas of extracellular space are presumably occupied
in vivo by amorphous matrix. Interestingly, whereas in the normal
monozygotic embryo a very small proportion of mesodermal cells
(fewer than 1%) possess a cilium, in the normal chimeras ciliated
cells comprise approximately 10% of the mesodermal population.
Each of these cilia has the 9 + 0 microtubule doublet substructure
typical of a non-motile cilium.

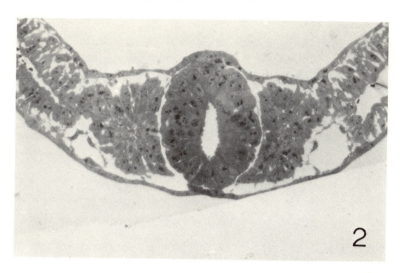

FIGURE 2. Transverse section through the mid-trunk region of a normal chimera showing well-formed neural tube, somites, and loose mesodermal cells. x250.

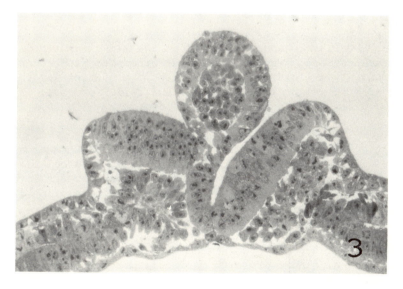

FIGURE 3. Transverse section through the mid-trunk region of a new abnormal chimera (left embryo of Figure 1) showing neural folds, somites, and loose mesodermal cells. Excess tissue is contiguous with the epithelium of one neural fold and contains a core of loose cells. x250.

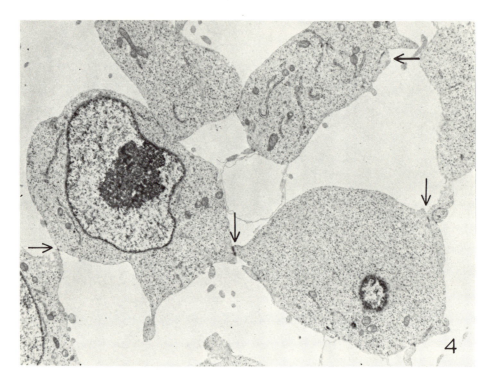

FIGURE 4. Stellate mesodermal cells in the mid-trunk region of a
    normal chimera. Tapering cellular processes project into the
    broad extracellular space and often form contact specializa-
    tions with neighboring processes and cells (*arrows*). x7,500.
    (Reduced 20% for purposes of reproduction)

Sections of t^{w18}-type chimeras reveal rounded mesodermal cells
that are densely packed together leaving little intercellular
space. As in the standard t^{w18} homozygote, very few small focal
contacts or gap junctions are seen between the neighboring lobose
pseudopods projecting from these cells (Fig. 5).

In contrast to the mesodermal cells of the standard homozygote, those of the t^{w18}-type chimera are rarely filled with large
residual bodies. There are also more cells per unit area in these
chimeras than in the homozygote. Furthermore, regions of stellate
cells joined by small focal junctions, as well as gap junctions,
are encountered in these chimeras, a situation rarely found in the
homozygote; these stellate cells may be normal cells originating
from the wild-type component of the chimera.

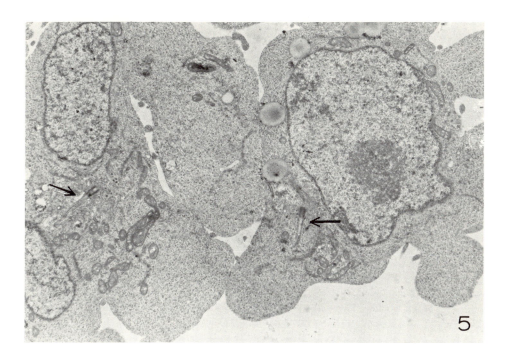

FIGURE 5. Rounded, clumped mesodermal cells in a t^{w18}-type chi-
     mera. Very few fine cellular processes are present in the
     narrow extracellular space; instead, broad lobopodia project
     from the cells. Several cells possess cilia (*arrows*) an-
     chored in a complex juxtanuclear zone. x7,500. (Reduced 20%
     for purposes of reproduction)

     One cellular characteristic of particular interest in meso-
dermal cells of the t^{w18}-type chimeras is the occurrence of bundles
of cytoplasmic filaments, each about 8–10 nm in diameter, close to
the nuclear envelope (Fig. 6). In addition, at least 25% of the
mesodermal cells in the t^{w18}-type chimeras are ciliated while fewer
than 1% of the cells in the standard t^{w18} homozygote possess cilia,
as in normal embryos (Fig. 5).

     Mesodermal cells located in the regions of a dorsal bulge of
excess tissue in the new abnormal chimeras usually have irregular
but smoothly contoured profiles (Fig. 7). There is a moderate
extracellular space, less than that seen in the normal chimeras but
greater than that seen in the t^{w18}-type chimeras. Neither finely
tapering cytoplasmic processes, typical of normal mesodermal cells,
nor broadly lobose pseudopods, usually found in the mutant mesoder
mal cells, are encountered in these zones of mesoderm; instead a
great many small finger-like cytoplasmic processes occupy the

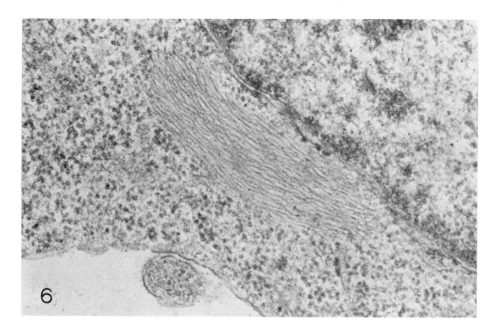

FIGURE 6. A bundle of 8—10 nm filaments near the nuclear envelope
in a mesodermal cell of a t^{w18}-type chimera. x61,000. (Reduced
20% for purposes of reproduction)

extracellular space and many form contact specializations with
one another.

Unlike the mesodermal cells of normal chimeras, of normal
monozygotic embryos, or of the t^{w18} homozygote, but like the mesodermal cells of the t^{w18}-type chimeras, mesodermal cells of the new
abnormal chimeras in these body regions of excessive growth possess bundles of 8—10 nm filaments (Fig. 8). In addition, the juxtanuclear zone in mesodermal cells of both the new abnormal and the
t^{w18}-type chimeras is characterized by a large Golgi apparatus,
numerous microtubules, and small dense bodies surrounded by many
profiles of granular endoplasmic reticulum and smooth vesicles.
As in the t^{w18}-type chimera, ciliated cells have been recorded in
25% of the mesodermal population of new abnormal chimeras.

Conclusions: Alteration of the t^{w18}/t^{w18} phenotype by chimerism

Although there are no cell markers to identify cell origin
unequivocally, since large numbers of unusual mesodermal cells are
seen only in those chimeric embryos that also have gross abnormalities, we believe the body regions showing protuberant growths are

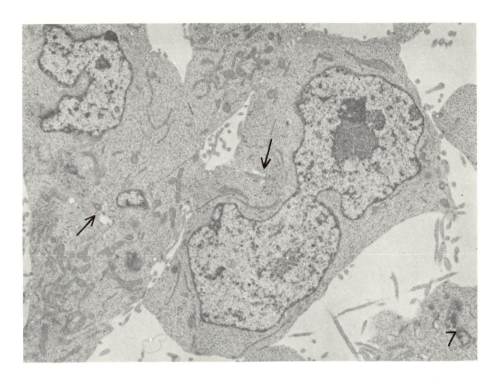

FIGURE 7. Mesodermal cells of irregular shape, with nuclei of
    irregular shape, in a new abnormal chimera. Many fine villous
    cytoplasmic processes occupy the extracellular space. In a
    number of cells, cilia (*arrows*) project from a complex juxta-
    nuclear zone. x7,500. (Reduced 20% for purposes of repro-
    duction)

probably populated by cells of t^{w18}/t^{w18} genotype. We offer the
following explanation for the intermediate morphology of the new
abnormal chimera.

    In the changed environment of a normal cell population, the
cells of mutant genotype are able to move out of the primitive
streak into the mesodermal location and in so doing they spread
out and assume stellate shapes. Quite possibly then, the cells
lack a signal component but can recognize and respond to signals
of the normal neighboring cells. However, while the cells of mutant origin now appear viable, they do not have a cell structure
identical to that of normal mesodermal cells. This atypical appearance may be due to, first, a release from the constraints imposed within a total population of mutant cells, but, second, a
persistent block in mesodermal differentiation.

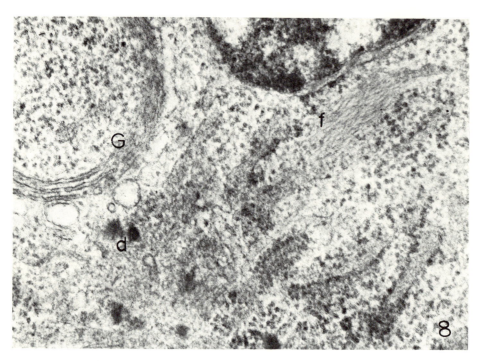

FIGURE 8. Part of the juxtanuclear zone of a mesodermal cell of
a new abnormal chimera showing a Golgi apparatus (*G*), dense
bodies (*d*), and a bundle of 8–10 nm filaments (*f*) in a background of polysomes and finely filamentous cytoplasm.
x61,000. (Reduced 20% for purposes of reproduction)

    The two distinctive classes of mutant↔normal chimeras proba-
bly result from a random variation in the distribution of cells of
the two genotypes within each chimeric embryo. It is likely, for
example, that in the t^{w18}-type chimera, most of the cells that
populate the primitive streak and mesoderm are of the mutant genotype and opportunities for interaction with normal neighbors are,
of course, limited; the chimeric embryo therefore closely resembles the standard t^{w18} homozygote. In the new abnormals, on the
other hand, a better balance of cells from the wild-type and mutant
partners probably permitted sufficient normal-cell-mutant-cell
interaction in the primitive streak and mesoderm. In these embryos,
presumably many cells of mutant origin became localized to a few
regions where they produced excessive tissue growths; a chimeric
embryo of nearly regular form but with some deviant structures,
in this case, resulted.

Ciliated mesodermal cells are of rare occurrence (approximately 1%) in monozygotic embryos, whether wild-type or t^{w18} mutants. It is puzzling that a significant increase (to approximately 10%) in this minor population is seen in normal chimeras, and that an even greater increase (to approximately 25%) is found in the mutant↔normal chimeras. We can only suggest that these ciliated cells may be less mature than the majority of mesodermal cells, since they are of greater frequency in the posterior trunk than at anterior levels. Possibly, these cells retain traits that are characteristic of their ectodermal progenitors. In this respect, it is noteworthy that other cellular traits shared by neural-epithelial cells are found in many mesodermal cells of the mutant↔normal chimeras. In addition to a cilium and a complex Golgi zone, these cells possess many microvillous-like cytoplasmic processes and bundles of filaments of the dimensions of tonofilaments.

Although detailed structure of mesodermal cells in t^4 and t^9 homozygotes has not been described, the gross morphology of these mutants, in the same complementation group with the t^{w18} mutation, resembles that of the new abnormal chimeras. These mutant embryos, at 8 days of gestation, have achieved more advanced development than the typical t^{w18} mutant and they exhibit an overproduction of ectoderm; but instead of a deficiency of mesoderm, as in t^{w18}/t^{w18} embryos, the mesoderm of t^4 and t^9 homozygotes fails to differentiate (Moser and Gluecksohn-Waelsch 1967). Similar regions of ectodermal overexpansion and arrested differentiation of mesoderm are evident in several new abnormal chimeras; these presumed mutant↔normal chimeras have advanced well beyond the point at which the t^{w18} homozygote is arrested.

It is possible that the genes t^4 and t^9 interrupt mesodermal differentiation, while the t^{w18} gene blocks an earlier transition from primitive streak to mesoderm. Lack of complementation between these mutations obviously does not imply gene identity. In the new abnormal chimeras mesodermal cells are abundant, but it is not clear if complete differentiation of their derivatives can occur, although several of these chimeras — unlike any of the homozygotes of this complementation group — possess somites.

We do not know if "rescue", strictly speaking, of the mutant cells can be effected. In some of the 8-day chimeric embryos it appears that cells of t^{w18}/t^{w18} genotype have been altered by the new environment. This observation may be akin to that seen when t^{w18} homozygotes transplanted to the testis of host mice produce numerous rosettes of embryonic neural epithelium and nests of undifferentiated cells (Artzt and Bennett 1972). Possibly, both in the teratomas and in the chimeras, where the new milieu contains normal cells, the t^{w18}/t^{w18} cells can proliferate and thrive but

nevertheless cannot differentiate mesodermal derivatives. This
question of rescue remains to be tested; in future experiments,
the tissues of chimeric mice at birth and later stages will be
analyzed for suitable enzyme markers linked to the t^{w18} gene.

THE t^{w32} MUTATION

Embryos homozygous for t^{w32} are arrested as morulae with a
constellation of cellular abnormalities mainly like those known
for homozygotes of the t^{12} gene, which is in the same complementation group. Again, in chimeras for t^{w32}/t^{w32} and wild-type, if
the cells of the mutant partner retained their phenotypes, we hoped
to have, in effect, a cell marker, since the defects for members
of this complementation group have been well studied (for t^{12} mutants, Smith 1956; Mintz 1964a; Calarco and Brown 1968; Hillman,
Hillman, and Wileman 1970; and for t^{w32} mutants, Hillman and Hillman 1975; Granholm and Johnson (1978). Since cells of the t^{12}/t^{12}
genotype in mutant↔normal chimeras are recognizable at the light-
microscope level (Mintz 1964b), we expected to be able to identify
and make electron-microscopic analysis of chimeric morulae and
blastocysts using the t^{w32} gene.

In contrast to their normal littermates, which are blastocysts
by the fourth day of development, arrested morulae homozygous for
either t^{w32} or t^{12} have large, round cells which contain fewer
polysomes, more accumulations of lipid droplets, including intra-
nuclear deposits, relatively pale nuclei with large, round, con-
tracted nucleoli, or sometimes fragmented nuclei. The arrested
morulae also appear less compact than normal morulae. The cells
retain cytoplasmic crystalloids and yolk bodies as well as small,
round mitochondria with arch-like cristae later than do normal
cells; mitochondria in cells of t^{w32} homozygotes also contain dense
material. The t^{w32} mutants become arrested and die at the early
morula stage, a bit earlier than the t^{12} homozygote, which dies at
the late morula stage. All of these features indicate an immaturity of cell structure in the mutant embryos; and indeed, retardation in the homozygotes is evident from early cleavage stages
(Hillman *et al.* 1970; Hillman and Hillman 1975).

During early compaction of the normal morula, cells maximize
their contacts with one another by spreading over one another,
interdigitating their cell surfaces, and forming numerous junctions
(Ducibella, Albertini, Anderson, and Biggers 1975; Calarco and
Epstein 1973; Magnuson, Demsey, and Stackpole 1977). We expected
that, in addition to the other identifying characteristics noted
above, we might detect atypical contacts where mutant and normal
cells abutted on each other in chimeric morulae and blastocysts if,
in fact, the mutant cells became incorporated into blastocysts.

Observations on embryos chimeric for the t^{w32}/t^{w32} *genotype*

Embryos at the 8-cell stage from *inter se* matings of $+/t^{w32}$ mice were paired with normal embryos using the methods of Mintz and Papaioannou as before. Aggregation chimeras using normal embryo pairs as controls were also made. After two days' growth *in vitro*, chimeric morulae and blastocysts, as well as some nonaggregated pairs, were fixed for light and electron microscopy.

A total of 25 control chimeras were retrieved (=control group), plus 3 nonaggregated pairs. In the potential mutant↔normal category (=experimental group), 37 chimeras were obtained, plus 8 nonaggregated pairs. The two groups differed markedly in the stages attained (Table 1).

Incomplete aggregation occurred among 27% of the chimeras in the experimental group. Moreover, in the experimentals, morulae were found among both the incomplete aggregants and nonaggregants

TABLE 1. Chimeras between t^{w32}/t^{w32} and wild-type genotypes

	Control group	Experimental group
Large blastocysts	11	17
Small blastocysts	13	9
Morulae	1	1
Incomplete aggregants ("dumbbells")		
blastocyst-blastocyst	0	0
blastocyst-morula	0	6
morula-morula	0	4
Non-aggregants (pairs)	3	8
blastocysts	(6)	(9)
morulae	(0)	(7)
Total number*	28	45

*Includes non-aggregant pairs

but were absent in these categories in the controls. Microscopi-
cally, all of the control chimeras, the large blastocysts in the
experimental group, and the nonaggregated blastocysts in both
groups, appear like the standard monozygotic embryos of the same
stages (Fig. 9). In the experimental group, three of the small
blastocysts and six incomplete aggregants have been confirmed as
mutant↔normal chimeras (Figs. 10, 11); five nonaggregant morulae
are mutants also. These numbers yield a total of 27% apparent
t^{w32}/t^{w32} embryos (nonaggregants included) which is somewhat lower
than the percent expected (38%).*

Cells of t^{w32}/t^{w32} genotype are readily recognized in these
chimeras by their relatively large size, pale staining nucleus
with a dense, round nucleolus, great lipid accumulations, and scant
polysome content (Figs. 10, 11, 12). Furthermore, the surface of
cells of mutant origin is relatively smooth, while that of normal
cells usually appears quite ruffled, with both fine and coarse
villous projections (Fig. 12). The normal cell surface has a
sturdy appearance, often having an outer coat of filamentous
material which is generally lacking on the mutant cell surface
(Figs. 13, 14). The subsurface cytoplasm of the normal cell always
contains a substantial feltwork of fine filaments (Figs. 13, 15,
16), whereas the mutant cell may sometimes have a similar cyto-
structure (Fig. 14) but more often does not (Figs. 15, 16).

Adjacent mutant-mutant and mutant-normal cells share relatively
few junctions compared to normal-normal cells. The lateral borders
of neighboring normal cells present an irregular profile of interdigitating cytoplasmic processes, but such an association is rarely
seen when one or both cells are of mutant type; contact surfaces of
mutant cells are usually quite flat (Figs. 15, 16).

In addition to the abnormalities already known for the t^{w32}
mutant, then, the cell surface appears affected: the cell coat is
not very robust, the surface contour is smooth, the number of cell
junctions is low, and the subsurface filamentous network is scant.
These traits, with several others cited earlier, are encountered
in early cleaving blastomeres. The mutant cells have remained
retarded even in the presence of normal cells in the chimera and
do not form normal cell-to-cell associations, perhaps because the
mutant cells are not developing in synchrony with the normal components. In this respect, it has been shown that normal embryo pairs
aggregate into chimeras when both members are at 8-cell to early
morula stages, but aggregate incompletely or not at all when one
or both embryos are late morulae or early blastocysts (Burgoyne
and Ducibella 1977).

*The gene t^{w32} has a high transmission ratio (average 0.75) through
males giving approximately 38% homozygotes when heterozygous mice
are mated (Bennett and Dunn 1971).

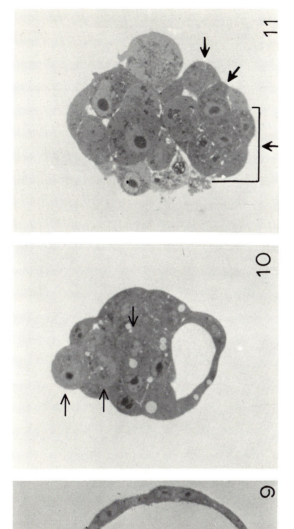
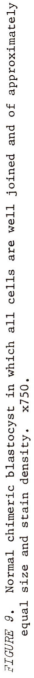

FIGURE 9. Normal chimeric blastocyst in which all cells are well joined and of approximately equal size and stain density. x750.

FIGURE 10. A *t^w32/t^w32* ↔ normal blastocyst with a small cavity. Several *mutant* cells (*arrow*) are evident in the inner cell mass and polar trophectoderm by their large size, pale staining, fragmented nuclei, and large round nucleolus. x750.

FIGURE 11. A *t^w32/t^w32* ↔ normal morula which appears poorly aggregated. Most of the cells are abnormal. A group of six *normal* cells (*arrow*) is recognizable at one pole by their small size, dark staining, irregular nucleoli, and relatively rough cell surfaces. x750.
(Figs. 9, 10 & 11 reduced 20% for purposes of reproduction)

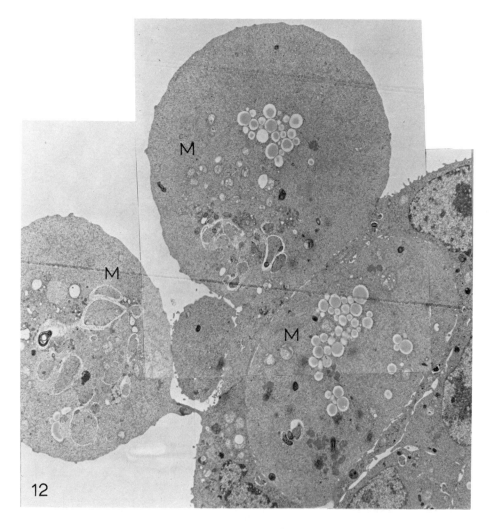

FIGURE 12.   Montage showing a portion of a mutant↔normal blastocyst.   Three mutant cells (M) are recognizable by their large
size, pale-staining cytoplasm, fragmented nuclei, accumulation of lipid droplets, Balbiani bodies, and relatively smooth
cell surfaces.   x5,000. (Reduced 30% for purposes of reproduction)

     Two further points are of interest.   In the mutant↔normal
chimeras the blastomeres of each of the two embryos paired usually
remain an intact group.   The same observation was made for chimeras
containing t^{12}/t^{12} cells (Mintz 1964b).   Whether intermingling of

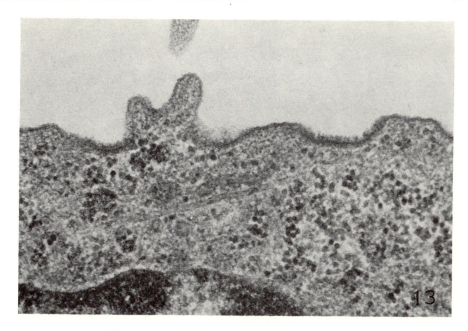

FIGURE 13. Portion of the cell surface of a normal outer cell in
a mutant↔normal blastocyst. The plasma membrane possesses
a number of microvilli, is markedly furrowed, and has a prominent cell coat. The subsurface cytoplasm contains a fine
filamentous network and microtubules. x85,000. (Reduced 25%
for purposes of reproduction)

blastomeres of two component normal embryos in a young aggregation
chimera occurs is not known.

Secondly, in the three mutant↔normal blastocysts we have not
found any cells of the mutant type comprising the mural trophectoderm. This observation is not consistent with that of Mintz
(1964b) for chimeric blastocysts with t^{12}/t^{12} cells, but our sample
is, obviously, extremely small.

Conclusions: Resistance of the t^{w32}/t^{w32} *phenotype to chimerism*

The immature phenotype of t^{w32} mutant cells persists in spite
of the proximity of normal cells in chimeric morulae and blastocysts. The asynchrony between the retarded and normal cells seems
to preclude integrated development of the two aggregated embryos.

The infrequency of blastocyst formation in these aggregates,
in contrast to the numbers of t^{12}/t^{12}↔normal chimeric blastocysts

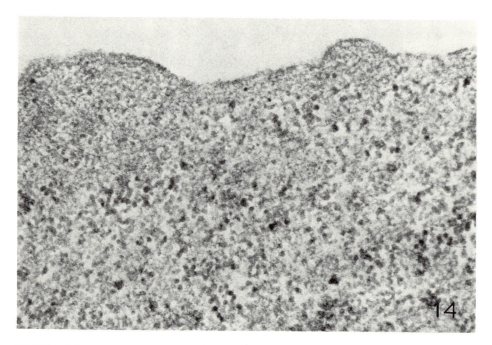

FIGURE 14. Portion of the cell surface of a mutant outer cell in
    a mutant↔normal blastocyst. In contrast with these features
    in the normal cell, microvilli are usually short and blunt,
    the surface is not very furrowed, and the cell coat is not
    robust. The subsurface cytoplasm of mutant cells is sometimes
    finely filamentous, as here.   x85,000. (Reduced 15% for purposes
    of reproduction)

produced by Mintz (1964b), may be due to the fact that t^{w32} homozygotes are arrested earlier than t^{12} homozygotes. Therefore, at
the 8-cell stage when embryo pairs are aggregated, the t^{w32} mutant
may already be defective and resist interactions with the normal
partner.

    Mintz (1964b) noted the relative immobility of the mutant
cells in chimeras, and the present fine-structural observations
provide a basis for this abnormality. Features of cells in arrested t^{w32}/t^{w32} morulae that are readily revealed by juxtaposition
to normal cells in chimeras are deficiencies of the cell coat and
of the subsurface filamentous network. It has been amply demonstrated that spreading of the cell surface, interdigitations of
adjacent cells, and formation of tight and gap junctions occur as
the morula becomes transformed into the blastocyst. In the mutant

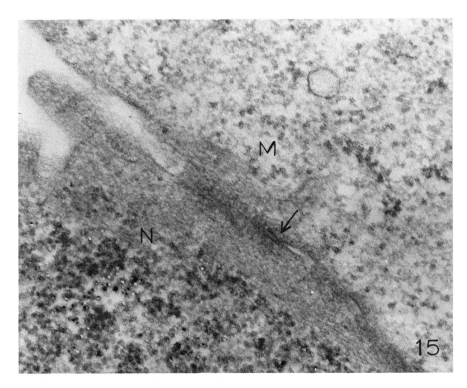

FIGURE 15. Adjacent normal and mutant cells (*N*, *M*) at their apical-lateral borders in the outer part of a chimera. Cell junctions (*arrow*) join the cells. A prominent subsurface band of fine filaments is seen in the normal cell, but, in the mutant cell, is present only at the region of contact between the two cells. There is a paucity of polysomes in the mutant cell. x85,000. (Reduced 20% for purposes of reproduction)

embryo, the deficiencies noted at the cell periphery may explain the reduction in interlocking villous cytoplasmic processes and the lack of stable cell associations. The failure of t^{w32} homozygotes to undergo blastocyst formation may be attributable to these defects.

Since these cellular interactions are essential to trophectoderm differentiation, it may be possible to induce cells of t^{w32}/t^{w32} phenotype to participate in blastocyst development in chimeras if the mutant cells can be excluded from the presumptive trophectoderm layer. We are attempting to test the viability and "rescue" of the mutant cells as components strictly of the inner cell mass by surrounding a single embryo from $+/t^{w32}$ x $+/t^{w32}$ litters with three wild-type embryos.

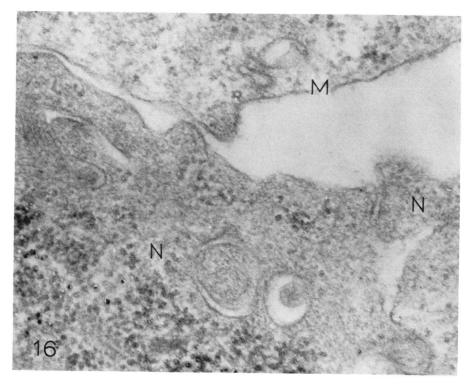

FIGURE 16. Neighboring normal and mutant cells (N, M) in the
     interior part of a chimera. The normal cell surfaces are
     characterized by many interdigitating folds, and a subsurface
     network of filaments is obvious. One villous projection is
     seen at the surface of the mutant cell, and very few subsur-
     face filaments are detectable. x85,000. (Reduced 15% for
     purposes of reproduction)

SUMMARY

     Some embryos believed to be chimeric for wild-type and t^{w18}/
t^{w18} genotypes appear grossly intermediate between normal 8-day
embryos and the typical mutant phenotype. At the cellular level,
no chimeric embryos contain mesodermal cells that are entirely
like those of the standard t^{w18} homozygote, thus suggesting an
alteration of the mutant phenotype.

     Morulae and blastocysts that are chimeric for wild-type and
t^{w32}/t^{w32} genotypes contain abnormal cells that possess the same
defects seen in the typical arrested mutant morula.

These projects required the joint efforts of several individuals, besides the author: D. Bennett, V. Papaioannou, K. Artzt, P. Marticorena, C. Calo, L. Divack, S. Dunn, and J. Babiarz.

This work was funded by NSF Grant number PCM 77-17835.

REFERENCES

Artzt, K. and D. Bennett. 1972. A genetically caused embryonal ectodermal tumor in the mouse. J. Natl. Cancer Inst. 48: 141-158.

Bennett, D. 1975. The T-locus of the mouse. Cell 6: 441-454.

Bennett, D. and L. C. Dunn. 1960. A lethal mutant (t^{w18}) in the house mouse showing partial duplication. J. exp. Zool. 143: 203-219.

Bennett, D. and L. C. Dunn. 1971. Transmission ratio distorting genes on chromosome IX and their interactions. In, Cell Interactions, L. Silvestri, Ed. Lepetit Coll. Biol. Med. 3.

Burgoyne, P. S. and T. Ducibella. 1977. Changes in the properties of the developing trophoblast of preimplantation mouse embryos as revealed by aggregation studies. J. Embryol. exp. Morph. 40: 143-157.

Calarco, P. G. and E. H. Brown. 1968. Cytological and ultrastructural comparisons of t^{12}/t^{12} and normal mouse morulae. J. exp. Zool. 168: 169-186.

Calarco, P. G. and C. J. Epstein. 1973. Cell surface changes during preimplantation development in the mouse. Devel. Biol. 32: 208-213.

Ducibella, T., D. F. Albertini, E. Anderson, and J. D. Biggers. 1975. The preimplantation mammalian embryo: characterization of intercellular junctions and their appearance during development. Devel. Biol. 45: 231-250.

Granholm, N. H. and P. M. Johnson. 1978. Identification of eight-cell t^{w32} homozygous lethal mutants by aberrant compaction. J. exp. Zool. 203: 81-88.

Hillman, N. and R. Hillman. 1975. Ultrastructural studies of t^{w32}/t^{w32} mouse embryos. J. Embryol. exp. Morph. 33: 685-695.

Hillman, N., R. Hillman, and G. Wileman. 1970. Ultrastructural studies of cleaving stage t^{12}/t^{12} mouse embryos. Am. J. Anat. 128: 311-340.

Magnuson, T., A. Demsey, and C. W. Stackpole. 1977. Characterization of intercellular junctions in the preimplantation mouse embryo
by freeze fracture and thin-section electron microscopy. Devel.
Biol. 61: 252-261.

Mintz, B. 1964a. Gene expression in the morula stage of mouse
embryos as observed during development of t^{12}/t^{12} lethal mutants
in vitro. J. exp. Zool. 157: 267-272.

Mintz, B. 1964b. Formation of genetically mosaic mouse embryos,
and early development of 'lethal (t^{12}/t^{12})-normal' mosaics. J.
exp. Zool. 61: 273-292.

Moser, G. C. and S. Glueksohn-Waelsch. 1967. Developmental genetics of a recessive allele at the complex T-locus in the mouse.
Devel. Biol. 16: 564-576.

Smith, L. J. 1956. A morphological and histochemical investigation of a preimplantation lethal (t^{12}) in the house mouse. J. exp.
Zool. 132: 51-83.

Spiegelman, M. and D. Bennett. 1974. Fine structural study of
cell migration in the early mesoderm of normal and mutant mouse
embryos (T-locus: t^{9}/t^{9}). J. Embryol. exp. Morph. 32: 723-738.

AN ANALYSIS OF DIFFERENTIATION IN COAGGREGATION CULTURES BETWEEN

MOUSE NEURONAL AND TUMOR CELLS

Leslie P. Kozak

The Jackson Laboratory, Bar Harbor, Maine 04609

Evidence exists that indicates interactions at the plasma-membrane surface of embryonic cells are involved in directing mor-phogenesis during early development (Saxen and Toivonen 1962). Consequently, a considerable effort has been directed at under-standing the molecular basis of specific cell-to-cell interactions, and in particular at identifying and characterizing specific mole-cules on the plasma-membrane surface that mediate or specify these interactions (Roth and Weston 1967; Steinberg 1970; Merrell and Glaser 1973; Hausman and Moscona 1975; Rutishauser, Thiery, Bracken-bury, Sela, and Edelman 1976). Although considerable progress has been made in characterizing macromolecules on the surface that affect cell adhesion, before an understanding of the molecular biology of cell-to-cell interactions and their role in differen-tiation can be achieved, specific genes must be identified whose expressions are modulated as a consequence of interactions at the cell surface.

In this paper I would like to describe a genetic locus in the mouse that, in certain cell types, appears to be regulated in part by the environment created when cells are tightly associated in a 3-dimensional array. This locus, *Gdc-1* located on Chromosome 15, which codes for the major isozyme of L-glycerol 3-phosphate dehydro-genase (α-GPDH) in adult tissue, and a related locus coding for the isozyme in the embryo, may provide us with a system to unravel the sequence of molecular events by which cellular interactions modulate the expression of specific nuclear genes during develop-ment. This description of the α-GPDH isozyme system will review studies on the genetics and protein structure of the isozymes, and on the regulation of isozyme expression in reaggregating cell cul-tures of mouse cerebellum and in mouse tumors grown *in vivo* and in tissue culture.

81

BIOCHEMICAL AND DEVELOPMENTAL CHARACTERISTICS OF L-GLYCEROL

3-PHOSPHATE DEHYDROGENASE ISOZYMES

The appearance of the isozymes of α-GPDH during development
of the mouse is schematically illustrated in Figure 1. According
to this scheme, there are two major isozymes expressed during
development. The earliest stage at which sufficient material
could be obtained to make the determinations was 8 days. In the
8-day embryo, an isozyme is detected that has a very rapid rate of
heat inactivation at 50°C ($t_{1/2} \sim 0.5$ min). The kinetics of heat
inactivation of the enzyme in the embryo suggested that it is the
major form present at this time (Kozak and Jensen 1974). By 10
days of gestation, a second isozyme is detected in extracts from
the whole embryo by separating the isozymes on isoelectric focusing (Rittman, Johnston, and Fondy 1977). When individual tissues
are analyzed by heat denaturation, it is apparent that there is
no uniform pattern of expression during development. Rather,
different tissues begin to accumulate the adult isozyme at different times: some tissues, such as liver, seem to express only the
adult isozyme even at the earliest time periods analyzed; whereas
other tissues, such as brain, continue to express the embryonic
isozyme even in adult tissues, although at low levels.

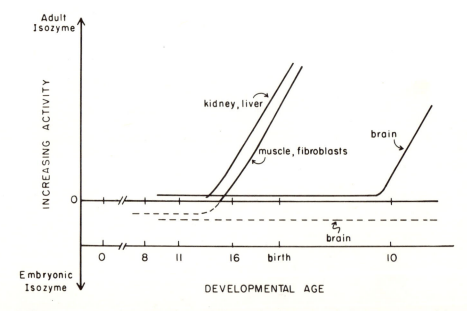

FIGURE 1. Developmental profiles of L-glycerol 3-phosphate dehy-
    drogenase: a schematic diagram illustrating the time of
    appearance of the embryonic (----) and adult (——) isozymes
    in the mouse.

In addition to these points, both isozymes can be expressed in the same cell as evidenced by the formation of heteropolymers. The heteropolymer is postulated to be a dimer composed of one subunit from each of the adult and embryonic homopolymers. Thus, the three isozymes can be separated by ion-exchange chromatography on DEAE-cellulose and are most readily detected in the brains of young mice, particularly at 11 to 12 days of age when the adult form has just started to increase (Fig. 2). This hybrid form (peak II) can also be generated *in vitro* by mixing the adult (peak I) and embryonic (peak III) isozymes together in the presence of high salt and sucrose, subsequently freezing and thawing, and then dialyzing against low ionic strength buffer (Kozak and Murphy 1976).

The observation that substantial amounts of a hybrid isozyme are present in brain has permitted us to obtain an antibody against the embryonic isozyme. Several early attempts to achieve this goal failed because insufficient enzyme was present in the fetal tissue from which the enzyme was extracted. An alternative approach was devised which depended first on purifying adult enzyme from muscle by a combination of affinity column chromatography on Blue Sepharose 6B and ion-exchange chromatography on DEAE-cellulose. This preparation of α-GPDH was injected into a rabbit and the antibodies produced were tested for their ability to immunoprecipitate the isozymes of α-GPDH found in postnatal brain. The α-GPDH activities represented by peaks I and II (Fig. 2) were both readily inactivated by the antisera, while the activity in peak III, the embryonic isozyme, was only slightly precipitated (Fig. 3). Since peak II was immunoprecipitable with anti-peak-I antisera, we reasoned that, if peak II was a hybrid of peak I and peak III isozymes, antisera produced against the peak II immune complex should react more strongly against peak III than the anti-peak-I antisera. When such an antiserum was produced, the postulated characteristics were observed, namely, the anti-peak-II antiserum precipitates peak III in addition to peaks I and II. Additional characteristics of the protein precipitated by anti-peak-II antisera were obtained by labeling the proteins in peaks I, II, and III with ^{125}I, immunoprecipitating with antisera, and separating the ^{125}I-labeled immunoprecipitated proteins on sodium dodecyl sulfate polyacrylamide gel electrophoresis. The major polypeptides present in each of the immunoprecipitates have identical molecular weights, and they migrate coincidentally with standard α-GPDH subunits.

A complicating feature of α-GPDH expression is that additional multiple forms of the enzyme can be demonstrated by chromatographic and isoelectric-focusing techniques. Although these forms seem to differ with respect to charge, little is known about their structural bases. The fact that these forms express the genetic structural variants, either electrophoretically or by heat denaturation,

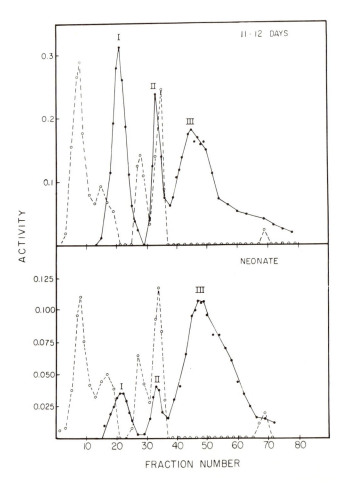

FIGURE 2.   Separation of isozymes of L-glycerol 3-phosphate dehy-
            drogenase on DEAE-cellulose ion-exchange chromatography.
            Brains from C57BL/6J mice were homogenized in 3 volumes of
            ice cold 10 mM Tris-HCl, pH 8.0 containing 1 mM EDTA, 2 mM
            dithiothreitol and 2 mM α-glycerol phosphate (buffer 1), and
            a 100,000 x g supernatant solution prepared. The enzyme solu-
            tions were dialyzed overnight against buffer 1 and applied to
            a (1 x 17.5 cm) DE-52 column (Whatman Co. Ltd.) that was equi
            equilibrated with buffer 1. The isozymes were eluted from
            the column with a 0 to 0.1 M linear 1-liter NaCl gradient in
            buffer 1. Fractions were assayed for protein by absorbance
            at 280 nm (0---0) and enzyme activity (●——●) by a spectro-
            photometric assay.

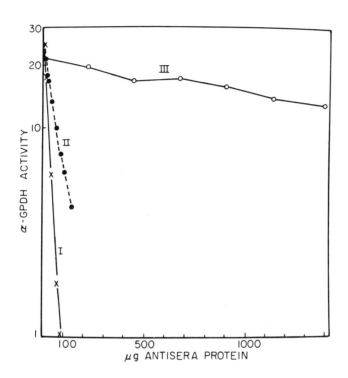

FIGURE 3. Immunoprecipitation of L-glycerol 3-phosphate dehydro-
    genase activity by antisera obtained from rabbits immunized
    with purified peak I enzyme. Immunoprecipitation was carried
    out in a reaction mixture containing 10 mM sodium phosphate,
    15 mM sodium chloride pH 7.5, approximately 20 mU of the
    designated isozyme and varying amounts of antisera. Each
    reaction mixture contains the same amount of serum protein,
    which is achieved by varying the amount of preimmune and
    immune sera added to the reaction. The reactions were incu-
    bated for 30 min at 37°C and then at 0–4°C overnight. The
    samples were centrifuged at 10,000 x g for 15 min and the
    supernatant solutions assayed for enzyme activity. Precipi-
    tin curves I, II, and III were obtained from the three peaks
    of activity separated on ion-exchange chromatography (Fig. 2).

suggests that they may arise by some type of posttranslational modification (Kozak and Erdelsky 1975).

The above results indicate that there are both similarities and differences in the embryonic and adult isozymes that could be equally well explained either by postulating that separate genetic structural loci code for each protein, or that the product of a single genetic locus is modified epigenetically. Genetic evidence suggests that there are probably two separate loci coding for the adult and embryonic isozyme. This evidence is that the three structural alleles that affect the electrophoretic and heat denaturation properties of adult α-GPDH do not cause similar modifications to the properties of the embryonic isozyme (Kozak and Jensen 1974).

THE EXPRESSION OF THE *Gdc-1* LOCUS IN REAGGREGATING CELLS

OF MOUSE CEREBELLUM

The cerebellum was selected as our model system for analyzing the effects of cell interactions on the differentiation of embryonic cells. The reasons for this selection were:

(1) The cerebellum has a population of proliferating undifferentiated cells in the external granule layer of 3- to 11-day-old mice present in the quantities required for tissue culture and biochemical analysis (Miale and Sidman 1961).

(2) The external granule layer cells go through a well-described phase of cell migration and sorting (Rakic 1971, 1973).

(3) Several mutants of the mouse have been described in which this sorting is abnormal (Sidman, Green, and Appel 1965; Rakic and Sidman 1973*a*, 1973*b*).

Reaggregating cell cultures of the cerebellum of 6-day-old mice were established by modification of methods developed by Moscona (Moscona 1961; Kozak 1977). The analysis of these cultures for α-GPDH expression indicated that, during the first few days, low amounts of enzyme activity were present that had the structural characteristics of the embryonic isozyme. Subsequently, there occurred an increase in activity, the time and extent of which depended on age of the mouse from which the cells were derived (Fig. 4). The timing of the increase was most striking in that it indicated that enzyme activity increased as a function of the chronological age of the cells and not of the length of time in culture (Fig. 5).

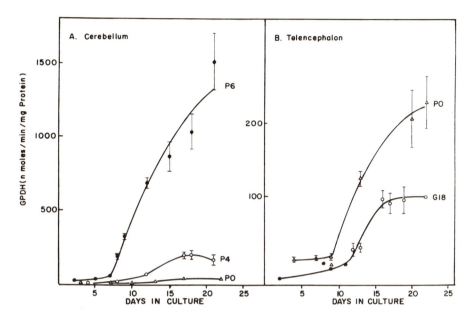

FIGURE 4. Development of L-glycerol 3-phosphate dehydrogenase in
reaggregating cell cultures from the cerebellum (A) and from
the telencephalon (B) of C57BL/6J mice of varying ages. P0,
P4, and P6 refer to Days 0, 4, and 6, respectively, after
birth; G18 refers to a fetus on the 18th day of gestation.
Each point with its error bars represents the mean ± the
standard error of three to six cultures.
[From Kozak 1977, by permission.]

    Information on the genetic mechanisms controlling the accumu-
lation of enzyme activity was obtained by measuring the rate of
enzyme synthesis during the culture period. Cultures were incubated with radioactively labeled amino acids, labeled enzyme protein was isolated by affinity column chromatography, and the rate
of α-GPDH synthesis relative to the synthesis of total cytoplasmic
trichloroacetic-acid-precipitable protein determined. A coincidence was observed between the measured rate of enzyme synthesis
and accumulation of enzyme activity, which indicates that the accumulation of activity is accomplished by an increase in enzyme synthesis (Kozak 1978*a*).

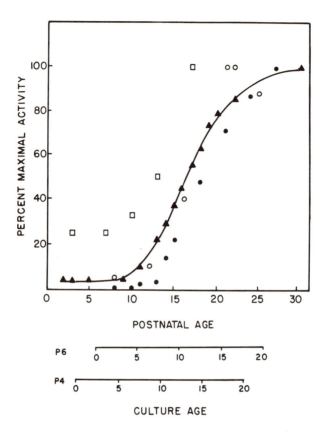

FIGURE 5. A comparison of the development of L-glycerol 3-phos-
     phate dehydrogenase *in vivo* (▲——▲) to development in reag-
     gregating cell cultures for cultures from the cerebellum (A).
     Cerebellar cells in the cultures were obtained from mice 0
     (□), 4 (o), and 6 (•) days of age. The data for aggre-
     gates from mice 0 days of age are plotted on the same scale
     as the *in vivo* data. [From Kozak 1977, by permission.]

     This observed accumulation of enzyme activity in culture
occurred only when cerebellar cells were cultured as aggregates.
Cells grown as monolayers in plastic tissue-culture flasks expressed very low levels of activity in which the predominant isozyme present had the heat-denaturation characteristics of the α-
GPDH present in fetal brain. These results on α-GPDH expression
in cerebellar cells in aggregate cultures indicate that a complex
biochemical differentiation occurs *in vitro* which involves differential expression of possibly distinct but related structural loci.
The regulation of this biochemical locus also adheres to a chrono-

logical time sequence, and genetic mechanisms that control the activity level of the enzyme also seem to be functioning in tissue culture. This biochemical differentiation of cerebellar cells *in vitro* is occurring simultaneously with an extensive morphological differentiation that include many features of the normal differentiation of granule cell neurons and glial cells (Kozak, Eppig, Dahl, and Bignami 1977).

THE EXPRESSION OF THE *Gdc-1* LOCUS IN TUMORS

The discussion in the preceding section indicated that *in vitro* conditions in which cell contact was maximized, i.e., aggregate cultures, facilitated the synthesis of the enzyme coded for by the *Gdc-1* locus. In the aggregation culture system, cell division is virtually absent; consequently, it is possible that expression of *Gdc-1* is initiated by a cessation of cell division, as was suggested recently by Rittmann *et al.* (1977) in their analysis of murine tumors. In a similar type of analysis of mouse tumors, we observed that solid tumors of the mouse invariably express the adult isozyme of α-GPDH, whereas ascites tumors express the embryonic isozyme (Kozak and Murphy 1976). From the variety of tumors analyzed, one tumor was selected for further analysis. This tumor, the 15091A mammary carcinoma, has been serially passaged since 1928; it grows extremely rapidly, whether in the ascites or solid form (passaged every 10 days). When this tumor was transplanted from the ascites form to the solid form, in alternate generations, the isozyme expressed was adult in the solid tumor and embryonic in the ascites form (Fig. 6).

In another experiment, a C1300 solid neuroblastoma expressing the adult isozyme was established in tissue culture and cloned. This cloned cell line expressed the embryonic isozyme in culture, and adult isozyme in the tumor when the cloned cells were injected subcutaneously into a mouse. The cloned cells in culture were submitted to conditions that not only arrest cell division but also cause a morphological differentiation *in vitro* (Augusti-Tocco and Sato 1969; Schubert, Humphreys, Baroni, and Cohn 1969; Schubert and Jacob 1970; Seeds, Gilman, Amano, and Nirenberg 1970). These conditions include treatments with cyclic AMP, bromodeoxyuridine, X irradiation, removal of serum, growth at high density, and growth as aggregates formed by gyratory motion in Erlenmeyer flasks. No culture conditions have been found that will promote expression of the adult isozyme in culture. Since these conditions include those that stop or slow down cell division, we conclude that cessation of cell division in culture is not a sufficient condition for synthesis of adult isozyme in the cell types being analyzed; rather, the form of growth is more critical in determining which type of isozyme will be expressed.

	SOLID TUMOR			ASCITES TUMOR	
Generation	Specific Activity	T½ in min.		Specific Activity	T½ in min.
1	35.4	4.6		2.4 ± 0.1	0.6
2	145.0	3.6		3.8 ± 0.1	0.7
3	49.3 ± 12.4	3.9		7.9 ± 0.8	0.6
4	not analyzed			9.9 ± 1.4	0.9
5	18.7	4.0		3.5 ± 0.3	0.5

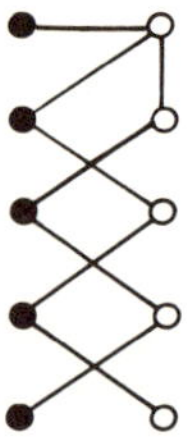

FIGURE 6. Changes in α-GPDH expression during interconversion of 15091A tumor. ●, solid tumors; O, ascites tumor. Specific activity is given in nmoles/min/mg protein. $t_{1/2}$ in min indicates the half-life of α-GPDH at 50°. [From Kozak and Murphy 1976, by permission.]

EXPRESSION OF THE *Gdc-1* LOCUS IN COAGGREGATION CULTURES OF

CEREBELLAR AND TUMOR CELLS

The fact that, under identical culture conditions, aggregates of cerebellar cells from 6-day-old mice can initiate the active synthesis of adult-type α-GPDH whereas neuroblastoma cells cannot suggests that, possibly, the cerebellar cells might provide the appropriate environment for α-GPDH synthesis in neuroblastoma cells if the two cell types were coaggregated together. When such cultures were set up and analyzed for α-GPDH expression, it was found that, not only did neuroblastoma cells not synthesize adult α-GPDH, but the cerebellar cells also stopped synthesizing adult enzyme. Table 1 summarizes the results on α-GPDH accumulation in a series of experiments in which we assessed the effects on neuroblastoma cells of X irradiation to stop cell division, freezing and thawing to destroy the integrity of the cell, and addition of conditioned medium from neuroblastoma cells to test for the presence of diffusible factor. The results indicate that even neuroblastoma cells fragmented by freezing and thawing are capable of blocking enzyme accumulation, but that conditioned medium from neuroblastoma cells contains nothing that blocks enzyme accumulation.

TABLE 1. Effect of tumor cells on the accumulation of L-glycerol 3-phosphate dehydrogenase in cultured mouse cerebellar cells

Expt.	Cell types	Days in culture	Cells per flask*	α-GPDH
				nmoles/min/mg protein
I	B6 CB P6	13	20 x 10^6	843.8 ± 36.1 (4)
	NB (X-irrad.)[†]	13	20 x 10^6	12.5 ± 0.9 (5)
	B6 CB P6 + NB (X irrad.)	13	25 x 10^6	66.4 ± 38.1 (5)
II	B6 CB P6	12	20 x 10^6	408.4 ± 94.6 (4)
	B6 CB P6 + NB (X irrad., F.-T.)	12	25 x 10^6	33.4 ± 4.2 (4)
III	B6 CB P6	10	20 x 10^6	145.6 ± 8.8 (5)
	B6 CB P6 + conditioned med.[‡]	10	20 x 10^6	200.9 ± 29.0 (7)
IV	B6 CB P6	11	20 x 10^6	260.9 ± 38.5 (6)
	B6 CB P6 + F9 (X irrad.)	11	25 x 10^6	68.9 ± 16.4 (6)

* When two cell types were coaggregated, there were 20 x 10^6 B6 CB P6 cells and 5 x 10^6 tumor cells.

[†] Neublastoma cells (NB) and F9 cells were X irradiated with 10,000 R and 1,000 R, respectively. NB cells were also frozen and thawed (F.-T.) in experiment II.

[‡] To obtain conditioned medium, neuroblastoma cells were cultured in BME + 15% horse serum for 24 hr; the cells were removed from the medium by centrifugation, and the cell-free medium was filtered through a 0.45 μ Nalgene filter and added immediately to cultured cerebellar aggregates. This procedure was repeated every 24 hr in order to keep the conditioned medium as fresh as possible.

The specificity of this effect by tumor cells on cerebellar cell differentiation in culture was assessed by coaggregating other tumor cells with the cerebellar cells. L-cells were found to be rather ineffective; however, F9 teratocarcinoma-derived cells (Bernstine, Hooper, Grandchamp, and Ephrussi 1973) are effective (Table 1). An interesting aspect of the experiment with F9 cells was that the X irradiation of F9 before the aggregation, in order to arrest cell division of the F9 cells, caused these cells eventually to fragment and lose their cytoplasm, as assessed by the disappearance of the F9 allozyme of the cytoplasmic glucose phosphate isomerase. Hence, it appears that these fragments, incorporated or retained in the aggregate with cerebellar cells (evident by electron microscopy), are still capable of blocking synthesis or accumulation of cerebellar α-GPDH (Kozak 1978b).

The mechanism underlying this phenomenon is unclear. The cerebellar cells still appear to be viable, as judged from microscopy and enzyme analysis, although a change in the type or morphology of the cerebellar cell in the aggregate has occurred. Whether a population of cells in the cerebellar aggregates has been eliminated or changed, or whether only a few genetic loci, such as the *Gdc-1* locus, have been repressed, must yet be determined.

CONCLUSIONS

That the differentiation of cerebellar cells in tissue culture is facilitated when cell contact is maximized, and that this differentiation is inhibited by neuroblastoma cells when the two cell types are associated in a mosaic relationship in an aggregate, suggests that interactions at the cell surface are important in this differentiation. It also suggests that, possibly, cell-surface components, or extracellular, nondiffusible material associated with neuroblastoma and teratocarcinoma cells, may block the differentiation of the cerebellar cells.

There is some evidence that addresses this point. Based upon the developmental profiles of hyaluronic acid in embryonic tissues as they proceed through phases of cell proliferation, migration, and finally terminal differentiation, Toole (1976) has postulated that because hyaluronic acid is high during periods of cell migration and decreases at the time of differentiation, hyaluronic acid might block the precocious differentiation of cells, and that the removal of hyaluronic acid by hyaluronidase would initiate terminal differentiation. Toole has also noted that the developing brain has periods of cell migration and sorting, and he cites evidence that the metabolism of hyaluronic acid in brain during these periods follows patterns similar to that of other embryonic tissues. Transformed cells are also known to synthesize hyaluronic acid (Satoh, Duff, Rapp, and Davidson 1973); consequently it would

be useful to assess the effects of hyaluronic acid on the differentiation of cerebellar cells in culture and thus test Toole's
model for the control of differentiation in this system.

In addition to extracellular matrix material, other possibly
more promising candidates for involvement in the phenomenon described in this paper are glycoproteins that are involved in mediating the interactions in a more direct manner than hyaluronic
acid, which, because of its hydration properties, acts by prevent-
ing cell contact. Glycoproteins have been identified that seem to
mediate adhesion between cells. Whether these or similar kinds of
molecules can modulate expression of specific genes must yet be
determined (Hausman and Moscona 1975; Rutishauser *et al.* 1976).

The essential message in this communication is that both neuroblastoma and primitive F9 embryonal carcinoma cells possess a
property that allows them to interact with cerebellar cells to
repress biochemical differentiation. Can one therefore identify
a molecular system that is involved in repressing differentiation,
which first becomes expressed during early embryonic development,
and which is intact and functional in the undifferentiated cerebellar cells of a 6-day-old mouse?

This research was supported by USPHS Grants HD 08431 and HD
06712. The Jackson Laboratory is fully accredited by the American
Association for Accreditation of Laboratory Animal Care.

REFERENCES

Augusti-Tocco, G., and G. Sato. 1969. Establishment of functional
clonal lines of neurons from mouse neuroblastoma. Proc. Natl.
Acad. Sci. USA 64: 311.

Bernstine, E. G., M. L. Hooper, S. Grandchamp and B. Ephrussi.
1973. Alkaline phosphatase activity in mouse teratoma. Proc.
Natl. Acad. Sci. USA 70: 3899.

Hausman, R. E. and A. A. Moscona. 1975. Purification and characterization of the retina-specific cell-aggregating factor. Proc.
Natl. Acad. Sci. USA 72: 916.

Kozak, L. P. 1977. The transition from embryonic to adult isozyme
expression in reaggregating cell cultures of mouse brain. Dev.
Biol. 55: 49.

Kozak, L. P. 1978*a*. Increased synthesis of L-glycerol 3-phos-
phate dehydrogenase during *in vitro* differentiation of reaggregating cerebellar cells. Dev. Biol., in press.

Kozak, L. P. 1978*b*. Coaggregation with tumor cells inhibits
expression by cerebellar cells of the adult isozyme locus, *Gdc-1*.
Dev. Biol., in press.

Kozak, L. P., J. J. Eppig, D. Dahl and A. Bignami. 1977. Ultrastructural and immunohistological characterization of a cell culture model for the study of neuronal-glial interactions. Dev.
Biol. 59: 206.

Kozak, L. P. and K. J. Erdelsky. 1975. The genetics and developmental regulation of L-glycerol 3-phosphate dehydrogenase. J.
Cell. Physiol. 85: 437.

Kozak, L. P. and J. T. Jensen. 1974. Genetic and developmental
control of multiple forms of L-glycerol 3-phosphate dehydrogenase.
J. Biol. Chem. 249: 7775.

Kozak, L. P. and E. D. Murphy. 1976. The reversible expression
of an adult isozyme locus, *Gdc-1*, in tumors of the mouse. Cancer
Res. 36: 3711.

Merrell, R. and L. Glaser. 1973. Specific recognition of plasma
membranes by embryonic cells. Proc. Natl. Acad. Sci. USA 70:
2794.

Miale, I. L. and R. L. Sidman. 1961. An autoradiographic analysis
of histogenesis in the mouse cerebellum. Exp. Neurol. 4: 277.

Moscona, A. A. 1961. Rotation-mediated histogenetic aggregation
of dissociated cells. Exp. Cell Res. 22: 455.

Rakic, P. 1971. Neuron-glia relationship during granule cell
migration in developing cerebellar cortex. A Golgi and electron-
microscopic study in *Macacus rhesus*. J. Comp. Neur. 141: 283.

Rakic, P. 1973. Kinetics of the proliferation and the latency
between final division and onset of differentiation of the cerebellar stellate and basket cells. J. Comp. Neur. 147: 523.

Rakic, P. and R. L. Sidman. 1973*a*. Sequence of developmental
abnormalities leading to granule cell deficit in cerebellar cortex
of Weaver mutant mice. J. Comp. Neur. 152: 103.

Rakic, P. and R. L. Sidman. 1973*b*. Organization of cerebellar
cortex secondary to deficit of granule cells in Weaver mutant
mice. J. Comp. Neur. 152: 133.

Rittman, L. S., S. M. Johnston and T. P. Fondy. 1977. Forms of cytosolic nicotinamide adenine dinucleotide-linked glycerol-3-dehydrogenase in normal and neoplastic mouse tissues. Cancer Res. 37: 2673.

Roth, S. and J. Weston. 1967. The measurement of intercellular adhesion. Proc. Natl. Acad. Sci. USA 58: 974.

Rutishauser, U., J. P. Thiery, R. Brackenbury, B. A. Sela and G. M. Edelman. 1976. Mechanisms of adhesion among cells from neural tissues of the chick embryo. Proc. Natl. Acad. Sci. USA 73: 577.

Satoh, C., R. Duff, F. Rapp and E. A. Davison. 1973. Production of mucopolysaccharides by normal and transformed cells. Proc. Natl. Acad. Sci. USA 70: 54.

Saxen, L. and S. Toivonen. 1962. Primary embryonic induction, pp. 1-271, Academic Press, London.

Schubert, D., S. Humphreys, C. Baroni and M. Cohn. 1969. *In vitro* differentiation of a mouse neuroblastoma. Proc. Natl. Acad. Sci. USA 64: 316.

Schubert, D. and F. Jacob. 1970. 5-Bromodeoxyuridine-induced differentiation of a neuroblastoma. Proc. Natl. Acad. Sci. USA 67: 247.

Seeds, N. W., A. G. Gilman, T. Amano and M. W. Nirenberg. 1970. Regulation of axon formation by clonal lines of a neural tumor. Proc. Natl. Acad. Sci. USA 66: 160.

Sidman, R. L., M. C. Green and S. H. Appel. 1965. Catalog of the neurological mutants of the mouse. Harvard University Press, Cambridge.

Steinberg, M. S. 1970. Does differential adhesion govern self-assembly processes in histogenesis? Equilibrium configurations and the emergence of a hierarchy among populations of embryonic cells. J. Exp. Zool. 173: 395.

Toole, B. P. 1976. Morphogenetic role of glycosaminoglycans (Acid Mucopolysaccharides) in brain and other tissues. In Neuronal Recognition, S. H. Barondes, Ed., Plenum Press, New York, pp. 275-329.

THE USE OF MOSAICS AND EXPERIMENTAL CHIMERAS TO STUDY THE PATHOGENESIS OF NEOPLASIA

Philip M. Iannaccone

University of California at San Diego, University
Hospital, 225 Dickinson, San Diego, California 92103

PAST STUDIES CONCERNING THE CELLULAR ORIGIN OF SPONTANEOUS AND INDUCED TUMORS

Electrophoretic variants of X-linked enzymes have been exploited to study the cellular origins of tumors (Fialkow 1976; Gartler 1974). Gartler and Linder first demonstrated that three lipomas, arising in females heterozygous for electrophoretic variants of Gd, the gene coding for glucose-6-phosphate dehydrogenase, were composed of cells that produced mainly one variant when both were expected (Gartler and Linder 1964).

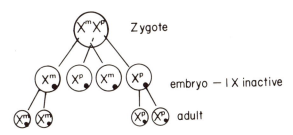

FIGURE 1. X inactivation in mammalian females. One X-chromosome is inactivated early in development. The inactivation is heritable, therefore adult tissues are comprised of small clones of cells with either maternal X (X^m) or paternal X (X^p) active.

The cells of placental females undergo random, heritable, and probably irreversible inactivation of one of their two X chromosomes early in embryonic development. As a result, females are mosaics composed of two cell types (Fig. 1), one with the maternal and the other with the paternal X chromosome active. The mosaicism can be demonstrated if the maternal and paternal X chromosomes are distinguishable. A suitable marker system is provided by any X-linked allelic polymorphism. Glucose-6-phosphate dehydrogenase, which is known to be X-linked (Ohno 1971), has a number of variants, the most useful of which can be demonstrated electrophoretically. Most Caucasian populations produce a cathodal isozyme (GD-B) that migrates slowly in an electrophoretic field. A proportion of African Negro males produce an anodal isozyme (GD-A) that migrates rapidly. Therefore, there is a proportion of the female population that is heterozygous for these variants. Since one X chromosome is inactivated early in development, these individuals are mosaics composed of cells which express Gd^A and cells which express Gd^B (Fig. 2). Linder and Gartler reasoned that if a tumor arising in these individuals had started from a large number of cells, then both cell types (Gd^A and Gd^B) would comprise the tumor. On the other hand, if one or a relatively small number of cells were responsible for

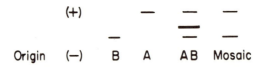

FIGURE 2. Electrophoretic patterns of glucose-6-phosphate dehydrogenase. The common electrophoretic variant of GD migrates slowly and is represented in the channel labeled "B". In addition, there is a rapidly migrating variant, GD-A, represented in the channel labeled "A". If both alleles were expressed in the same cell, one might expect the pattern depicted in the channel labeled "AB". Here, both A and B isozymes are shown and a hybrid band representing a heteropolymer (formed by the interaction of A and B subunits) is shown in a position of intermediate mobility. In fact, tissue homogenates from heterozygous females have an electrophoretic pattern represented in the channel labeled "mosaic," showing only the A and B isozymes. This pattern demonstrates that the two alleles are not active in the same cell. Cloning experiments have shown that the adult tissues of female heterozygotes are composed of two populations of cells, one expressing the Gd^A and the other expressing the Gd^B allele.

the production of the tumor, then the tumor would be composed of
only one cell type. Thus it was concluded that the lipomas had
arisen from one cell or, at most, a few cells. This observation
was extended to leiomyomata of the uterus (Linder and Gartler 1965).
With several hundred tumors studied, virtually all were demonstrated
to contain a single type of glucose-6-dehydrogenase. Many other
neoplastic conditions were studied with this marker in subsequent
years (Fialkow 1976). In general, all adequately studied tumors
were found to contain one of the two variants present in the smallest samples of normal tissue. Some interesting exceptions include
multiple neurofibromatosis. This autosomal dominant condition pre-
disposes afflicted persons to the development of multiple neurofibromas. Although the tumor masses are histologically homogeneous,
they contain both Gd^A and Gd^B cells in the heterozygous females
studied (Fialkow, Sagebiel, Gartler, and Rimoin 1971). This suggests that there is some heritable change, originating as a germ
line mutation, which affects a large number of cells. Then some
second event starts the tumor off, affecting the large number of
susceptible cells. While it is true that only a specific tissue
is involved in this process, it is possible that the initial event
affects a tissue-specific process, for example, a mutation in DNA-
repair mechanisms that is relevant to that tissue only.

There are other lines of evidence that suggest human spontaneous tumors are clonal growths. If a tumor is composed of cells
that all contain a common chromosomal structural aberration, this
suggests that all of the tumor cells have arisen from the same cell.
The probability is very small that all of the tumor cells would
have the same aberration by chance alone. Several tumors have been
demonstrated to have common marker chromosomes. Chronic myelogenous
leukemia (CML), for example, is frequently associated with the so-
called Philadelphia chromosome. The nearly ubiquitous presence of
this marker in CML suggests that the alteration of chromosome structure may be causally related to the disease, though this remains a
controversial issue. Tumors that are composed of cells capable of
producing immunoglubulins, in general, produce only a single type
of immunoglobulin — which again suggests the tumor is composed of
a clone of cells. In addition, a number of tumors have been shown
to be composed of cells expressing a single electrophoretic variant
of Gd and a single type of immunoglobulin (Fialkow 1976).

There has been a great deal of interest in the interaction of
carcinogens and cellular components since the earliest induction of
specific tumors in experimental animals. Interest in these interactions has narrowed to determining which of the various cellular
macromolecules are capable of covalent reaction with chemical carcinogens. The hope was, and is, that this information would impli-
cate the site(s) of key interaction(s), and allow the mechanism of
action to be deduced.

Two theories of chemical carcinogenesis which are now competing are: (1) that carcinogens cause structural changes in DNA through covalent bonding and that these changes result in the neoplastic phenotype; and (2) that carcinogens modify controlling proteins which can, by themselves, result in the expression of the neoplastic phenotype. The ubiquitous nature of covalent interaction between carcinogens and cellular macromolecules does not allow us to choose between these two possibilities.

In this context, it would be useful to know if the interactions that cause the formation of tumors are rare. If the neoplasia were found to arise from a rare event, a mutational theory of the origin of these tumors would be supported, since one might expect effects on controlling proteins to be more general. Mutational theories are supported by the fact that, at the cellular level, the malignant phenotype is heritable.

The first suggestion that alteration in the chromosome comple-ment of the cell could be responsible for expression of neoplastic phenotype is found in Theodor Boveri's monograph, "On the Problem of the Origin of Malignant Tumors" (1914). Boveri sets forth a theory of the origin of tumors based on his early observations of atypical mitotic activity. He suggests that aberrations in cyto-kinetic mechanisms can result in cells with more than the appropri-ate number of chromosomes, as well as cells with fewer than the appropriate number. Boveri then proposes that aberrant cells may occasionally survive, and that a rare cell may be capable of un-checked growth. He suggests that an absolute consequence of this theory is that the resulting tumor grows as a clone of cells, each carrying the aberrant chromosome complement, and that "...every theory of cancer is wrong which does not take into account its uni-cellular origin." This concept of a chromosomal origin of cancer later became embodied in the somatic-mutation theory of cancer, first published by Bauer in 1928, but suggested by Morgan and Bridges in a recounting of Boveri's work in 1919. In the 1930's, a concept known as the field theory was formulated by Willis and other researchers (Willis 1967). The field theory suggested that tumors arose as the result of generalized effects in entire tissues, or at least in a large segment of tissues. This "field" of cells is transformed by carcinogenic stimulus and grows into the tumor. The somatic-mutation and field theory parallel theories of carcino-gen interaction with DNA and protein, respectively.

THE USE OF EXPERIMENTAL CHIMERAS TO STUDY CELLULAR ORIGIN OF INDUCED TUMORS

To study the question of the clonality of chemically induced tumors, we need a system analogous to X-linked mosaicism of humans in an experimental animal. However, suitable X-linked polymorphisms

in common laboratory rodents were not available until recently.
We have attempted to reproduce such a system with experimental chimeras. Our chimeras were produced by amalgamating embryos of mouse
strains that expressed different electrophoretic variants of glucose
phosphate isomerase (GPI-1; E.C.5.3.1.9), a dimeric enzyme coded
for by a single known autosomal locus (Chapman, Whitten, and Ruddle
1971). Two forms of the enzyme are known: a slowly migrating
anodal variant (GPI-1A) and a rapidly migrating cathodal variant
(GPI-1B; Fig. 3).

Combinations of Swiss albino mice expressing GPI-1A and Swiss
albino mice expressing GPI-1B were made by microinjection of inner
cell masses (Gardner, in press), or by morula aggregation. The
inner cell masses were removed from donor embryos by microsurgery
or by treatment with rabbit antimouse antiserum, followed by guinea-
pig complement to lyse the trophoblast. In addition, combinations

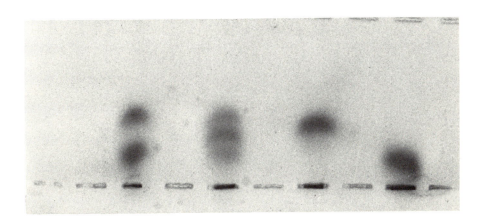

FIGURE 3. Electrophoretic patterns of glucose phosphate isomerase.
    From right to left: hemolysate from a homozygous $Gpi-1^a/Gpi-1^a$
    animal; hemolysate from a homozygous $Gpi-1^b/Gpi-1^b$ animal;
    hemolysate from a heterozygous $Gpi-1^a/Gpi-1^b$ animal (note he-
    teropolymeric band of intermediate mobility and greater inten-
    sity); homogenate of chimeric tissue, showing both a and b
    isozymes. The horizontal electrophoresis was done using
    12% starch gels (w/v in a 1:20 dilution of tank buffer). The
    tank buffer was 0.2 M Triscitrate pH 6.4. A current of 8—12
    ma was applied across a 6 cm gap for three hours at 4°C.
    (From Iannaccone et al. 1978. Reproduced by permission of
    J. Cell. Science.)

of embryos between Swiss albino (Gpi-1^a/Gpi-1^a) and CBA/HT6T6 (which are Gpi-1^b/Gpi-1^b), were made by microinjection of CBA inner cell masses obtained by microsurgery (Fig. 4; Iannaccone, Gardner, and Harris 1978).

Tumors were induced by topical application of 7,12-dimethyl-benz[a]anthracene (DMBA), followed by twice weekly applications of croton oil (C.O.) or 12-0-tetradecanoylphorbol-13-acetate(TPA). Tumors were also induced by topical application of 20-methylcholanthrene (MCA), followed by application of TPA twice weekly and injection of MCA subcutaneously. These various treatments resulted in the formation of squamous cell carcinomas, a basal cell carcinoma, and fibrosarcomas (Fig. 5), as well as of benign papillomas (Fig. 6). A total of 96 primary tumors and 13 recurrences were obtained (Table 1). The tumors were removed either surgically or shortly after death and then homogenized in tris lysis buffer. The homogenate was centrifuged and the supernatant was subjected to electrophoresis.

Of the 96 tumor homogenates studied, 46 contained greater than ninety-five per cent GPI-1A activity and 43 contained greater than ninety-five per cent GPI-1B activity (Fig. 7). The 13 recurrences gave the same results as the primary tumors, with the exception of two tumors containing both isozymes while the primary tumors

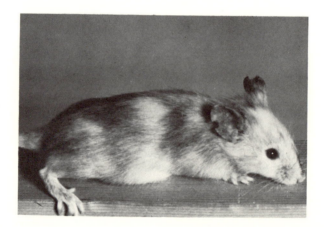

FIGURE 4. Chimera C56 was produced by injecting the inner cell mass from a CBA/HT6T6, Gpi-1^b/Gpi-1^b blastocyst into the blastocoele of a Swiss albino Gpi-1^a/Gpi-1^a blastocyst. CBA/HT6T6 mice have agouti coats. The adult chimera has broad bands of pigmentation, extending to the tail, which result from the clonal derivation of melanocyte precursors. This pattern of coat pigmentation is not related to variegation of epidermal cells. Both eyes of this individual contained pigment.

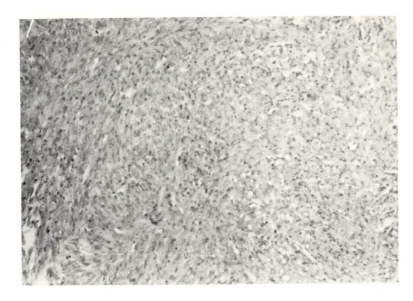

FIGURE 5. Fibrosarcoma T339 from chimeric mouse C87. This tumor
was produced by a single subcutaneous injection of 2.5 mg of
methylcholanthrene in olive oil. The tissue was analyzed 16
weeks after injection of the carcinogen.

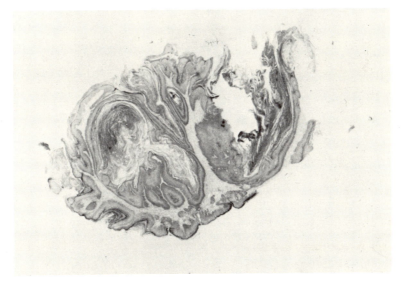

FIGURE 6. This papilloma (T319) was induced in chimeric mouse C70
with DMBA and is composed of abnormal epidermal proliferation
over a small core of loose, fibrous connective tissue.

TABLE 1. Glucose phosphate isomerase isozyme banding patterns in chimeric tissues and tumors derived from them (From Iannaccone *et al.* 1978)

	No. animals	No. of samples showing banding patterns		
		GPI-1A	GPI-1B	GPI-1A & B
Normal epidermis	28	14	25	456
Normal dermis	22	2	17	398
Normal subcutaneous tissue	4	0	0	25
Tumors	21	46(9)*	43(2)*	7(2)

*The numbers in parentheses refer to additional analyses done on tumors that recurred after surgical removal of the primary tumor.

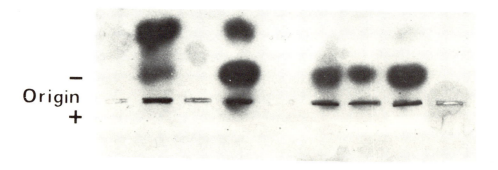

FIGURE 7. Electrophoretic pattern of tumor homogenates and standard blood mixtures. From left to right: the first channel with a pattern is a hemolysate from a $Gpi\text{-}1^b/Gpi\text{-}1^b$ animal with 5% (V/V) $Gpi\text{-}1^a/Gpi\text{-}1^a$ blood added; the second is a homogenate of a small piece of normal tissue adjacent to tumor T263; the third, fourth and fifth are homogenates of three individual samples from different areas of tumor T263, a subcutaneous fibrosarcoma. The normal tissue contains both isozymes, while the tumor contains only one. Tissue was homogenized in 10 mM lysate buffer at pH 7.4. (From Iannaccone *et al.* 1978. Reproduced by permission of J. Cell. Science.)

had been shown to contain only one. Seven of the 96 primary tumors
resulted in homogenates which contained both activities. In these
cases we have circumstantial evidence of coalescence between two
or more primary tumors, or of tumor contamination by host tissues.
We may therefore conclude that none of the primary tumors produced
both isozymic variants. A total of 495 small pieces of isolated
epidermis were homogenized and subjected to electrophoresis. All
but 39 contained both variants of GPI-1. Mouse epidermis was isolated by cold trypsinization (Fig. 8a and 8b; Iannaccone *et al.*
1978). Small samples of dermis were studied (417 samples) in the
same way and all but 19 demonstrated both variants (Fig. 9, Table
1). These data suggest that the tumors arose from a small number
of cells.

The possibility remains, however, that the cells of the tumor
express a single isozyme because of selection. The selection might
be a result of the carcinogen affecting only one of the two cell
types, although both cell types have been shown to form tumors.
The selection might be a result of one population of cells having
a growth advantage over the other cell type. However, there are
seven animals that have both types of tumors, i.e., tumors comprised
of cells producing only GPI-1A isozyme and other tumors comprised
of cells that produce only GPI-1B isozyme. It is difficult to con-
ceive of a mechanism that, within the same animal, would result in
selective growth advantage of one cell type for one tumor and then
selective growth advantage of the other cell type for the next
tumor. Moreover, there should be a point early in the development
of the tumor when both isozymes are present, reflecting the presence
of both cell types. This is not the case, since tumors studied at
1 to 32 weeks of age have given the same results of a single isozyme expressed by the tumor cells. In addition, samples from different parts of the same large tumor (hence, of different ages of
the same tumor) all show the same single isozyme.

The tumor might have contained only one isozyme and yet have
arisen from a large number of cells if the target tissue was composed of large contiguous areas of cells of the same *Gpi-1* type.
That is, the tumors might have arisen from a nonmosaic field. This
issue can be resolved by studying small samples of normal tissue to
derive an estimate of the patch and clone size.

Nesbitt (1974) has described patches and clones by using the
analogy of a checkerboard in which squares are assigned black or
white (i.e. the cell types of the chimera) by flipping a coin. Each
individual square then represents a clone of cells. Several adjacent squares will be the same color and the areas of a single color
are patches. During embryogenesis there is considerable cell mixing. Therefore, following the amalgamation of two embryos, the
positions of cells will be randomized, at least in the inner cell

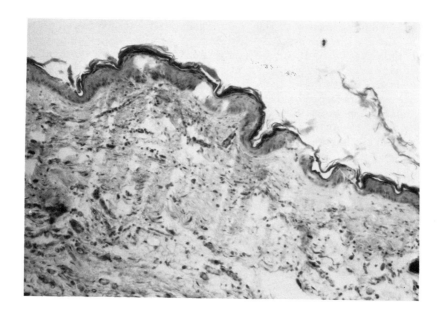

FIGURE 8a. Normal chimeric mouse skin.

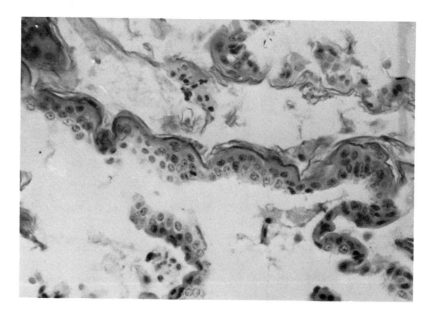

FIGURE 8b. Chimeric epidermis isolated by treatment of whole skin
            with 1% tripsin (W/V in phosphate buffered saline) at 4°C
            overnight. The epidermis was removed with fine forceps as a
            sheet.

mass. At some point in embryogenesis, the cells become fixed and
descendant cells remain contiguous, which procudes a clone. Adjacent clones of the same cell type form a larger contiguous area,
called a patch.*

     The relative frequency of the two cell types affects the number
of clones in a patch. As the proportion of one cell type increases,
a point is reached where the cells of that type form one large
patch. This critical proportion has been estimated to be eighty
per cent (West 1975), but others suggest that it occurs at a lower
level (Domb and Sykes 1960). When the critical proportion is
reached, the chimeric tissue can be considered as a sea of the major
cell type with islands of the minor cell type.

     The clone size can be estimated by measuring the variation in
proportion of cell types in a large number of very small samples
(Linder and Gartler 1965a). In our work with the GPI-1 chimeras,
the proportions were determined by visual comparison of the isozyme
band intensity to standard gels (Fig. 9). A distribution of the
proportions was developed and the number of clones per sample estimated by the analysis of means and variance as described by Wegmann
(1970). This led to the estimate that the chimeric epidermis studied had approximately 600 cells per clone. For animals with equal
numbers of the two types of cells, West's computer model (1975)
suggests there are approximately 25 clones per patch, leading to

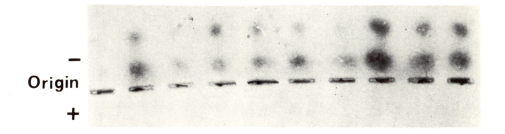

Origin

FIGURE 9. Electrophoretic pattern of normal epidermis. Contiguous
     pieces of normal isolated epidermis (less than 1.0 mm^2) were
     teased free of the main sheet of epidermis and placed on small
     pieces of cellulose acetate. After freezing, they were sub-
     jected to electrophoresis. Both isozymes are present in these
     samples, but in varying proportions. The variation in these
     proportions is used to estimate clone size.

---

*See also papers by West and by Whitten, this volume (editor).

the conclusion that there approximately 15,000 epidermal cells per
average patch. Using an analysis developed by Hutchinson (1973)
and later modified by Friedman and Fialkow (1976), we have estimated
that our tumors could have arisen from no more than eight cells.
The most probable interpretation of these data is that the chemically induced tumors discussed here are clonal growths.

If tumors arise from mutational events, then the causal interactions would be rare between the chemicals responsible and the
target tissue cells. A specific prediction of this hypothesis is
that chemically induced tumors are clonal growths. This explanation gains support from the observation that most carcinogens are
effective mutagens, and, as far as can be tested, nonmutagenic com-
pounds are not carcinogenic.

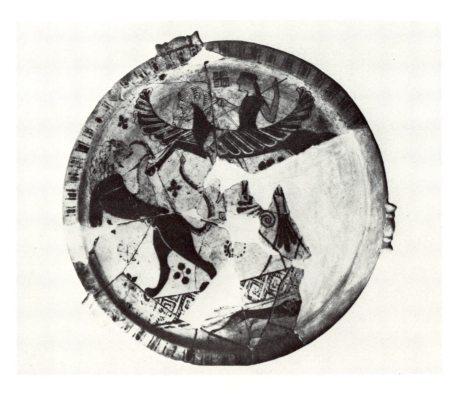

FIGURE 10. The Homeric legend of the Chimera is depicted on this
    plate from Thasos made in the mid-7th century, B.C. Bellero-
    phon is shown on the winged horse Pegasus attacking the Chi-
    mera. The Chimera was originally described in the Iliad as
    a she-monster composed of a lion in front, a goat in the mid-
    dle and a serpent behind. (Reproduced by permission of École
    Francaise d'Archéologie, Athens, Greece.)

REFERENCES

Bauer, K. H. 1928. Mutationstheorie der Geschwulstentstehung. Springer-Verlag, Berlin.

Boveri, T. 1914. Zur Frage der Entstehung maligner Tumoren. Gustav Fisher (Jena), translated by Boveri, M. (1929). Williams & Wilkins (Baltimore).

Chapman, V. M., W. K. Whitten and F. H. Ruddle. 1971. Expression of paternal glucose phosphate isomerase-1 (Gpi-1) in preimplantation stages of mouse embryos. Devel. Biol. 26: 153-158.

Domb, C. and M. F. Sykes. 1960. Cluster size in random mixtures and percolation processes. Phys. Rev. 122: 77-78.

Fialkow, P. J. 1976. Clonal origin of human tumors. Biochim. Biophys. Acta 458: 283-321.

Fialkow, P. J., R. W. Sagebiel, S. M. Gartler and D. L. Rimoin. 1971. Multiple cell origin of hereditary neurofibromas. New England J. Med. 284: 298-300.

Friedman, J. M. and P. J. Fialkow. 1976. Viral "tumorigenesis" in man: cell markers in *Condyloma accuminata*. Int. J. Cancer 17: 57-61.

Gardner, R. L. Production of chimeras by injecting cells or tissue into the blastocyst. In Methods in Mammalian Embryology, Vol. II (in press).

Gartler, S. M. 1974. Utilization of mosaic systems in the study of the origin and progression of tumors. In Chromosomes and Cancer, J. German, Ed., pp. 313-334. Wiley, New York.

Gartler, S. M. and D. Linder. 1964. Selection in mammalian mosaic cell populations. Cold Spring Harbor Symp. Quant. Biol. 29: 253-260.

Hutchison, H. T. 1973. A model for estimating the extent of variegation in mosaic tissues. J. Theor. Biol. 38: 61-79.

Iannaccone, P. M., R. L. Gardner and H. Harris. 1978. The cellular origin of chemically induced tumors. J. Cell Science 29: 249-269.

Linder, D. and S. M. Gartler. 1965. Problem of single cell versus multi-cell origin of a tumor. Proc. 5th Berkeley Symp. on Math. Statis. and Probab. 625-633.

Linder, D. and S. M. Gartler. 1965a. Glucose-6-phosphate dehydrogenase mosaicism: utilization as a cell marker in the study of
leiomyomas. Science 150: 67-69.

Morgan, T. H. and C. B. Bridges. 1919. Contributions to the genetics of *Drosophila melanogaster*. The Carnegie Institution (Washington) p. 108.

Nesbitt, M. N. 1974. Chimeras vs. X inactivation mosaics: significance of differences in pigment distribution. Develop. Biol.
38: 202-207.

Ohno, S. 1971. Genetic implication of karyological instability of
malignant somatic cells. Physiol. Rev. 51: 496-526: see p. 500.

Wegmann, T. G. 1970. Enzyme patterns in tetraparental mouse liver.
Nature 225: 462-463.

West, J. D. 1975. A theoretical approach to the relation between
patch size and clone size in chimeric tissue. J. Theor. Biol. 50:
153-160.

Willis, R. A. 1967. Pathology of Tumours. 4th edition. Butter-
worths, London.

ANTIBODIES TO ALLOZYMES AS POTENTIAL CELL MARKERS FOR CHIMERIC

MOUSE STUDIES

John Gearhart and Mary Lou Oster-Granite

Department of Anatomy, University of Maryland, School
of Medicine, Baltimore, Maryland 21201

INTRODUCTION

The limiting factor in the use of mouse chimeras for the revelation of detailed fate maps during embryogenesis is the lack of
suitable cell marker systems. This limitation is evident when the
list of available chimeric or mosaic markers is examined and compared to the criteria for an ideal marker system. An ideal cell
marker should (1) be expressed in all descendants of a cell; (2)
be present in all cells of a tissue or organism; (3) be cell autonomous; (4) be cell localized; (5) exist in variant forms which are
selectively neutral; (6) have variant forms which can be detected
in histologic sections; and (7) have variants which are expressed
early in embryogenesis.

McLaren (1976) has discussed many of the available chimeric
marker systems in the mouse, pointing out their limitations. While
some of the existing marker systems meet several of the ideal requirements, they are often severely lacking in others. Three examples of the most frequently used marker systems illustrate some of
these problems. (For a more complete coverage of marker systems,
the reader is referred to McLaren 1976.)

Genetic variants of β-glucuronidase activity (Swank, Paigen,
and Ganschow 1973) have been used in studies of chimeras (Condamine,
Custer, and Mintz 1971; Mullen 1977, 1978). However, two disadvantages of this system make for equivocal interpretation of results.
First, the enzyme is not detectably present in many tissues, although Mullen and colleagues (Herrup and Mullen 1977) have recently
partially overcome this objection. Second, the enzyme is transferred amongst cells, creating a third phenotypic class of cells in

111

chimeras that is intermediate between the high- and low-activity
phenotypes (Feder 1976). Feder (1976) has demonstrated that this
intermediate class may be of either high- or low-activity genotype.

Several disadvantages also exist for use of the pigmentary
system in the mouse (Mintz 1974) as an overt marker of chimerism.
First, there is lack of cell autonomy, since some melanocytes will
not function in hair follicles of certain genotypes. Second, there
is a lack of cellular localization, since hair pigmentation is not
localized within cells. Third, pigmentation is limited to only a
few tissues, such as skin, the pigmented retina of the eye, the
choroid of the eye, and the inner ear.

Genetic electrophoretic variants have also been employed in
studies of mouse chimeras. Glucosephosphate isomerase (GPI) is
the most common example of this group of markers that has been used
extensively. Variants of GPI are expressed early in embryogenesis
(Chapman, Whitten, and Ruddle 1971), and the enzyme is ubiquitous.
But it has one great disadvantage: its variants are only revealed
following the destruction of the cells or tissues. Thus, the GPI
marker system meets most of the ideal requirements, but fails mainly
because it cannot be revealed in histologic sections of intact
organs.

In the quest for an ideal marker system, several alternatives
exist. First, new genetic variants may be found in feral populations of mice. For example, Padua, Bulfield, and Peters (1976)
recently reported finding two new alleles of GPI affecting electrophoretic mobility. One of these alleles results in lower GPI activity in red blood cells. This activity is further reduced by heat
treatment. Second, mutagenic treatments may be employed to produce
genetic variants. This procedure is obviously time consuming and
expensive. The third alternative is to adapt existing marker systems in order to better fulfill the ideal requirements. We have
chosen to take this latter approach and to obtain antisera that are
allozyme-specific for genetic electrophoretic variants of enzymes.
These antisera, when coupled to labeled antibodies, can be used to
reveal chimerism in histologic sections.

USE OF GLUCOSEPHOSPHATE ISOMERASE ALLOZYMES

The genetic polymorphism for glucosephosphate isomerase (GPI,
E.C.5.3.1.9) has been used frequently to reveal chimeric tissues in
the mouse. GPI has a key function in glycolysis and gluconeogene-
sis, where it catalyzes reversible aldose-ketose isomerizations of
glucose-6-phosphate and fructose-6-phosphate with one of the highest
catalytic rates of all the glycolytic enzymes. Until recently,
studies on GPI have been limited by the lack of a suitable method
for isolation of the enzyme. Dr. Robert Gracy and his colleagues

at North Texas State University have recently developed a simple
isolation procedure for human and rabbit GPI that involves a single
step elution from the ion exchanger cellulose phosphate (Phillips,
Talent, and Gracy 1976). With minor modifications, we have used
this procedure to isolate GPI from mouse tissues.

The genetic electrophoretic variants of mouse GPI result from
different alleles at the autosomal *Gpi-1* locus (DeLorenzo and
Ruddle 1969). The slow migrating form of the enzyme is designated
as GPI-1A (structural allele, *Gpi-1^a*); and the fast or cathodal
form of the enzyme is GPI-1B (*Gpi-1^b* allele). Since this enzyme
is a dimer composed of two monomers of approximately 70,000 m.w.,
a heterodimer is generated in tissues of F_1 mice having two different homodimer parents and in the muscles of chimeras formed between
two different homodimer parents (Gearhart and Mintz 1972). Recently, Padua *et al.* (1978) have found two new alleles of the structural
locus in wild populations of mice and have designated these *Gpi-1^c*
and *Gpi-1^d*. GPI-1C has a greater electrophoretic mobility than does
GPI-1B, while GPI-1D appears to have a slower mobility than GPI-1A.

We here report the isolation of the homodimers GPI-1A and GPI-
1B from several tissues of different mouse strains, the production
of allozyme-specific antisera against GPI-1B, and the use of such
antisera in histologic sections.

EXTRACTION, ISOLATION, AND HOMOGENEITY OF GPI

GPI was isolated from skeletal muscle, brain, and liver of
C57BL/6J, C57BL/6-*bg^j*, C57BL/6-*pcd*, BALB/c, AKR/J, and A/J male and
female adult mice by a modification of the procedure of Phillips
et al. (1976) (Gearhart and Oster-Granite 1978). Briefly, this procedure consists of extracting GPI in triethanolamine containing 1 mM
EDTA and 0.1% 2-mercaptoethanol at pH 8.2. The ratio of buffer volume to tissue wet weight is 5 : 1. Following overnight dialysis at
pH 7.0, the supernatant of a low-speed centrifugation is stirred
with cellulose phosphate that has been equilibrated at pH 7.0. The
cellulose phosphate is then washed free of unbound protein at pH
7.0 and at pH 7.4 before being packed into a column under nitrogen
pressure. The enzyme is eluted with 3 mM fructose-6-phosphate in
10 mM imidazole, 0.1% 2-mercaptoethanol at pH 7.4. All steps are
carried out at 0—4°C. The eluted enzyme is concentrated by membrane filtration and dialyzed against saturated $(NH_4)_2SO_4$ in 25 mM
imidazole with EDTA and mercaptoethanol.

From 100 grams of tissue, generally 20 mg of enzyme is recovered from skeletal muscle, 15 mg from liver, and 5 mg from whole
brain. The specific activity of enzyme recovered from the muscle
is over 1000 U, while that recovered from liver and brain is 350 U.
Table 1 shows the results of a purification of GPI-1A from AKR skeletal muscle.

TABLE 1. Isolation of GPI-1A from AKR-J mouse skeletal muscle

Fraction	Total activity (units)*	Total protein (mg)	Specific activity	Purification	% recovery
Tissue extract	70482	7735	9	(1)	(100)
Sample added to CP	42250	3198	13	1.5	60 (100)
pH 7.0 wash	[1294]	—	—	—	[2] [3]
pH 7.4 wash	[204]	—	—	—	[<1] [<1]
Substrate elution	34287	29	1172	130	49 81
Concentration	21303	20	1065	117	30 50

*Units represent the μmoles of fructose-6-phosphate converted to glucose-6-phosphate min^{-1} at 30°C.

Homogeneity was assessed by standard polyacrylamide gel electrophoresis, SDS gel electrophoresis, and analytical thin-layer
isoelectricfocusing (Fig. 1).

IMMUNIZATIONS AND ANTIBODY PRODUCTION

Goats were immunized with 4 mg of purified GPI-1A or GPI-1B
by intradermal injections in complete Freund's adjuvant. Antibodies
to GPI and the allozymes of GPI were detected by double diffusion
precipitin reactions (Fig. 2) in agar gels and by radioimmune assays
(Fig. 3). Goat sera were fractionated with $(NH_4)_2SO_4$ (50%) in
borate-buffered saline at pH 8.3. Purified GPI allozymes were
labeled with ^{125}I using chloramine-T (Hunter and Greenwood 1962).
Radioimmune assays were performed using the method of Askenase and
Leonard (1970) (see legend for Fig. 4).

The goat immunized with GPI-1A produced a high titer of anti-
GPI antibody that appears to be nonspecific for the GPI allozymes.
The goat immunized with GPI-1B produced a lower titer of antibody
to GPI (Fig. 3), but some of these antibodies appear specific for
GPI-1B (Table 2). For absorptions, the purified enzymes were conjugated to Sepharose 4B (Cuatrecasas 1970) at concentrations of 5
mg of enzyme per gram dry weight Sepharose. Complete absorption
of anti-GPI antibodies resulted in the loss of precipitin bands in
the double diffusion assay and in the loss of ^{125}I binding in the
radioimmune assay.

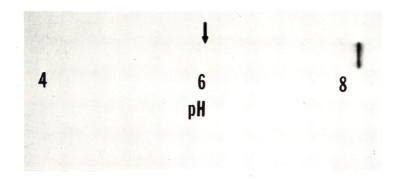

FIGURE 1. Thin-layer polyacrylamide isoelectric focusing of GPI-1A
     isolated from AKR/J skeletal muscle. 15 µg of enzyme was ap-
     plied (arrow) to the gel in which a 3.5—10.5 pH gradient was
     established with 1 M H_3PO_4 at the anode and 1 N NaOH at the
     cathode. The gels were stained with Coomassie Blue R for pro-
     tein, and with nitroblue tetrazolium for GPI activity (Gear-
     hart and Mintz 1972).

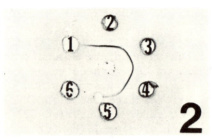

FIGURE 2. Double diffusion precipitin gels. Center well: GPI-1B, 10 µl of 1 mg/ml concentration. Well 1: preimmune serum. Wells 2-4: successive bleeds of immune serum. Wells 5 and 6: incompletely (5) and completely (6) absorbed anti-GPI-1B on GPI-1B-conjugated Sepharose.

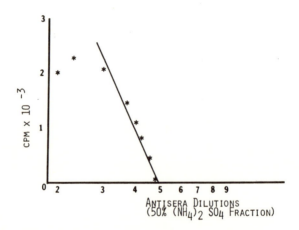

FIGURE 3. Binding of ^{125}I-GPI-1B to goat antisera. Dilutions of goat anti-GPI antisera are aliquotted into polystyrene tubes, and ^{125}I-GPI is then reacted with the bound antibodies. See legend of Fig. 4 for details of the radioimmune assay.

TABLE 2. Absorptions of goat anti-GPI-1B antisera*

	Dilutions	CPM	% Maximum
50% $(NH_4)_2SO_4$ Serum Fraction	200 1000	2520 2146	100 100

Serum absorbed with
    GPI-1A conjugated
    Sepharose†
	200
	1000
		442
		464
			18
			20

Serum absorbed with
    GPI-1B conjugated
    Sepharose†
	200
	1000
		90
		148
			3
			6

* Fractionated goat anti-GPI-1B serum was diluted (1/200, 1/1000) and reacted with Sepharose conjugated to GPI-3A or GPI-1B. The binding of ^{125}I-GPI-1B by absorbed serum is measured according to the procedure described in the legend of Fig. 4.

† 5 mg of enzyme conjugated/ml of Sepharose.

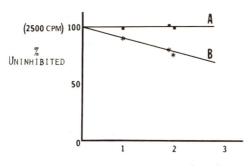

NANOGRAMS "COLD" ENZYME

FIGURE 4. Specific inhibition of ^{125}I-GPI-1B binding to GPI-1A absorbed sera. Anti-GPI-1B antisera are absorbed on GPI-1A conjugated Sepharose. Absorbed antisera are then bound to polystyrene tubes. The tubes are washed with phosphate-buffered saline (PBS), and 1% bovine serum albumin (BSA) in PBS is added. The tubes are then incubated for 30 min and the BSA-PBS is aspirated. 50 µl of cold enzyme is added, followed by 1 ml of ^{125}I-GPI (0.5 mCi/50 µg GPI) diluted to 40,000 cpm. The tubes are vortexed and incubated overnight at 37°C. A = 50 µl of cold GPI-1A is added before ^{125}I-GPI-1B. B = cold GPI-1B is added before ^{125}I-GPI-1B.

To confirm the allozyme specificity of anti-GPI-1B, inhibition
tests were performed using uniodinated (cold) GPI-1A and GPI-1B in
the radioimmune assay. Figure 4 shows that the cold GPI-1B continues to inhibit the binding of hot (iodinated) GPI-1B to antibody-
coated tubes, while GPI-1A does not. The absorbed anti-GPI-1B sera
were used for the immunocytochemical revelation of GPI in tissue
sections.

IMMUNOFLUORESCENCE STUDIES ON PURE-STRAIN TISSUES

Mice were perfused with cold 95% ethanol or 96% ethanol containing 1% glacial acetic acid. Tissues were removed in the cold
and processed by the method of Sainte-Marie (1962). Serial sections, 6 μ thick, were oriented on glass slides, stored in the cold,
and deparaffinized in cold solutions. After incubation in phosphate-buffered saline (PBS), sections were incubated for 30 minutes
with normal rabbit serum, washed twice with PBS, and reacted with
goat sera. Following a 30-minute incubation, the sections were
washed with PBS and reacted with fluorescein-conjugated rabbit anti-
goat antibodies. Slides were mounted in PBS-buffered polyvinyl
alcohol and glycerine (Rodriguez and Deinhardt 1960) and observed
under an Olympus AH microscope equipped with a vertical fluorescence
illuminator. Slides were coded for the scoring of fluorescence.
Controls consisted of staining with preimmune sera, or sera that had
been cross-absorbed with the appropriate purified enzyme conjugated
to Sepharose.

The photomicrographs in Figure 5 show the specificity of anti-
GPI-1B for pure-strain tissues from mice carrying the *Gpi-1^b* allele.
The tissues in the photograph on the left of each pair are of the
Gpi-1^a genotype. They have been reacted with anti-GPI-1B antisera
that were absorbed on GPI-1A-conjugated Sepharose. The tissue in
the photomicrographs on the right side of each pair are of *Gpi-1^b*
genotype. They have been reacted with anti-GPI-1B that was absorbed
on GPI-1A-conjugated Sepharose. The positive- and negative-staining

--→

FIGURE 5. Photomicrographs of tissues stained by an indirect
      method for GPI using anti-GPI-1B antibodies and fluorescein-
      conjugated rabbit anti-goat antibodies (7S). The right mem-
      ber of each pair demonstrates anti-GPI-1B (absorbed on GPI-
      1A-conjugated Sepharose) reacted with tissue from a mouse of
      the *Gpi-1^a* genotype. The left member of each pair demonstrates
      the same anti-GPI-1B reacted with tissue from a mouse of the
      Gpi-1^b genotype. Magnification: 50x (Reduced 20% for purposes
      of reproduction) A, B: Quadriceps femoris pars intermedias;
      C, D: liver; E, F: cerebellar cortex

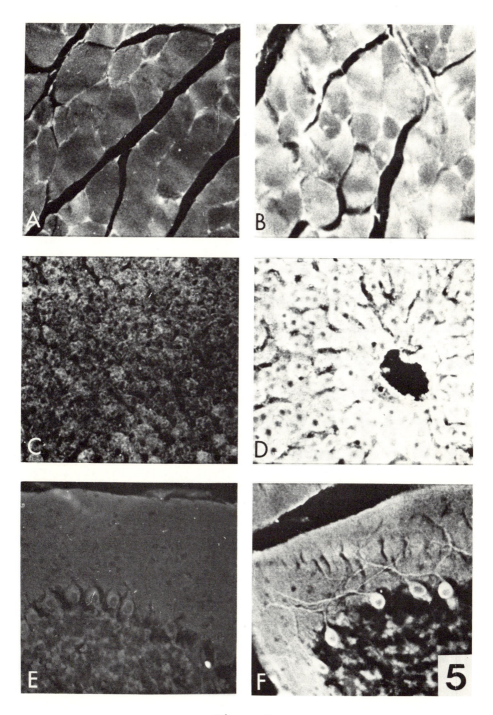

Figure 5

fibers of the quadriceps femoris pars intermedius in Figure 5B indicate the possible presence of high- and low-glycolytic-activity fibers in this predominantly fast muscle (Yellin and Guth 1970). The perimysium and endomysium generally fluoresce quite brilliantly in this staining system.

As shown in Figure 5D, the fluorescence in liver was generally uniform throughout the tissue, with increased intensity surrounding the central veins. We are currently investigating the histochemical localization of GPI in the liver to confirm this observation.

The Purkinje cell bodies in the cerebellar cortex have a low level of autofluorescence (Fig. 5E), but the difference between this low-level and positive staining is dramatic (Fig. 5F). The cell bodies and dendrites fluoresce brilliantly, while the nucleus within the cell body does not. Contrary to the conclusions of Dewey et $al.$ (1976), the cell body does appear, both histochemically and immunocytochemically, to contain GPI. All cell types in the cerebellar cortex, and their processes, stain for GPI. These include the basket, stellate, granule, Golgi, Purkinje, and Bergmann glial cells. Additionally, many other parts of the nervous system also stain brilliantly for GPI. These include the deep cerebellar nuclei, the axons contained within the cerebellar peduncles, and the neurons and processes of the hippocampal formation.

SUMMARY

Glucosephosphate isomerase is a ubiquitous enzyme that exists in several electrophoretically distinct allozymic forms in different mouse strains. This genetic polymorphism meets many of the requirements for cell markers in chimeric or mosaic systems. Two of the variants, GPI-1A and GPI-1B, have been purified and used to raise antisera in goats. Antibody specific for GPI-1B has been obtained, and has been found to react specifically by fluorescent staining in sectioned tissues from pure-strain adult mice carrying the $Gpi-1^b$ allele. We are now testing this immunohistochemical system on embryonic and fetal tissues, and in tissues composed of both $Gpi-1^a$ and $Gpi-1^b$ components developed from aggregation chimeras.

Due to the lack of an antiserum specific for GPI-1A, the staining for GPI-1B must initially be correlated with other chimeric cell markers (e.g., β-glucuronidase in liver) before it can be used as a reliable cell marker in chimeras. Additionally, a horse-radish peroxidase-conjugated system for cellular localization of GPI at the electron microscope level is being developed.

This research was supported by a grant from the National Science Foundation (PCM-16763) and from the Paralyzed Veterans of America. JG is the recipient of a Basil O'Connor Research Award from the National Foundation-March of Dimes. MLOG is an Alfred Sloan Foundation Fellow. We acknowledge the assistance of Ms. Anne Hartman.

REFERENCES

Askenase, P. W. and E. J. Leonard. 1970. Solid phase radioimmuno-assay of human β-1C globulin. Immunochem. 7: 29-41.

Chapman, V. M., W. K. Whitten and F. H. Ruddle. 1971. Expression of paternal glucosephosphate isomerase-1 (*GPI-1*) in preimplantation mouse embryos. Devel. Biol. 26: 153-158.

Condamine, H., R. P. Custer and B. Mintz. 1971. Pure-strain and genetically mosaic liver tumors histochemically identified with the β-glucuronidase marker in allophenic mice. Proc. Nat. Acad. Sci., USA 68: 2032-2036.

Cuatrecasas, P. 1970. Protein purification by affinity chromato-graphy. Derivations of agarose and polyacrylamide beads. J. Biol. Chem. 245: 3059-3065.

DeLorenzo, R. J. and F. H. Ruddle. 1969. Genetic control of two electrophoretic variants of glucosephosphate isomerase in the mouse (*Mus musculus*). Biochem. Genet. 3: 151-162.

Dewey, M. J., A. G. Gervais and B. Mintz. 1976. Brain and ganglion development from two genotypic classes of cells in allophenic mice. Devel. Biol. 50: 68-81.

Feder, N. 1976. Solitary cells and enzyme exchange in tetraparen-tal mice. Nature 263: 67-69.

Gearhart, J. D. and B. Mintz. 1972. Clonal origins of somites and their muscle derivatives: Evidence from allophenic mice. Devel. Biol. 29: 27-37.

Gearhart, J. and M. L. Oster-Granite. 1978. Isolation of glucose-phosphate isomerase from mouse tissues and the obtainment of anti-GPI antisera. Submitted for publication.

Herrup, K. and R. J. Mullen. 1977. Biochemical and genetic factors in the heat inactivation of murine-β-glucuronidase. Biochem. Genet. 15: 641-653.

Hunter, W. M. and F. C. Greenwood. 1962. Preparation of iodine-131 labeled human growth hormone of high specific activity. Nature 194: 495-496.

McLaren, A. 1976. Mammalian Chimaeras. Cambridge University Press, Cambridge, Great Britain.

Mintz, B. 1974. Gene control of mammalian differentiation. Ann. Rev. Genet. 8: 411-470.

Mullen, R. J. 1977. Genetic dissection of the CNS with mutant-normal mouse and rat chimeras, In Soc. Neurosci. Symp. 2: 47-65. W. M. Cowan and J. A. Ferendelli, eds.

Mullen, R. J. 1978. Presented at this conference.

Padua, R. A., G. Bulfield and J. Peters. 1978. Biochemical genetics of a new glucosephosphate isomerase allele (*Gpi-1^c*) from wild mice. Biochem. Genet. 16: 127-143.

Phillips, T. L., J. M. Talent and R. W. Gracy. 1976. Isolation of rabbit glucosephosphate isomerase by a single-step substrate elution. Biochem. Biophys. Acta 429: 624-628.

Rodriguez, J. and F. Deinhardt. 1960. Preparation of a semipermanent mounting medium for fluorescent antibody studies. Virology 12: 316-317.

Sainte-Marie, G. 1962. A paraffin embedding technique for studies employing immunofluorescence. J. Histochem. Cytochem. 10: 250-256.

Swank, R. T., K. Paigen and R. E. Ganschow. 1974. Genetic control of glucuronidase induction in mice. J. Mol. Biol. 81: 225-243.

Yellin, H. and L. Guth. 1970. The histochemical classification of muscle fibers. Exper. Neurol. 26: 424-432.

Use of Chimeras and Mutational or Disjunctional Mosaics to Study Gamete Differentiation, Sexual Development, and Origin of the Germline

REPRODUCTION IN SINGLE-SEX CHIMERAS

Anne McLaren

MRC Mammalian Development Unit, Wolfson House,
(University College London), London NW1 2HE, England

Chimeras can be either of mixed chromosomal sex, XX ↔ XY, or they can be single-sex, XX ↔ XX or XY ↔ XY. If the sex ratio at the time of chimera formation is unity, mixed-sex and single-sex chimeras will be expected to occur in equal numbers. The data available from chromosomal sexing of chimera components suggest that this expectation is fulfilled (McLaren 1976). The problems of XX ↔ XY animals, both from the point of view of sexual differentiation, and as regards the fate of their germ cells, are considered elsewhere in this volume. In this paper I shall restrict myself to single-sex chimeras and their germ cells.

The gonad contains not only germ cells but also somatic cells. The mammalian gonad, both female and male, is characterized by very intimate connections between the germ cells and the somatic cells.

In the female, the cumulus cells that surround the developing oocyte have processes that penetrate through the zona pellucida and terminate on the surface of the vitellus. Gap junctions link the somatic and the germ cell surfaces (Anderson and Albertini 1976), and electrophysiological studies have shown zero electrical resistance between the two cell types. The gap junctions persist up to the time that LH-induced oocyte maturation begins (Szöllösi *et al.* 1978). Their function is unknown. In insects, somatic nurse cells pump RNA and other substances into the developing oocytes. In mammals, it seems unlikely that any information-carrying molecules pass across the gap junctions, but transfer of signalling molecules like cyclic AMP, or various ions, from the follicle cells into the oocyte cannot be ruled out.

    In the male too there are very intimate connections between
the germ cells and the somatic cells. The spermatid develops with
its head completely embedded in the giant Sertoli cell (Nagano
1968), and indeed it has been suggested that the shape of the sperm
head is determined by mechanical forces exerted by the Sertoli cell
(Phillips 1970; but see Fawcett, Anderson, and Phillips 1971).
There are also cytoplasmic processes connecting one spermatogonium
with another; we do not know for certain whether these link only
the two products of a cell division, or whether they can be formed
between unrelated germ cells.

    In chimeras, the gonad potentially contains two genetically
distinct populations of somatic cells and two populations of germ
cells; and because the germ cells have migrated into the gonad from
outside, any given germ cell is just as likely to be associated
with somatic cells (follicle cells in the female, Sertoli cells in
the male) of contrasting genetic type as it is to be associated
with cells of its own genetic type. We may therefore enquire
whether the development of the germ cells is affected in any way
by the genetic constitution of the neighbouring somatic cells.

                CAN THE GERM-CELL GENOTYPE BE MODIFIED?

    First, is the genotype of the germ cells ever modified, for
example by some infective process akin to transformation or trans-
duction in bacteria, or do they always "breed true" to their initial
genotype? With radiation chimeras, a claim has been made that genetic material from the donor strain can become incorporated into the
genome of the sperm, so that the immunological properties of the
progeny are modified (Kanazawa and Imai 1974). For aggregation chimeras, there are surprisingly few published data on this question.
Progeny classified for only a single gene difference, for example
a coat color gene, yield no relevant evidence: to spot such an
effect, one needs to score more than one gene difference.

    I therefore looked at the progeny of male chimeras whose com-
ponent strains differed by some nine different genetic characters,
arguing that the more differences one was dealing with, the more
chance there might be of seeing some effect (McLaren 1975a). One
component carried the nine recessive alleles, the other the corresponding dominants. Of 1851 progeny from 20 chimeric mice, 1092
inherited the entire package of recessive alleles, the other 759
the entire package of dominants. There was no evidence that any
gamete carried say eight recessives and one dominant allele. For
the one character that was scored quantitatively, namely tail
length, the expression of the mutant gene was identical whether the
gamete carrying it had developed in a chimeric mouse, or in a normal
mutant animal. So although one can never rule out the possibility

that modification of the germ-cell genotype might occur if one
looked at larger numbers, or at different genes, I certainly found
no evidence of it.

IS THE GERM-CELL PHENOTYPE MODIFIED BY NEIGHBOURING SOMATIC CELLS?

What about modification of sperm phenotype? For any cell type,
chimeras offer an approach to the question of whether the phenotype
of the cell is determined by its own genotype or by the genotype of
the neighbouring cells, that is, by its cellular environment. For
a germ cell, this means the neighbouring somatic cells, with which
as we have seen it may be in very intimate contact.

The genetic basis of sperm phenotype was first explored for the
mouse by Beatty and Sharma (1960), who showed that such characters
as head length, head breadth, and midpiece length differed significantly from one inbred strain to another. For example, Burgoyne
(1975) compared C3H with C57BL sperm, and showed that the C57BL
sperm have shorter and broader heads but longer midpieces. By cal-
culating a discriminant function based on all three characters, it
became possible to classify a single unknown sperm as either C3H
or C57BL with only a 2% chance of error.

Studies by Beatty and his colleagues (Beatty 1969; Williams,
Beatty, and Burgoyne 1970) on the sperm of F_1 males had already
shown that the haploid genotype of the sperm was unlikely to be involved in the determination of sperm shape. To distinguish between
the effect of the genotype of the sperm's diploid spermatogonial
precursor, and the genotype of the enveloping Sertoli cell, Burgoyne
(1975) studied sperm shape in C3H $\leftrightarrow$ C57BL chimeras. The genotype
of the spermatogonium and the genotype of the neighbouring Sertoli
cells are of course identical in normal males, but not necessarily
so in chimeras.

Burgoyne argued as follows. In a chimera with equal contributions from the two components to the somatic tissue, any given
spermatid is equally likely to be associated with a Sertoli cell
of same genotype as with one of different genotype. In gonads
where all the spermatids are derived from one component, as in an
XX $\leftrightarrow$ XY chimera, if sperm genotype determines sperm shape there
will be a single peak, as in control males. If shape is imposed
entirely by the Sertoli cell, one would expect two peaks, corresponding to the two peaks of the two component strains. If both
factors play a part, there will again be two peaks but one will
now be intermediate, or there may be a single peak but widened in
the direction of the other strain. In gonads where spermatids are
derived from both components, then whether sperm shape is determined entirely by sperm genotype or entirely by Sertoli cell genotype, we should see two peaks, corresponding to the two peaks of

the component strains; but if both factors play a part, an intermediate population or populations will appear, or at least the two
peaks will be extended towards one another. Whether or not both
components contribute to the sperm population can be determined by
breeding tests.

Burgoyne examined samples of sperm from chimeric males, and
found no evidence at all for any influence of the somatic cells on
sperm shape. For example, a C57BL-XX ↔ C3H-XY male, who was breeding entirely from his C3H component, yielded sperm that all fell in
a single peak corresponding to that of control C3H sperm, with no
indication of any sperm of C57BL or intermediate shape.

So far we've seen no evidence of any influence of the somatic
cells on the developing gametes. Is this a general finding? An
interesting counter-example was investigated recently by Mary Lyon
and her colleagues (Lyon, Glenister, and Lamoreux 1975).

This concerns the X-linked mutant testicular feminization, *Tfm*.
XY mice carrying *Tfm* on their X chromosome develop a testis that
secretes androgen, but because their tissues fail to respond to
androgen the rest of the phenotype is female. Spermatogenesis is
arrested at the first meiotic division, and one can again ask
whether it is the genotype of the germ cell or the genotype of the
surrounding somatic cells that is responsible for this arrest.
When chimeras were made between XY embryos with and without the *Tfm*
gene, the resulting males produced two sorts of progeny, one corresponding to the normal component and the other to the *Tfm* component.
This result suggests that the genetically normal population of somatic cells was able to support the development of *Tfm*-bearing sperm
as well as normal sperm. In other words, the failure of spermatogenesis in *Tfm* mice seems to be due to the androgen-resistance of
the somatic cells of the testis, not to any gene action exerted in
the germ cells themselves. Which somatic cells are involved is not
yet clear, but either the Sertoli cells or the tubular epithelial
cells seem likely candidates.

Other examples of apparent genetic effects on sperm characteristics are known in mice: for example, Weir (1976) has studied a
case where both the capacity to sire litters in a competitive situation and the sex ratio of the progeny have been shown to be influenced by the Y chromosome. Krzanowska (1976) has shown that the Y
chromosome plays an important role in determining the incidence of
abnormalities of sperm head shape. Appropriate chimera studies
could reveal whether these Y chromosome effects are exerted through
the germ cells themselves or through the somatic cells.

REPRESENTATION OF CHIMERA COMPONENTS IN THE GONAD

We now turn to the actual representation of the two chimera components in the gonad. As far as the somatic tissue is concerned, enzyme determinations suggest that the gonads of a chimera are much like all other organs of the body, with both genetic components almost always present, but with one tending to predominate in certain strain combinations. In C3H ↔ C57BL male chimeras, for example, GPI assays show that the C57BL component is usually more strongly represented in the testis than is the C3H.

As far as the germ cells are concerned, although both genetic components can be represented in the gonads of a single individual, it is by no means true that they are always both present. For a start, up to two thirds of males are likely to be XX ↔ XY chimeras and, since the XX germ cells fail to give rise to functional sperm even though they reach the fetal testis, one does not expect two types of offspring from such males.

But what about single-sex chimeras, XY ↔ XY males and XX ↔ XX females? In theory there seems no reason why both populations of germ cells should not reach the developing gonads and give rise to functional germ cells, so one would expect appropriate breeding tests to give rise to mixed litters. In practice, the proportion of chimeras producing two types of progeny seems to vary from one strain combination to another. Table 1 lists some published data. Among the males, bearing in mind that up to two thirds of each sample may be XX ↔ XY animals, only the last three samples give evidence that single-sex chimeras are producing single progenies. Of the McLaren (1975b) males, five were shown to be XY ↔ XY by chromosome sexing, and in the "unbalanced" group of Mullen and Whitten (1971) up to 50% may have been XY ↔ XY because the sex ratio was close to one. Among the females, every sample shows a fair proportion of single-progeny animals, and only the "unbalanced" combinations would be likely to include fertile XX ↔ XY chimeras.

So we have the problem that the population of functional germ cells, unlike most other tissues of the body, seems quite often to be drawn from only one of the two chimera components. Why should this be? One possible explanation is that, at least in some strain combinations, one or the other cell line is often by chance excluded from the germ-cell population. This could be because the number of cells initially set aside to become primordial germ cells is very small, so that the chance of them all being from one component or the other is quite high; or it could be because the two components were not randomly mixed at the time of allocation. Another type of explanation involves cell selection, i.e., the more rapid proliferation of germ cells of the one component than of the other.

TABLE 1. Published data on the breeding performance of overt chimeras.*

Sex	Source	Total no. of progenies (no. chromosomally sexed)	% single progenies overall	% single progenies among XX ↔ XX or XY ↔ XY only
♀	Mullen and Whitten (1971)			
	"Balanced"	19 (0)	31.6	—
	"Unbalanced"	17 (0)	58.8	—
	Ford et al. (1975)	4 (3)	25.0	0.0
	McLaren (1975b)	4 (3)	100.0	100.0
♂	Mystkowska and Tarkowski (1968)	5 (4)	60.0	0.0
	Mintz (1969)	23 (0)	60.9	—
	Mullen and Whitten (1971)			
	"Balanced"	46 (0)	76.1	—
	"Unbalanced"	17 (0)	94.1	—
	Ford et al. (1975)	7 (5)	57.1	33.0
	McLaren (1975b)	16 (11)	93.7	80.0

*Where progeny sizes are published, those of less than 13 young have been omitted.

Mintz (1968) pointed out that in the female, where the diploid mitotic proliferative phase of gametogenesis is completed well before birth, the germ-cell population in the adult should be stable; but that in the male, where spermatogonial proliferation continues throughout life, one might expect to see a progressive shift in the proportions of the two types of progeny as the chimeric males aged. She published an intriguing graph, of breeding performance in a C3H ↔ C57BL male chimera, which fully confirms this prediction (Mintz 1968, Fig. 7). In the first 10 litters from C57BL females, the male fathered 15% black and 85% agouti young; in the next 10 litters, only 1% black, 99% agouti; and thereafter only agouti. The results from the 11 other breeding males of this strain combination are not published in detail, but are reported to show the same pattern. If the 50 litters illustrated came from 50 different C57BL females, all of about the same age at the time of mating, then the point is established unequivocally. But if the chimeric male was mated to only 10 females, each of which produced 5 litters, then as Burgoyne (1973) has pointed out, it could be that in the first 10 litters, which would comprise the first litter from each female, the inbred C57BL progeny survived better relative to the F_1 agouti progeny than they did in the older females.

Since even a minute difference in mitotic rate in a mitotically active tissue will lead to one cell population outgrowing the other, germ-cell selection must be expected to occur in some strain combinations. In a given strain combination, it should always lead to the same component predominating, for example, C3H in C3H ↔ C57BL chimeras. But in some of the samples in which there seemed to be too many chimeras of both sexes producing single-type progenies, neither component predominated, but rather some of the single-type progenies were from the one component and some from the other. I therefore return to the suggestion of a founder effect, namely, that the initial number of primordial germ cells might be so small, or the cell mixing to which they were subjected might be so incomplete, that they would often by chance be all of the one component or all of the other.

One final observation, from our own work. In the series of chimeras reported by McLaren (1975b), the few males that sired mixed progenies showed highly significant heterogeneity in the proportions of the two components from one litter to the next. Table 2 shows a series of 12 litters from a single male. The proportions of the two types of young are highly variable, so that of two litters born on successive days, and therefore conceived very close together in time, one litter could be all of the one component and the other almost all of the other component. The effect seems unrelated to the individual females used, or to their age or parity, or to the age of the male. Again one wonders about the possibility of some founder effect, producing different proportions of the two germ cell

TABLE 2.   Segregation of progeny in 12 litters sired by a male
     chimera paired with 6 females (a-f) of the recessive stock.*

| Date of birth | | Number of progeny | |
of litter	Female	'Recessive'	'Dominant'
21 Apr 1972	a	0	6
12 Jun 1972	a	4	0
16 Oct 1972	b	7	0
6 Nov 1972	b	5	1
20 Dec 1972	c	5	1
25 Dec 1972	d	5	1
21 Jan 1973	e	7	0
8 Mar 1973	b	0	6
9 Mar 1973	c	6	0
22 Mar 1973	d	1	1
29 Apr 1973	b	8	0
5 May 1973	f	0	3

*From McLaren (1975a)

populations either in the two testes, or in the individual testis
tubules. Little is known about the origin of sperm in a single
ejaculate.

     The two components in this particular strain combination were
genetically quite unrelated to one another. In a series of chimeras
between genetically very closely related embryos, CBA and CBA-T6,
there was no significant heterogeneity among the different litters
sired by each chimeric male, so that the proportions of the two

types of progeny looked as if all the germ cells had been drawn from a single randomly distributed population (Mystkowska, personal communication).

Clearly we need more data, for a variety of different strain combinations, on the proportion of mixed versus single progenies, on the proportion of the two types of progeny in successive litters from individual males and females, and on the effect of age on these proportions. I urge all who are raising chimeras for whatever purpose, to mate them up appropriately, keep records of their litters, and publish all their breeding data *in extenso*.

REFERENCES

Anderson, E. and D. F. Albertini. 1976. Gap junctions between the oocyte and companion follicle cells in the mammalian ovary. J. Cell Biol. 71: 680–686.

Beatty, R. A. 1969. A genetic study of spermatozoan dimensions in mice selected for body weight. Ind. J. Hered. 1: 2–21.

Beatty, R. A. and K. N. Sharma. 1960. Genetics of gametes. III Strain differences in spermatozoa from eight inbred strains of mice. Proc. Roy. Soc. Edinburgh B, 68: 25–53.

Burgoyne, P. S. 1973. The genetic control of germ cell differentiation in mice. Ph.D. Thesis, University of Edinburgh.

Burgoyne, P. S. 1975. Sperm phenotype and its relationship to somatic and germ line genotype: a study using mouse aggregation chimeras. Dev. Biol. 44: 63–76.

Fawcett, D. W., W. A. Anderson and D. M. Phillips. 1971. Morphogenetic factors influencing the shape of the sperm head. Dev. Biol. 26: 220–251.

Ford, C. E., E. P. Evans, M. D. Burtenshaw, H. M. Clegg, M. Tuffrey and R. D. Barnes. 1975. A functional 'sex-reversed' oocyte in the mouse. Proc. Roy. Soc. Lond. B. 190: 187–197.

Kanazawa, K. and A. Imai. 1974. Parasexual-sexual hybridization — heritable transformation of germ cells in chimeric mice. Jap. J. Exp. Med. 44: 227–234.

Krzanowska, H. 1976. Inheritance of sperm head abnormality types in mice — the role of the Y chromosome. Genet. Res. 28: 189–198.

Lyon, M. F., P. H. Glenister and M. L. Lamoreux. 1975. Normal
spermatozoa from androgen-resistant germ cells of chimaeric mice
and the role of androgen in spermatogenesis. Nature 258: 620-622.

McLaren, A. 1975a. The independence of germ-cell genotype from
somatic influence in chimaeric mice. Genet. Res. 25: 83-87.

McLaren, A. 1975b. Sex chimaerism and germ cell distribution in
a series of chimaeric mice. J. Embryol. exp. Morph. 33: 205-216.

McLaren, A. 1976. Mammalian Chimaeras. Cambridge University
Press.

Mintz, B. 1968. Hermaphrodism, sex chromosomal mosaicism and germ
cell selection in allophenic mice. J. Anim. Sci. (Suppl. 1), 27:
51-60.

Mintz, B. 1969. Developmental mechanisms found in allophenic mice
with sex chromosomal and pigmentary mosaicism. Birth Defects:
Original Article Series 5: 11-22. In: First Conference on the
Clinical Delineation of Birth Defects, ed. D. Bergsma and V.
McKusick. New York: National Foundation.

Mullen, R. J. and W. K. Whitten. 1971. Relationship of genotype
and degree of chimerism in coat color to sex ratios and gametogenesis in chimeric mice. J. exp. Zool. 178: 165-176.

Mystkowska, E. T. and A. K. Tarkowski. 1968. Observations on
CBA-p/CBA-T6T6 mouse chimaeras. J. Embryol. exp. Morph. 20: 33-52.

Nagano, T. 1968. Fine structural relation between the Sertoli cell
and the differentiating spermatid in the human testis. Z. Zell-
forsch. 89: 39-43.

Phillips, D. M. 1970. Development of spermatozoa in the woolly
opossum with special reference to the shaping of the sperm head.
J. Ultrastruct. Res. 33: 369-380.

Szöllösi, D., M. Gérard, Y. Ménézo and C. Thibault. 1978. Per-
meability of ovarian follicle; corona cell-oocyte relationship in
mammals. Ann. Biol. anim. Biochem. Biophys. 18(2), in press.

Weir, J. A. 1976. Allosomal and autosomal control of sex ratio
in PHH and PHL mice. Genetics 84: 755-764.

Williams, D. A., R. A. Beatty and P. S. Burgoyne. 1970. Multivariate analysis in the genetics of spermatozoan dimensions in mice.
Proc. Roy. Soc., B 175: 313-331.

GERM CELLS IN XX ↔ XY MOUSE CHIMERAS

Andrzej K. Tarkowski

Department of Embryology, Institute of Zoology, University of Warsaw, Poland

Despite the fact that cells of both genetic sexes coexist in sex-chromosome chimeras, the sexual differentiation of these individuals tends to be canalized into a male (predominantly) or a female direction, rather than leading to a hermaphroditic condition. This creates an opportunity for approaching the problem of whether or not the germ cells of the mouse can undergo functional sex reversal. Up to the time when experimental mouse chimeras became available (Tarkowski 1961; Mintz 1962), this question remained unanswered, because all attempts to reverse sexual differentiation in placental mammals were unsuccessful. Since then, results obtained by breeding XX ↔ XY mouse chimeras have led to the conclusion that the XX chromosomal constitution precludes differentiation of germ cells into spermatozoa; and they have provided some evidence that the XY constitution may be compatible with oogenesis.

Although sex-chromosome chimeras have proved extremely useful in studying this particular problem, they do not represent the ideal experimental model. There are two main reasons for this. First, the gonads of such individuals consist of a mixture of four types of cells — germ cells of opposite genetic sex, and somatic cells of opposite genetic sex; and, second, the primary contribution to the gonad of these four cell populations varies from individual to individual, as well as between the gonads of the same individual. Because both the contribution and the distribution of these cells within the gonads are variable, each animal is to a certain extent unique. The ideal situation for studying functional sex reversal of germ cells is when the gonads consist of only two components — germ cells of one genetic sex and somatic tissue that is either of the opposite sex (both genetically and phenotypically), or of the same genetic sex but undergoing differentiation characteristic of

135

the opposite sex. Both situations have been experimentally created
in lower vertebrates; and the second one may also occur due to mutation causing sex reversal. Such mutation is known to occur in
the goat (see Short 1972) and in the mouse (Cattanach, Pollard,
and Hawkes 1971). Despite the above-mentioned shortcomings, experimental chimerism has been one of the most fruitful and most
extensively exploited approaches in studies on functional sex
reversal of germ cells in mammals.

Because the conclusions regarding the ability or inability of
primordial germ cells to differentiate into gametes characteristic
of the opposite sex are based on breeding data, it is of importance
to know whether, and how often, the germinal tissue displays mixed
composition when the two components are of the same genetic sex.
There is abundant evidence that overt chimeras can produce gametes
of both genetic types (Mystkowska and Tarkowski 1968; Mintz 1968,
1969; Mullen and Whitten 1971; Ford, Evans, Burtenshaw, Clegg,
Tuffrey, and Barnes 1975; McLaren 1975, 1978); but this is not a
rule, and, in some strain combinations, more animals produce single-
type progeny than mixed progeny. However, for the problem under
consideration more meaningful information comes from the breeding
data of those animals whose single-sex chimerism was karyologically
confirmed. In the studies of Mystkowska and Tarkowski (1968), Ford
et al. (1975), and McLaren (1975), 3 out of 3, 4 out of 6, and 1 out
of 8 such chimeras, respectively, produced mixed progenies. It may
be of importance that in our own studies, the two strains used for
the construction of chimeras (CBA-p and CBA-T6T6) were genetically
very closely related — probably more related than the strains used
in any other study. Complete absence of germ cells of one genetic
type means that either the whole germ-cell population was derived
exclusively from one component, or that there has been a selection
against one type of germ cell. Such a selection can occur as early
as during migration of primordial germ cells into the genital
ridges, and as late as at the time of fertilization.

XX ↔ XY MALES

Breeding tests of overt chimeras whose XX ↔ XY chimerism was
cytogenetically confirmed (Mystkowska and Tarkowski 1968; Mintz
1968; McLaren 1975; Ford *et al*. 1975) showed that such animals produced spermatozoa of only one genetic type which invariably corresponded to the XY component. Indirect evidence in favour of the
view that XX germ cells cannot undergo functional sex reversal has
also been provided by Mintz (1968), who showed that, in a large
sample of progeny of chimeras, the sex ratio was not distorted in a
female direction. This conclusion is in agreement with observations that, in the testes of intersexual XX goats (see Short 1972)
and in sex-reversed female mice carrying the *Sxr* gene (Cattanach *et
al*. 1971), spermatogenesis never occurs: in fact, the germ cells

degenerate in late embryogenesis (goat) or shortly after birth
(mouse). The XX;*Sxr* germ cells appear to be unable to undergo
spermatogenesis even in male chimeras in which the other component
is a genetically normal XY (Gordon 1976). In XO genetic females
carrying the *Sxr* gene, spermatogenesis does occur, although spermatozoa are abnormal and immobile (Cattanach *et al.* 1971).

All the above observations strongly suggest that it is the
presence of two X chromosomes, rather than the absence of the Y
chromosome, that precludes spermatogenesis. The Y chromosome may
be important for the normal course of spermiogenesis; but it does
not appear to be indispensable — at least in this particular
situation — for the occurrence of spermatogenesis.

If the XX germ cells in the testes of sex-chromosome chimeras
do not form spermatozoa, what happens to them? Unless there is
selection against these cells in the pre-gonadal period, they
should contribute equally with XY primordial germ cells to the
initial population of germ cells in the gonads. In a first step
toward elucidating the fate of the XX cells Mystkowska and Tarkowski (1968) examined cytogenetically the primary spermatocytes at
metaphase I in 3 XX ↔ XY chimeras (2 males, 1 hermaphrodite) in
which one component (CBA-T6T6) carried chromosomal markers. It
was thought that XX germ cells might have been able to initiate
spermatogenesis but that they degenerated later, during spermiogenesis. This supposition was not confirmed: all primary spermatocytes proved to be XY. Clearly, elimination of XX germ cells
must have occurred earlier. The next step was stimulated by a
single and curious observation of a group of small oocytes situated
within the sex cords, and side by side with typical prespermatogonia (gonocytes), in the otherwise normal testis of a 5-day-old
chimeric male. Because, by structure and size, these oocytes
corresponded to oocytes in normal ovaries of the same age, they
must have originated from cells which began meiotic prophase on
the normal time schedule characteristic for females. This observation prompted us to study histologically the gonads of chimeric
male embryos at the age of 16—17 days, i.e. at the time when germ
cells in the ovary are mostly in pachytene (Mystkowska and Tarkowski 1970). In 5 out of 11 embryos examined, meiotic germ cells
were observed in testes. Three of these 5 embryos were examined
karyologically and proved to be sex-chromosome chimeras. The incidence of meiotic germ cells per gonad varied from 0.08% to 38.6%;
in three embryos it was similar on both sides, and in two different. Are these cells XX, XY, or both? The most obvious explanation is that the cells in question are of XX consitution, and that
they behave autonomously and enter into meiotic prophase on a time
schedule normal for XX. This explanation is favoured by McLaren
on the basis of cytogenetic studies that she and her colleagues
performed on 16½- to 18½-day chimeric male fetuses (McLaren,

Chandley, and Kofman-Alfara 1972). These investigators could not
detect the sex vesicle with the XY bivalent in meiotic germ cells.
Furthermore, the ^{3}H-thymidine labeling pattern did not resemble
that found in the meiotic prophase of male germ cells. By day $18\frac{1}{2}$,
all these cells were degenerating. In our own studies (Mystkowska
and Tarkowski 1970), we also investigated 12 chimeric males at 8—
20 days of postnatal life, but we did not find any other case of
oocytes growing in testes. Either this phenomenon is sporadic; or,
such oocytes degenerate during the first few days of postnatal
life.

For various reasons, we do not favour the concept that the
meiotic germ cells in embryonic testes are exclusively XX and that
they represent the whole population of genetically female germ
cells (which logically follows from the idea that initiation of
meiosis is an autonomous process). First, meiotic germ cells
usually constitute only a small fraction of the germ-cell population, and their incidence is much lower than the incidence of XX
somatic cells, as estimated from the liver. Second, the incidence
of meiotic cells may be strikingly different in the two gonads of
the same embryo. Third, in regions of the testis where meiotic
cells are more numerous, the structure of the testicular tissue
is atypical — with sex cords not clearly differentiated. Finally,
in the ovaries of XX ↔ XY female embryos (Mystkowska and Tarkowski, unpublished observations), and in the ovarian parts of ovotestes of newly born chimeras (Tarkowski 1964), all germ cells start
meiosis prenatally and are not accompanied by gonocytes. These
various observations suggest, on the one hand, that in the testes
of chimeric embryos only some of the XX germ cells begin meiosis;
and, on the other, that the prenatal initiation of meiosis is in
some way influenced by the surrounding somatic tissue. This influence might be either inductive or simply permissive.

Three other interesting observations are also pertinent to
this problem. First, it was shown by Ożdżeński (1972) that when
early testes from normal mouse embryos are transplanted to ectopic
sites, some germ cells initiate meiosis at the time characteristic
for ovaries — that is, long before meiosis normally begins in testes. Second, as shown by Ford et al. (1975) and by Evans, Ford,
and Lyon (1977), genetically male germ cells appear to be able to
complete oogenesis in the ovary of chimeric females. Since all
oocytes are formed prenatally, these particular male germ cells
must have entered meiosis precociously, and together with XX germ
cells. Third, according to Byskov and Saxen (1976), germ cells in
the young testis of the mouse can be forced to initiate meiosis
precociously under the influence of the older embryonic ovary. In
view of the above observations, I find it even more difficult to
accept the view that, in chimeric testes, only XX germ cells can
begin meiosis prenatally. The alternative interpretation, which

we have put forward earlier (Tarkowski 1970; Mystkowska and Tarkowski 1970), is that initiation of meiosis in the embryonic testes
of XX ↔ XY male chimeras depends on local environmental conditions
to which germ cells are exposed (and, because the distribution of
XX and XY somatic cells in the gonad is very likely to be uneven,
these conditions may vary from place to place), rather than on
their genetic sex. According to this concept, those XX germ cells
which have not begun meiosis on the normal time schedule remain
"hidden" among prespermatogonia (gonocytes) and probably degenerate
before, or at the time when, definitive spermatogonia are formed
shortly after birth. This interpretation finds support in the fact
that, in the testes of intersexual goats (Short 1972) and sex-
reversed mice (Cattanach et al. 1971), XX germ cells display all
features characteristic of typical prespermatogonia, and die prenatally or shortly after birth. It is also worth remembering that
in these animals XX germ cells do not enter into meiosis during
embryogenesis, as might be expected if this process were fully
autonomous and triggered independently of the type of gonadal
tissue surrounding the germ cells.

The next, and perhaps far more important, question is why
some germ cells in embryonic chimeric testes (and all germ cells
in normal ovary) begin meiosis at all. Are they induced to enter
into meiotic prophase, or simply permitted to do so? In our earlier papers (Tarkowski 1970; Mystkowska and Tarkowski 1970), we
favoured the latter explanation, i.e., that at a certain phase of
the life history of germ cells (for instance after a certain definite number of gonial divisions), they start meiosis — provided
they are in a permissive environment, which is the ovarian environment (or, in the case of XX ↔ XY testes, the regions in which XX
somatic cells dominate). In embryonic testes, the germ cells are
not permitted to begin meiosis, although potentially they are able
to do so, as shown by the work of Ożdżeński, Ford et al., and Evans
et al. referred to earlier in this paper. That they do not start
meiosis is not surprising, because at approximately the same time
as meiosis begins in the ovary, gonial divisions in testes become
exceedingly rare — if they occur at all. If mitoses are in some
way prevented, then meiotic prophase also cannot be initiated.
Although this concept satisfactorily explains behavior of germ
cells in sex-chromosome chimeras and in normal development, it is
highly speculative and based only on indirect evidence.

The recent work of Byskov (1974), Byskov and Saxen (1976),
and O and Baker (1976) appears to favour the first alternative,
namely, that meiosis in ovaries is induced, and that the meiosis-
inducing factor comes from rete ovarii. Although, in the light of
these studies, the "inductive" hypothesis appears to be more plausible than the "permissive" one, there are facts that cannot be
easily explained in this way, such as, for instance, Ożdżeński's
observations (loc. cit.) on the precocious initiation of meiosis

in normal embryonic testes transplanted to ectopic sites. From
where could the meiosis inducing factor come in this case?

XX ↔ XY FEMALES

Until quite recently, there has been no evidence for the functional sex reversal of XY germ cells in the mouse and for their
differentiation into oocytes. The work of Ford *et al.* (1975) on
the XXY animal borne by an XX ↔ XY chimeric female (the available
evidence implied that the oocyte had originated from the XY component), and the description of an XY oocyte undergoing first meiotic
division (Evans *et al.* 1977), demonstrates that this is possible.
However, there are three reasons why development beyond birth from
an XY oocyte may be an extremely rare event.

First, development of the female phenotype on the background
of sex-chromosome chimerism occurs relatively rarely. Second, although XO germ cells in the mouse can complete oogenesis (Welshons
and Russell 1959), it appears that the viability of embryos derived
from oocytes containing only one X chromosome is subnormal (Cattanach 1962; Morris 1968; Burgoyne and Biggers 1976). This makes
it likely that the viability of embryos originating from XY oocytes
would be decreased also. Third, in comparison to males, females
produce relatively few young during their life span, and this further reduces the chance of detecting XY oocytes by breeding tests.

REFERENCES

Burgoyne, P. S. and J. D. Biggers. 1976. The consequences of X-
dosage deficiency in the germ line: impaired development in vitro
of preimplantation embryos from XO mice. Develop. Biol. 51: 109-
117.

Byskov, A. G. 1974. Does the rete ovarii act as a trigger for
the onset of meiosis. Nature (London) 252: 396-397.

Byskov, A. G. and L. Saxen. 1976. Induction of meiosis in fetal
mouse testis in vitro. Develop. Biol. 52: 193-200.

Cattanach, B. M. 1962. XO mice. Genet. Res. (Cambridge) 3: 487-
490.

Cattanach, B. M., C. E. Pollard and S. G. Hawkes. 1971. Sex reversed mice: XX and XO males. Cytogenetics 10: 318-337.

Evans, E. P., C. F. Ford and M. F. Lyon. 1977. Direct evidence
of the capacity of the XY germ cell in the mouse to become an
oocyte. Nature (London) 267: 430-431.

Ford, C. E., E. P. Evans, M. D. Burtenshaw, H. M. Clegg, M. Tuffrey and R. D. Barnes. 1975. A functional 'sex-reversed' oocyte in the mouse. Proc. Roy. Soc. Lond. B 190: 187-197.

Gordon, J. 1976. Failure of XX cells containing the sex reversed gene to produce gametes in allophenic mice. J. Exp. Zool. 198: 367-373.

McLaren, A. 1975. Sex chimaerism and germ cell distribution in a series of chimaeric mice. J. Embryol. exp. Morph. 33: 205-216.

McLaren, A. 1978. Reproduction in single-sex chimeras. In Genetic Mosaics and Chimeras in Mammals, Liane B. Russell, Ed., Plenum Press, New York and London.

McLaren, A., A. C. Chandley and S. Kofman-Alfaro. 1972. A study of meiotic germ cells in the gonads of foetal mouse chimaeras. J. Embryol. exp. Morph. 27: 515-524.

Mintz, B. 1962. Formation of genotypically mosaic mouse embryos. Amer. Zool. 2: 432 (abstract).

Mintz, B. 1968. Hermaphroditism, sex chromosomal mosaicism and germ cell selection in allophenic mice. J. Anim. Sci. (Suppl. 1) 27: 51-60.

Mintz, B. 1969. Developmental mechanisms found in allophenic mice with sex chromosomal and pigmentary mosaicism. Birth Defects: Original Article Series 5: 11-22. In First Conference on the Clinical Delineation of Birth Defects, D. Gergsma and V. McKusick, Eds., National Foundation, New York.

Morris, T. 1968. The XO and OY chromosome constitutions in the mouse. Genet. Res. (Cambridge) 12: 125-137.

Mullen, R. J. and W. K. Whitten. 1971. Relationship of genotype and degree of chimerism in coat color to sex ratios and gametogenesis in chimeric mice. J. exp. Zool. 178: 165-176.

Mystkowska, E. T. and A. K. Tarkowski. 1968. Observations on CBA-p/CBA-T6T6 mouse chimaeras. J. Embryol. exp. Morph. 20: 33-52.

Mystkowska, E. T. and A. K. Tarkowski. 1970. Behaviour of germ cells and sexual differentiation in late embryonic and early postnatal mouse chimaeras. J. Embryol. exp. Morph. 23: 395-405.

O, W. and T. G. Baker. 1976. Initiation and control of meiosis in hamster gonads in vitro. J. Reprod. Fert. 48: 399-401.

Ożdżeński, W. 1972. Differentiation of the genital ridges of mouse embryos in the kidney of adult mice. Arch. Anat. micr. 61: 267-278.

Short, R. V. 1972. Germ cell sex. In The Genetics of the Spermatozoon, R. A. Beatty and S. Gluecksohn-Waelsch, Eds., pp. 325-345. Edinburgh and New York.

Tarkowski, A. K. 1961. Mouse chimaeras developed from fused eggs. Nature (London) 190: 857-860.

Tarkowski, A. K. 1964. True hermaphroditism in chimaeric mice. J. Embryol. exp. Morph. 12: 735-757.

Tarkowski, A. K. 1970. Are the genetic factors controlling sexual differentiation of somatic and germinal tissues of a mammalian gonad stable or labile? Fogarty International Center Proceedings No. 2. Environmental Influences on Genetic Expression. Biological and Behavioral Aspects of Sexual Differentiation. U.S. Government Printing Office.

Welshons, W. J. and L. B. Russell. 1959. The Y-chromosome as the bearer of male determining factors in the mouse. Proc. Nat. Acad. Sci. USA 45: 560-566.

USE OF THE *SEX REVERSED* GENE (*Sxr*) TO INVESTIGATE FUNCTIONAL SEX

REVERSAL AND GONADAL DETERMINATION IN MAMMALS

Jon Gordon

Department of Biology, Yale University, New Haven,
Connecticut 06520

Functional sex reversal is a well established phenomenon in
many classes of organisms and demonstrates that sex determination
in those organisms is influenced by the extra-embryonic environment. Experimental reversal of chromosomally male *Xenopus laevis*
embryos to functional females has been accomplished by adding estrogens to the water in which these embryos develop (Chang and Witschi
1955; Gallien 1955). Chromosomally male embryos of the fish *Oryzias
latipes* have been similarly reversed by estrogens (Yamamoto 1953,
1955), and female embryos of this same species have been reversed
to functional males with testosterone (Yamamoto 1958). Other experiments have reversed males of *Amblystoma maculatum* (Foote 1940,
1941) and of the urodele, *Pleurodeles waltlii* (Gallien 1950, 1951).

In contrast, modification of the environment with steroids has
been unsuccessful in completely reversing the sex of many mammalian
species, including guinea pigs (Dantchakoff 1936), mice (Turner
1939, 1940), rats (Greene 1942), hamsters (Bruner and Witschi 1946),
rabbits (Jost 1947), and monkeys (Wells and van Wagenen 1954). The
bovine freemartin co-twin also provides evidence that, in mammals,
primary sex determination depends not on the hormonal environment
of the embryo but on the genetic makeup of that embryo. Freemartinism occurs when dizygotic-twin bovine embryos of the opposite genetic sex develop placental anastomoses and exchange cells or hormones. The female twin is masculinized. This masculinization has
been shown not to depend on testosterone (Jost, Chodkiewicz and
Mauleon 1963; Jost 1965) but is always correlated with the presence
of XY cells in the blood or in other tissues of the female twin
(Owen 1945; Ohno, Trijillo, Stenius, Christian and Teplitz 1962;
Goodfellow, Strong, and Stewart 1965). Thus, in mammals, it is the

143

genetic sex of the embryo which determines its gonadal differentiation, and not the environment.

From these data it is evident that the genetic sex of a mammalian embryo must be mixed in order to study functional sex
reversal and sex determination. The technique of embryo aggregation (Tarkowski 1961; Mintz 1962) provided a means whereby XY ↔
XX mouse chimeras could be produced in large numbers. These allophenic mice enable the experimenter to produce sex chimerism during
early cleavage and thus to mix the genetic sexes of all cell populations which contribute to sex differentiation. One would expect
such mice to provide a solution to the problem of functional sex
reversal in mammals and thus an elucidation of the cell type(s)
responsible for gonad determination. In my view, the most startling
observation yet made on allophenic mice is that they have not supplied these solutions.

Experiments with chimeric mice have thus far indicated that
although the somatic component of the mouse gonad is capable of
functionally reversing, the germ-cell component is not. Mintz
(1969) produced a chimeric male mouse whose testes contained over
95% XX cells; all of the germ cells, however, were derived from XY
cells. Ford, Evans, Burtenshaw, Clegg, Barnes, and Tuffrey (1974)
described a female chimera with an ovarian follicle containing over
98% XY follicle cells. These experiments have established that the
somatic cells of the gonad can be functionally reversed in an
environment of genetic mosaicism.

Investigating the possibility that XX cells might become sperm
in chimeric mice, Mintz (1968) bred 288 chimeras and scored the sex
ratio of the more than 29,000 offspring produced. She reasoned that
if XX cells were becoming sperm in these chimeras the sex ratio of
their offspring would be distorted in favor of females. No such s
sex ratio distortion was observed. Mystkowska and Tarkowski (1968,
1970), Tarkowski (1969), and McLaren, Chandley, and Kofman-Alfaro
(1972) examined the gonads of fetal mouse chimeras and observed germ
cells entering meiosis in embryonic testes at a time corresponding
to the onset of meiosis in oogenesis. These workers interpreted
their results to mean that XX primordial germ cells (pgcs) were not
reversed by the testicular environment. Data concerning the fate
of XY pgcs in XY ↔ XX chimeras which become females is less clear.
Because chimeras produced between strains of comparable developmental vigor ("balanced" chimeras) more often develop as males (Tarkowski 1963; McLaren 1972; Mullen and Whitten 1971), fewer females
have been available for analysis. Nonetheless, thousands of chimeric mice have now been constructed, and not one female chimera
has produced offspring from Y-chromosome bearing oocytes. Indirect
evidence of oocytes derived from XY cells has, however, been reported. Ford *et al*. (1975) identified an XXY mouse bearing the

coat-color marker of the XY component of its XY ↔ XX chimeric
female parent. The chimera, however, was not available for further
breeding. Evans, Ford, and Lyon (1977) later karyotyped oocytes in
female chimeras and found one which was apparently XY. Unfortunately, this method of analysis precluded further progeny testing of
the chimera. At the moment, therefore, the ability of the germ
cells to undergo sex reversal remains unproven.

Several hypotheses have been put forward to explain the apparent irreversibility of the germ cells of mammals. Lifschytz and
Lindsley (1972, 1974) have pointed out that in the XY primary
spermatocyte, the single X chromosome becomes inactivated. In an
XX primary spermatocyte, an additional X chromosome is present and
presumably remains active. The failure to inactivate this additional X may prevent XX spermatocytes from undergoing meiosis.
This view is supported by observations on the autosomal dominant
gene *Sex reversed* (*Sxr*) in mice. This gene confers a male phenotype on XX mice, but these XX;*Sxr*/+* males are sterile (Cattanach,
Pollard, and Hawkes 1971), and postmeiotic cells cannot be seen
histologically in their testes (Figure 1). On the other hand,
meiosis occasionally proceeds in XO;*Sxr* mice (Mittwoch and Buehr
1973) and results in abnormal sperm. Since the only difference
between XO;*Sxr* and XX;*Sxr* mice is the X chromosome dosage, the
presence of a second X chromosome is strongly implicated as a barrier to meiosis in the male.

Aberrant X-chromosome dosage may also explain why XY cells
function poorly as oocytes. Evidence exists from studies in mice
(Epstein 1969; Kozak, McLean, and Eicher 1974) and humans (Gartler,
Liskay, and Campbell 1972; Gartler, Liskay, and Gant 1973) that
both X chromosomes are active in normal XX primary oocytes. The
apparent sterility of XO humans and the reduced fertile lifespan
of XO mice (Lyon and Hawkes 1973) are in accord with the view that
a single X results in a deficiency of X-linked enzymes, which im-
pairs the function of oocytes. Circumstantial evidence also exists
which suggests that the presence of a Y chromosome may itself present a barrier to oogenesis. In the wood lemming, *Myopus schisticolor*, fertile females have been observed in which every somatic
cell is XY (Gropp, Winking, Frank, Noack, and Fredga 1976). Yet,
in the germ line, the Y chromosome is lost, and all oocytes produced contain an X chromosome (Fredga, Gropp, Winking, and Frank
1976). These oocytes, when fertilized by Y-bearing sperm from
normal XY males, all develop as females. This result shows that
the defect in these animals cannot be related to their Y chromosome:
it is the X chromosome that is most likely affected (Fredga, Gropp,

---

Sxr is never present in homozygous condition, since it can be
transmitted only by one sex, namely XY;*Sxr*/+ males. Throughout
this chapter, the genotype *Sxr*/+ is abbreviated as *Sxr*

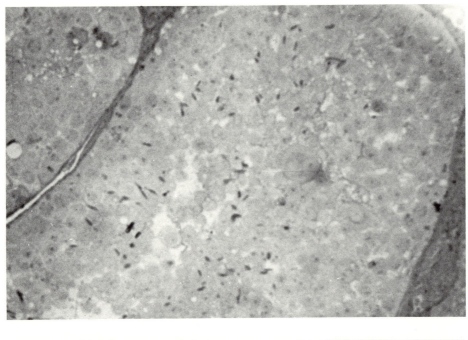

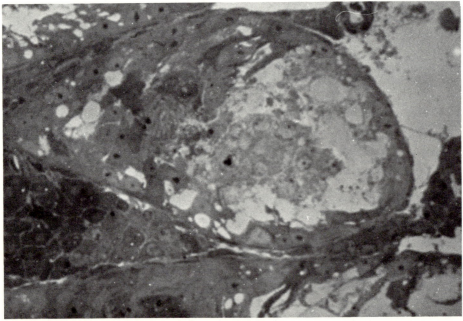

Figure 1

FIGURE 1. Top: Histological section of a normal mouse testis.
The postmeiotic spermatid nuclei are easily seen as densely
staining, elongate elements.
Bottom: Section from the testis of an XX;*Sxr* mouse. The
tubule lumen contains only Sertoli cell nuclei. No postmeiotic cells are seen.

Winking, and Frank 1977). An obvious interpretation of this phenomenon is that the Y chromosome is lost in the germ lines of the
XY females in response to a selective pressure for maintenance of
fertility. Thus, XY cells may for several reasons be unable to
differentiate as oocytes.

Another explanation exists, however, for the failure to observe
germ-cell sex reversal in mammals: the germ cells may contribute
to the determination of the gonad phenotype. If this were the case,
one would fail to observe reversal not because the germ cells are
genetically unable to reverse, but because germ cells might always
induce adjacent somatic cells to differentiate in accordance with
their own genotype. If this local differentiation does not correspond to the final phenotype of the gonad, these groups of cells may
die out and leave behind only those germ cells whose genotype agrees
with the final gonad phenotype. Against this proposal are the observations that embryos deprived of pgcs by genetic or teratogenic
means still develop normal gonads. For example, mice homozygous
for the dominant spotting (*W*) gene produce pgcs that migrate poorly
and that do not divide en route to the genital ridge. The result
is a gonad with almost no germ cells (Mintz and Russell 1957).
Despite the absence of germ cells, however, the gonad develops normally (Coulombre and Russell 1954). Embryonic rats whose pgcs are
destroyed by injections of the alkylating agent Busulfan into pregnant females also develop germ cell-free gonads that are otherwise
normal (Hemsworth and Jackson 1963; Merchant 1975). These observations imply that the germ cell has no necessary role in gonad determination; but they do not rule out the possibility that, when present, the germ cells exert an effect on gonad development.

ANALYSIS OF CHIMERAS HAVING AN *Sxr* COMPONENT

We have produced allophenic mice designed to maximize the
possibility of obtaining functional sex reversal, and thus to test
the explanations that have been offered for the failure to observe
sex reversal. These experiments involved the aggregation of XX
embryos carrying the autosomal dominant for *sex reversed* (*Sxr*),
with normal XX and XY embryos, marked by albino, *cc* (Gordon 1976).
We reasoned that XX cells carrying male-determining genes such as

Sxr might be better equipped than ordinary XX cells to undergo spermatogenesis in an XX;*Sxr* ↔ XY chimera that developed as a normal male. Such spermatogenesis would be easily detected by breeding these males. If XX;*Sxr* cells differentiated into sperm, all offspring carrying the pigment marker characteristic of the XX;*Sxr* cells would be either XX or XX;*Sxr*; both of these phenotypes are readily distinguishable from XY mice. Such a result would une-quivocally prove that cells with two X chromosomes can undergo spermatogenesis. A similar progeny test can be applied to XX;*Sxr* ↔ XX mice which become fertile females. If XX;*Sxr* cells differen-tiated into oocytes, the *Sxr* gene would be passed through the female and be detected among the progeny. This result would prove that male-determining genes do not prevent oogenesis and would favor the notion that X-chromosome dosage is important to this process.

In our initial report (Gordon 1976), 24 of 37 such chimeras had been progeny tested. Two mice were sterile hermaphrodites, and these had not been analyzed further. Since that time, we have progeny tested the remaining chimeras and have analyzed the gonads of the hermaphrodites histologically. A sample of the final breed-ing data is summarized in Table 1. The mice selected for this table illustrate several important features of this experiment. First, these chimeras were of the balanced type; most of them were males. Second, the strain carrying the *Sxr* gene was not excluded from the germ line in single-sex chimeras. Mice #s 31, 25, and 7 illustrate this fact. We know from these examples, therefore, that the strain background of the *Sxr*-bearing cells did not prevent them from popu-lating the germ line and attempting gametogenesis. Finally, XX;*Sxr* progeny were produced but resulted only from sperm derived from XY;*Sxr* pgcs. When XX;*Sxr* progeny were present, XY littermates were always found that carried the same coat-color markers. Mice #s 8 and 33 demonstrate this point. These updated data are thus consis-tent with our original results and suggest that XX cells carrying male-determining genes cannot differentiate either as spermatocytes or as oocytes.

It should be recognized that, although suggestive, negative data such as these can never be conclusive. Although the single-sex chimeras demonstrate comparable developmental vigor between the two strains employed in these aggregations, the possibility that XX;*Sxr* cells are, by virtue of the presence of the *Sxr* gene, developmen-tally less vigorous cannot be ruled out. These cells may simply be eliminated by competition with the normal pgcs of the albino strain, and may never reach the gonad. Such a competitive difference would have to be related to the presence of the *Sxr* gene alone, since the genetic backgrounds of the aggregated strains have already been shown to be developmentally comparable. But we have since demon-strated (Gordon 1977) that a single allelic change can profoundly affect the competitive ability of cells in chimeras; thus, the *Sxr* gene may be acting in this way.

TABLE 1. Summary of breeding from allophenic mice produced by aggregation of XY;Sxr+;CC x XX;++;cc embryos with XY;++;cc x XX;++;CC embryos

Mouse no.	Sex*	Coat color cc %	Coat color CC %	cc progeny M	cc progeny F	Cc progeny M	Cc progeny F	Cc progeny XX;Sxr	Genotype†
1	H	30	70	sterile		—	—	—	XX ↔ XX;Sxr
2	M	25	75	30	32	0	0	0	XY ↔ XX;(Sxr)
5	M	15	85	4	3	10	10	0	XY ↔ XY
7	F	50	50	42	42	3	3	0	XX ↔ XX
8	M	20	80	14	16	23	6	4	XY ↔ XY;Sxr
9	M	50	50	37	39	0	0	0	XY ↔ XX;(Sxr)
10	H	50	50	sterile		—	—	—	XX ↔ XX;Sxr
11	M	15	85	0	0	7	3	0	XX ↔ XY
18	M	15	85	52	50	0	0	0	XY ↔ XX;(Sxr)
19	M	65	35	33	47	0	0	0	XY ↔ XX;(Sxr)
20	F	75	25	13	10	0	0	0	XX ↔ XX;(Sxr)
25	F	45	55	21	18	7	4	0	XX ↔ XX
27	M	90	10	17	6	12	18	0	XY ↔ XY
31	M	70	30	3	6	20	35	0	XY ↔ XY
33	M	5	95	0	0	9	7	7	XX ↔ XY;Sxr

*M = Male, F = Female, H = Hermaphrodite.

†Parentheses indicate that the presence of the Sxr gene in these chimeras could not be proved or disproved by progeny testing.

Another possibility is that the number of allophenic mice produced was inadequate to investigate effectively the fertility of XX;Sxr cells. This objection can be applied particularly well to the female chimeras, which numbered only eight. Against this argument are the facts that, in balanced chimeras such as these, most females are XX ↔ XX, and that in our single-sex chimeras we readily observed both cell strains in the germ line. Yet several of our females produced oocytes only from the albino strain. This result is unexpected for such chimeric females, and indicates that these mice were XX;Sxr ↔ XX mosaics which developed as females but which could not produce oocytes from the XX;Sxr pgcs. At this point, therefore, our data support the view that mammalian pgcs are not functionally reversible.

In order to determine the genotypes of the two hermaphroditic chimeras, we have subjected their gonads to histological analysis. The presence of ovarian tissue on gross examination was taken as evidence that one of the components of both chimeras was XX; testicular tissue indicated that the other component was XY;Sxr, XY, or XX;Sxr. For our purposes, it was important only to distinguish the XX;Sxr male component from the other two, since we already knew that XY and XY;Sxr cells could produce normal gametes and induce a male phenotype in mixed-sex chimeras. A karyotype that failed to reveal XY cells would not distinguish between these possibilities. Since XX cells were known to be present in the chimeras, a karyotype revealing only XX cells might easily represent a sample of cells which were all XX and would not prove that a chimera was XX;Sxr ↔ XX. Histological evaluation, however, afforded the possibility of distinguishing the XX;Sxr ↔ XX mouse from the other two sex chimeras. In XY ↔ XX (and presumably also XY;Sxr ↔ XX) chimeric hermaphrodites, spermatogenesis is often seen and occasionally results in mature sperm (Tarkowski 1964; Mintz 1965; McLaren 1975). XX;Sxr pgcs in XX;Sxr ↔ XX chimeras would not be expected to undergo spermatogenesis, however, since in XX;Sxr mice spermatogenesis does not proceed beyond the primary spermatocyte stage. Thus, the failure to detect spermatogenesis in our hermaphrodites would not prove, but would strongly suggest that these mice were XX;Sxr ↔ XX. Sections of the gonads of one of our hermaphrodites are shown in Figure

————————————————————➔

FIGURE 2. Top: Histological section of the testicular portion of the gonad of an XX;Sxr ↔ XX hermaphrodite. The tubule lumen contains only Sertoli cells, indicating that the male portion of the mosaic was XX;Sxr.
Bottom: Histological section of an ovarian portion of the gonad from the same mouse. The tissue is mostly stroma; a single seminiferous tubule in cross section is indicated by the arrows. No spermatogenic elements are seen in this tubule.

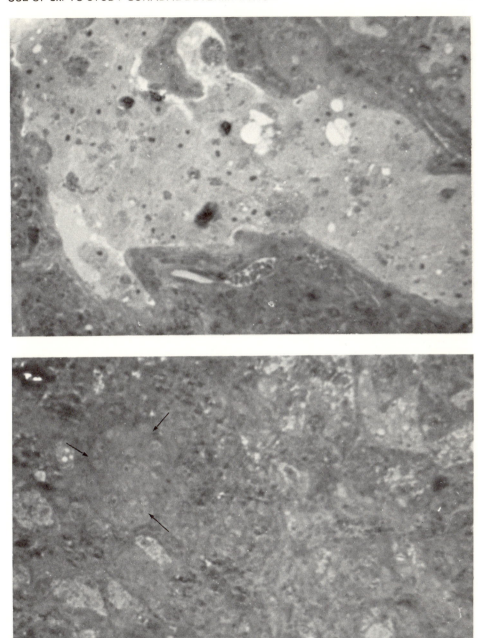

Figure 2

2. This figure illustrates that the testicular tissue in both gonads was totally devoid of spermatogenic elements. Sections from the other hermaphrodite were similar in appearance. We have thus concluded that both of these hermaphrodites were XX;*Sxr* ↔ XX.

The importance of this conclusion is underscored when it is considered together with the observation that none of the chimeras produced in this series unambiguously displayed the XX;*Sxr* pheno-type. This fact stands in sharp contrast to our expectations. XY ↔ XX mice usually develop phenotypes indistinguishable from either XY or XX mice. XX;*Sxr* ↔ XX mice would also, therefore, be expected to develop a phenotype indistinguishable from either XX;*Sxr* or XX mice. Yet this did not occur; these mice became either females or hermaphrodites.

This observation can be explained in two ways. First, the *Sxr* gene may not produce, quantitatively or qualitatively, all of the male-determining elements elaborated in the presence of a normal Y chromosome. In this case, XX cells in XX;*Sxr* ↔ XX gonads might not be so strongly influenced to develop into testicular cells by neighboring XX;*Sxr* cells. The fact that XX;*Sxr* testes are identical histologically to XY testes lacking germ cells suggests that, if the *Sxr* gene is deficient, the deficiency resides in the quantity of male-determining elements produced and not their quality. Histologi-cal analysis is crude, however, and the possibility that XX;*Sxr* testes have defects not revealed by this method must be considered. In either case, a uniformly XX;*Sxr* gonad would result in exposure of every gonadal cell to the male-determining products of the *Sxr* gene. This exposure might obscure the deficiencies of *Sxr* with respect to testis induction. In XX;*Sxr* ↔ XX chimeras, the XX cells would produce no male-determining substance. Their presence might therefore reduce the total amount of testis-determining gene product below a threshold that reveals deficiencies in the *Sxr* gene, as com-pared with a Y chromosome. Whether or not the aberrant sexual development of our XX;*Sxr* ↔ XX chimeras is based on a deficiency in the *Sxr* gene will be known when all male-determining gene products are better characterized and quantitated.

A second explanation for the absence of chimeras identical in phenotype to XX;*Sxr* mice is that the *Sxr* gene is equivalent to a Y chromosome, but XX;*Sxr* and XX cells compete much more equally than do XY and XX cells to populate those tissues which determine gonad sex. This possibility rests on the assumption that a competitive difference exists between cells in chimeric embryos with respect to populating of the gonad-determining tissues. Evidence indeed exists to support this assumption. When balanced chimeras are produced, normal males most often result (Tarkowski 1961; McLaren 1972; Mullen and Whitten 1971). This observation suggests that, all other things being equal, XY cells will win out in competition with XX cells in sex chimeras, and will dominate the sex-determining tissues. If this advantage of XY cells is superseded by placing the XX cells on a more vigorous genetic background, the sex chimeras develop into females as often as into males (Mullen and Whitten 1971). This result is consistent with the hypothesis that the precursor pool of sex-determining cells is small, that XY cells in this precursor pool win out in competition with any XX cells that might also be present, and that, if the XX cells are on a superior genetic background, they will often become the exclusive occupants of that small sex-determining pool of cells and produce a female chimera. That all of our XX;*Sxr* ↔ XX mice became females or hermaphrodites agrees with the notion that XX;*Sxr* and XX cells compete more equally than do XY and XX cells. When the precursor pool of cells was populated by both XX;*Sxr* and XX cells, hermaphrodites resulted instead of males, and the increased ability of the XX cells to become sole members of the pool accounts for the large numbers of females in the XX;*Sxr* ↔ XX group. Also in agreement with this explanation is the fact that all of the XY ↔ XX;*Sxr* chimeras developed as normal males and not as XX;*Sxr* sterile males. If the behavior of XX;*Sxr* cells is similar to that of XX cells in balanced chimeras such as these, XY ↔ XX;*Sxr* mice should develop similarly to XY ↔ XX mice; that is, as normal males. For these reasons we favor the view that the absence of chimeras corresponding in phenotype to XX;*Sxr* mice is based on differential competition between XY and XX;*Sxr* cells to occupy those tissues which direct gonad differentiation. A competitive difference between XY and XX;*Sxr* or XX cells might well be based on X-chromosome dosage. A single X chromosome might give XY cells a proliferative advantage, a migratory advantage, or both.

Our data are thus in accord with the view that the absence of hermaphroditism in XY ↔ XX chimeras is based on differential competition between XY and XX cells with respect to populating the gonad-determining tissues, with the XY cells usually being competitively superior. Once these cells have directed the differentiation of the gonad, the question still remains as to the fate of the pgcs of the opposite sex genotype. Can the germ cells undergo functional sex reversal or not? It is my assertion that they cannot, because in sex chimeras the pgc population and the gonad-determining cell population are one and the same.

A MODEL FOR GONAD DETERMINATION

This hypothesis appears to conflict with the large body of data alluded to previously which shows that gonads deprived of pgcs are able to differentiate normally. A simple model for gonad determination can be constructed, however, which explains this observation and the facts that most sex chimeras become normal males, that XY sperm can develop in an XX testis and XX oocytes in an XY ovary, and that functional sex reversal is not observed in mammals.

This model is based on the differential expression of genes coding for the H-Y male antigen and the receptor for that antigen. The H-Y antigen was discovered when skin from male mice grafted to syngeneic females was found to be rejected (Eichwald and Silmser 1955). This antigen has since been invariably correlated with development of a testis. For example, XY mice hemizygous for *testicular feminization* (*tfm*) have a female external sex phenotype but develop testes which are retained in the inguinal canal (Lyon and Hawkes 1970). These mice express the H-Y antigen (Bennett, Boyse, Lyon, Matheson, Scheid, and Yanagisawa 1975). XO mole-voles, which develop testes despite their XO karyotype, also express the H-Y antigen (Nagai and Ohno 1977), as do XX;*Sxr* sterile male mice (Bennett, Matheson, Scheid, Yanagisawa, Boyse, Wachtel, and Cattanach 1977). These observations have led many workers to propose that the H-Y antigen is the testis-determining substance (Wachtel, Ohno, Koo, and Boyse 1975; Ohno, Christian, Wachtel, and Koo 1976; Silvers and Wachtel 1977; Wachtel 1977). Of course, to have such an effect, the H-Y antigen must interact with a receptor. Ohno (1976) has proposed that all gonial cells, be they XX or XY, have H-Y receptors, and that all XY cells express the H-Y antigen. This model explains well how chimeric mice can have testes composed largely of XX cells: H-Y antigen expressed by the few XY cells interacts with receptor on the XX cells and causes them to organize into a testis. Figure 3a illustrates how an XY pgc can exert such an effect on many XX cells. Ohno's model does not explain the observation of Ford *et al.* (1974), however, that an XX oocyte can be surrounded by XY cells and still develop as an oocyte. Why did not the H-Y antigen on those XY cells interact with receptors on that oocyte and cause it to attempt spermatogenesis?

The following model is based on three simple premises and can answer this question as well as the others raised previously. The three premises are as follows: (1) all XY cells express the H-Y antigen; (2) all somatic cells (particularly gonadal somatic cells) have H-Y receptors; and (3) primordial germ cells do not have H-Y receptors. The third assumption constitutes the distinguishing feature of this model and explains why primordial germ cells are so important to gonad development in sex chimeras. I shall now apply this model to each of the observations previously listed and demonstrate how it explains them.

Gonads deprived of pgcs differentiate normally. In a uniformly XY or XX animal, pgcs are irrelevant to gonad determination. If the embryo is XY, all gonadal somatic cells will express the H-Y antigen, and all of the cells will have H-Y receptors which will interact with that antigen. Thus, the gonadal somatic cells will "induce themselves" to form a testis. If the embryo is XX,

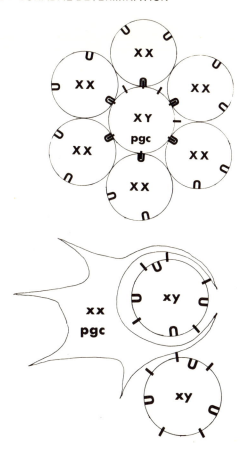

FIGURE 3. Top: Diagram illustrating the potent masculinizing
    effect of an XY cell in a mosaic gonad. Receptors for H-Y
    antigen on several surrounding XX cells interact with H-Y
    antigen on a single XY cell, in this case a primordial germ
    cell.
    Bottom: Diagram showing how an XX primordial germ cell, by
    virtue of not containing H-Y antigen or its receptor, can
    prevent H-Y receptors on somatic cells from interacting with
    H-Y antigen. The result is local ovarian differentiation.

none of the cells will express H-Y antigen. Thus, despite the
presence of H-Y receptors on the gonadal somatic cells the absence
of antigen will result in ovarian differentiation.

*XY sperm can develop in an XX testis, and XX oocytes can
develop in an XY ovary.* XY pgcs, expressing H-Y antigen, arrive
in an XX genital ridge. They interact with numerous XX somatic

cells which have receptors (see Fig. 3a) and induce these cells to
form seminiferous tubules. When XX pgcs arrive at an XY genital
ridge, they are not expressing H-Y antigen, nor do they have receptors for the antigen. Thus, they can intercalate themselves
between the XY somatic cells and prevent the H-Y receptors on these
cells from interacting with H-Y antigen. Because they are denied
interaction with H-Y antigen, the XY somatic cells develop into
ovarian tissue. This scheme is illustrated in Figure 3b. These
XY ovarian cells then proliferate and, in response to FSH, form
follicles such as the one observed by Ford and his coworkers
(1974). That such XY follicles may arise from relatively few XY
cells which later proliferate has been previously proposed by
McLaren (1976).

   Functional sex reversal is not observed in mammals. Functional sex reversal is not observed because pgcs, by virtue of not
utilizing the H-Y antigen system for their own differentiation,
cause local organization of gonadal somatic cells in accordance
with their own genotypes. XY cells express the H-Y antigen and
induce somatic cells to form seminiferous tubules. Thus, XY pgcs
cannot be placed in an ovarian environment because they will create
a testicular environment. Similarly, XX pgcs cannot be placed in
a testicular environment because they cause local ovarian development as illustrated in Figure 3b. If most of the gonad is populated by XY pgcs, primordial follicles would find themselves located in a testis and would be expected to degenerate. The observation that such degenerating follicles can often be seen in the
testes of embryonic mouse chimeras (Mystkowska and Tarkowski 1968,
1970; McLaren *et al.* 1972) is in agreement with this prediction.

   Most sex chimeras become normal males. In a balanced sex
chimera, the gonadal somatic cells are both XX and XY, as are the
pgcs. The XY somatic cells and pgcs are equally capable of inducing neighboring cells to form seminiferous tubules. As illustrated
in Figure 3a, a single XY cell may induce many of its neighbors to
form tubules. An XX pgc, though capable of inducing local ovarian
differentiation, must physically disrupt patches of XY cells and
prevent the H-Y receptor on these cells from interacting with antigen. The fact that the XX pgc must do more than simply contact XY
cells makes the XX pgc a less potent determiner of gonadal sex than
any XY cell. Moreover, XY pgcs have a potential competitive advantage over XX pgcs. Pgcs must migrate and proliferate extensively
en route to the gonad and, as already described, this behavior may
allow for selection in favor of the XY pgcs. These two factors
thus lead to a predominance of males among balanced chimeras. In
unbalanced chimeras, XX pgcs are on a vigorous genetic background
which increases the statistical chance that all of the pgcs arising
in the yolk sac will be XX. In this situation, the genital ridge
is also likely to contain more XX cells. Thus, the chances of H-Y
receptors being blocked or of not contacting H-Y antigen is much
greater and ovaries more often result.

If this model is correct, then our XY ↔ XX;*Sxr* chimeras constitute the best test so far of the ability of XX cells to become
sperm. Since XX;*Sxr* cells express the H-Y antigen, they induce
testicular differentiation. Therefore, this gene permits the
experimenter to place XX;*Sxr* cells in a testis environment and to
associate these XX;*Sxr* cells with normal XY somatic cells. For
these reasons, we interpret our failure to observe sperm derived
from XX;*Sxr* pgcs as the strongest evidence presented thus far that
XX cells are genetically incapable of producing sperm. By the same
reasoning, however, we must conclude that XX;*Sxr* ↔ XX chimeras
are in no way a better test of the ability of cells containing
male-determining genes to produce oocytes than were previous experiments with chimeric mice. Our model predicts that H-Y antigen
on XX;*Sxr* pgcs will cause local testicular differentiation and prevent XX;*Sxr* pgcs from exposure to an ovarian environment.

One intriguing prediction arising from this model is that an
XY pgc that did not express the H-Y antigen would behave exactly
like an XX pgc; it would induce ovarian differentiation. In this
hypothetical situation the ability of XY cells to produce oocytes
would be tested. The XY oocyte in diakinesis observed by Evans
et al. (1977) may, in fact, represent the observation of an XY
cell which failed to express H-Y.

This model also predicts that genital ridges in XY ↔ XX chimeras which are deprived of pgcs might more often become ovotestes.
This expectation arises from the fact that pgcs migrate through the
genital ridge tissue and undoubtedly break up patches of cells. An
XY pgc might in this way expose XX cells in the center of an XX
patch to H-Y antigen and commit them to testicular differentiation.
Such patches of XX cells might be more likely to remain intact in
an embryo without pgcs and develop into ovary. Preliminary attempts to construct sex mosaics without pgcs in our laboratory have
met with little success, but the preliminary results indicate that
pgc-deprived gonads in XY ↔ XX mosaics are more likely to become
ovotestes. Pursuit of this and other related experiments should
lead to a more complete understanding of mammalian sex determination and germ-cell differentiation.

SUMMARY

We have produced large numbers of allophenic mice by aggregating embryos homozygous for albino with normally pigmented embryos
carrying the autosomal dominant gene *Sex reversed* (*Sxr*). These
chimeras were bred to albino mice of the opposite sex, and 35 of
37 produced progeny. However, none of the offspring were derived
from gametes arising from XX;*Sxr* primordial germ cells. These
results provide evidence that XX cells do not differentiate into
sperm, even when provided with male-determining genes, and that XX

cells containing male-determining genes likewise do not differentiate into oocytes. These data further support the notion that
functional sex reversal does not occur in mammals.

Histological analyses of two hermaphroditic chimeras indicate
that these mice were XX;*Sxr* ↔ XX. Moreover, none of the mosaics
produced were phenotypically XX;*Sxr*, as might have been expected
for most XX;*Sxr* ↔ XX chimeras. These observations suggest that
the male-determining capacity of the *Sxr* gene is not as great as
that of the Y chromosome; or, that XX;*Sxr* cells in XX;*Sxr* ↔ XX
mosaics do not compete against XX cells in populating the gonad-
determining tissues as well as do XY cells in XY ↔ XX mosaics.

This latter interpretation is consistent with the hypothesis
that the primordial germ cell is capable of influencing its local
environment in the genital ridge in such a way as to induce a
gonad phenotype concordant with its own genotype. We provide here
a model for gonad determination that incorporates this hypothesis,
and that also explains the observations that hermaphroditism in
allophenic mice is a rare occurrence, and that uniformly XY and XX
gonads deprived of primordial germ cells are able to differentiate
normally into testes and ovaries.

This work was supported by NIH grant 5 R01 HD 07741-05, NSF
grant PCM76-23036, and is from a thesis submitted in partial ful-
fillment of the requirements for the degree of Doctor of Philoso-
phy at Yale University.

REFERENCES

Bennett, D., E. A. Boyse, M. F. Lyon, B. J. Matheson, M. Scheid
and K. Yanagisawa. 1975. Expression of H-Y (male) antigen in
phenotypically female Tfm/Y mice. Nature 257: 236.

Bennett, D., B. J. Matheson, M. Scheid, K. Yanagisawa, E. A. Boyse,
S. Wachtel and B. M. Cattanach. 1977. Serological evidence for
H-Y antigen in Sxr, XX sex-reversed phenotypic males. Nature 263:
255.

Bruner, J. A. and E. Witschi. 1946. Testosterone-induced modifications of sex development in female hamsters. Am. J. Anat. 79:
293.

Cattanach, B. M., C. E. Pollard and S. G. Hawkes. 1971. Sex-
reversed mice: XX and XO males. Cytogenet. 10: 318.

Chang, C. Y. and E. Witschi. 1955. Breeding of sex-reversed males of *Xenopus laevis* Daudin. Proc. Soc. Exp. Biol. Med. 89: 150.

Coulombre, J. C. and E. S. Russell. 1954. Analysis of the pleiotropism at the W-locus in the mouse. The effects of W and W^v substitution upon postnatal development of germ cells. J. Exp. Zool. 126: 277.

Danchakoff, V. 1936. Realisation du sexe a volonte par inductions hormonales. I. Inversion du sexe dans un embryon genetiquement male. Bull. Biol. France et Bergique 70: 241.

Eichwald, E. J. and C. R. Silmser. 1955. Communication. Trans. Bull. 2: 154.

Epstein, C. J. 1969. Mammalian oocytes: X chromosome activity. Science 163: 1078.

Evans, E. P., C. E. Ford and M. F. Lyon. 1977. Direct evidence of the capacity of the XY germ cell in the mouse to become an oocyte. Nature 267: 430.

Foote, C. L. 1940. Response of gonads and gonaducts of Ambystoma larvae to treatment with sex hormones. Proc. Soc. Exp. Biol. Med. 43: 519.

Foote, C. L. 1941. Modification of sex development in the marbled salamander by administration of synthetic sex hormones. J. Exp. Zool. 86: 271.

Ford, C. E., E. P. Evans, M. D. Burtenshaw, H. Clegg, R. D. Barnes and M. Tuffrey. 1974. Marker chromosome analysis of tetraparental AKR ↔ CBA-T6 mouse chimaeras. Differentiation 2: 321.

Ford, C. E., F. R. S. Evans, E. P. Burtenshaw, M. D. Clegg, H. M. Tuffrey and R. D. Barnes. 1975. A functional "sex-reversed" oocyte in the mouse. Proc. Roy. Soc. Lond. 190: 1-7.

Fredga, K., A. Gropp, H. Winking and F. Frank. 1976. Fertile XX and XY type females in the wood lemming *Myopus schisticolor*. Nature 261: 225.

Fredga, K., A. Gropp, H. Winking and F. Frank. 1977. A hypothesis explaining the exceptional sex ratio in the wood lemming (*Myopus schisticolor*). Hereditas 85: 101

Gallien, M. L. 1950. Inversion du sexe (feminisation) chez l'Urodele *Pleurodeles waltlii* Michah., traite par le benzoate d'oestradiol. C. rend. Acad. Sci. 231: 919.

Gallien, M. L. 1951. Sur la descendance unisexule d'une femelle
de *Pleurodeles waltlii* Michah. ayant subi, pendant sa phase larvaire, l'actien gynogene du benzoate d'oest radiol. C. rend.
Acad. Sci. 233: 828.

Gallien, M. L. 1955. Descendence unisexule d'une femelle de
Xenopus laevis daud ayant subi, pendant sa phase larvaire, l'action gynogene du benzoate d'oest radiol. C. rend. Acad. Sci. 240:
913.

Gartler, S. M., R. M. Liskay, B. K. Campbell, R. Sparks and N.
Gant. 1972. Evidence for two functional X chromosomes in human
oocytes. Cell Differ. 1: 215.

Gartler, S. M., R. M. Liskay, and N. Gant. 1973. Two functional
X-chromosomes in human foetal oocytes. Exp. Cell Res. 82: 464.

Goodfellow, S. A., S. J. Strong and J. S. S. Stewart. 1965.
Bovine freemartins and true hermaphroditism. Lancet i: 1040.

Gordon, J. 1976. Failure of XX cells containing the sex reversed
gene to produce gametes in allophenic mice. J. Exp. Zool. 198:
367.

Gordon, J. 1977. Modification of pigmentation patterns in allophenic mice by the W gene. Differentiation 9: 19.

Greene, R. R. 1942. Hormonal factors in sex inversion: the
effects of sex hormones on embryonic sexual structures of the rat.
Biological Symposia 9: 105.

Gropp, A., H. Winking, F. Frank, G. Noack and K. Fredga. 1976.
Sex-chromosome aberrations in wood lemmings. Cytogenet. Cell Genet.
17: 343.

Hemsworth, B. N. and H. Jackson. 1963. Effect of busulphan on
the developing gonad of the male rat. J. Reprod. Fertil. 5: 187.

Jost, A. 1947. Recherches sur la differenciation de l'embryon de
lapin. II. Action des androgenes synthese sur l'histogenese
genitale. Arch. Anat. microscop. et Morphol. exper. 36: 242.

Jost, A. 1965. In Organogenesis, R. L. deHaan and H. Ursprung,
Eds., pp. 611. Holt, Rinehart, and Milano, New York.

Jost, A., M. Chodkiewicz and P. Mauleon. 1963. Intersexulaite
du foetus de Veau produite par des androgenes. Comparison entre
l'hormone foetale responsable du free-martinisme et l'hormone tes-
ticulaire adulte. C. r. hebd. Seanc. Acad. Sci., Paris 256: 274.

Kozak, L. P., G. K. McLean and E. M. Eicher. 1974. X linkage of phosphoglycerate kinase in the mouse. Biochem. Genet. 11: 41.

Lifschytz, E. and D. L. Lindsley. 1972. The role of X chromosome inactivation during spermatogenesis. Proc. Nat. Acad. Sci. 69: 182.

Lifschytz, E. and D. L. Lindsley. 1974. Sex chromosome activation during spermatogenesis. Genetics 78: 323.

Lyon, M. F. and S. G. Hawkes. 1970. X-linked gene for testicular feminization in the mouse. Nature 227: 1217.

Lyon, M. F. and S. G. Hawkes. 1973. Reproductive lifespan in irradiated and unirradiated chromosomally XO mice. Genet. Res., Camb. 21: 185.

McLaren, A. 1972. Germ cell differentiation in artificial chimeras of mice. In The Genetics of the Spermatozoon, R. A. Beatty and S. Gluecksohn-Waelsh, Eds., p. 313. Edinburgh and New York.

McLaren, A. 1975. Sex chimarism and germ cell distribution in a series of chimaeric mice. J. Embryol. exp. Morph. 33: 205.

McLaren, A. 1976. Mammalian Chimaeras. M. Abercrombie, D. Newth and J. G. Torrey, Eds. Cambridge University Press, Cambridge, London, New York, Melbourne.

McLaren, A., A. C. Chandley and S. Kofman-Alfaro. 1972. A study of meiotic germ cells in the gonads of foetal mouse chimaeras. J. Embryol. exp. Morph. 27: 515.

Merchant, H. 1975. Rat gonadal and ovarian organogenesis with and without germ cells. An ultrastructural study. Develop. Biol. 44: 1.

Mintz, B. 1962. Formation of genotypically mosaic mouse embryos. Amer. Zool. 2: 432 (abstr.).

Mintz, B. 1965. Experimental genetic mosaicism in the mouse. In Preimplantation Stages of Pregnancy, G. E. W. Wolstenholme and M. O'Connor, Eds., p. 194. Churchill, London.

Mintz, B. 1968. Hermaphroditism, sex chromosomal mosaicism, and germ cell selection in allophenic mice. J. Anim. Sci. (Suppl. 1) 27: 51.

Mintz, B. 1969. Developmental mechanisms found in allophenic mice with sex chromosomal and pigmentary mosaicism. Original Article Series 5: 11-22. In First Conference on the Clinical Delineation of Birth Defects, D. Bergsma and V. McKusick, Eds. National Foundation, New York.

Mintz, B. and E. S. Russell. 1957. Gene-induced embryological modifications of primordial germ cells in the mouse. J. Exp. Zool. 134: 207.

Mittwoch, V. and M. Buehr. 1973. Gonadal growth in embryos of sex reversed mice. Differentiation 1: 219.

Mullen, R. J. and W. K. Whitten. 1971. Relationship of genotype and degree of chimerism in coat color to sex ratios and gametogenesis in chimeric mice. J. Exp. Zool. 178: 165.

Mystkowska, E. T. and A. K. Tarkowski. 1968. Observations on CBA-p/CBA-T6T6 mouse chimeras. J. Embryol. exp. Morphol. 20: 33.

Mystkowska, E. T. and A. K. Tarkowski. 1970. Behavior of germ cells and sexual differentiation in late embryonic and early postnatal mouse chimeras. J. Embryol. exp. Morph. 23: 395.

Nagai, Y. and S. Ohno. 1977. Testis-determining H-Y antigen in XO males of the mole-vole (Ellobius lutescens). Cell 10: 729.

Ohno, S. 1976. Major regulatory genes for mammalian sexual development. Cell 7: 315.

Ohno, S., L. C. Christian, S. S. Wachtel and G. C. Koo. 1976. Hormone-like role of H-Y antigen in bovine freemartin gonad. Nature 261: 597.

Ohno, S., J. M. Trijillo, C. Stenius, L. C. Christian and R. L. Teplitz. 1962. Possible germ cell chimaeras among newborn dizygotic twin calves (Bos taurus). Cytogenet. 1: 258.

Owen, R. D. 1945. Immunogenetic consequences of vascular anastomoses between bovine twins. Science 102: 400.

Silvers, W. K. and S. S. Wachtel. 1977. H-Y antigen: Behavior and function. Science 195: 956.

Tarkowski, A. K. 1961. Mouse chimaeras developed from fused eggs. Nature, Lond. 190: 857.

Tarkowski, A. K. 1963. Studies on mouse chimaeras developed from eggs fused in vitro. Natl. Cancer Inst. Monograph. 11: 51.

Tarkowski, A. K. 1964. True hermaphroditism in chimaeric mice. J. Embryol. exp. Morph. 12: 735.

Tarkowski, A. K. 1969. Germ cells in natural and experimental chimeras in mammals. Phil. Trans. Roy. Soc. Lond. B. 259: 107.

Turner, C. D. 1939. The modification of sexual differentiation in genetic female mice by the prenatal administration of testosterone propionate. J. Morphol. 65: 353.

Turner. C. D. 1940. The influence of testosterone propionate upon sexual differentiation in genetic female mice: Postnatal androgen alone and in combination with prenatal treatments. J. Exp. Zool. 83: 1.

Wachtel, S. S. 1977. H-Y antigen and the genetics of sex determination. Science 198: 797.

Wachtel, S. S., S. Ohno, G. C. Koo and E. A. Boyse. 1975. Possible role for H-Y antigen in the primary determination of sex. Nature 257: 235.

Wells, L. J. and G. van Wagenen. 1954. Androgen-induced female pseudohermaphroditism in the monkey (*Macaca mulatta*); anatomy of the reproductive organs. Contr. Embryol. Carnegie Inst. Washington 35: 93.

Yamamoto, T. 1953. Artificially induced sex-reversal in genotypic males of the medaka (*Oryzias latipes*). J. Exp. Zool. 123: 571.

Yamamoto, T. 1955. Progeny of artificially induced sex-reversals of male genotype (XY) in the medaka (*Oryzias latipes*) with special reference to the YY male. Genetics 40: 406.

WHY NOT ANDROGYNES AMONG MAMMALS?

Susumu Ohno

Department of Biology, City of Hope National Medical
Center, Duarte, California 91010

It is a curious fact that man through the ages appears to
have been fascinated by the idea of finding a creature who is made
of the right half of a man and the left half of a woman fused into
one. In medieval drawings and paintings, such a creature was
called an androgyne (Fig. 1). Although, on rare occasions, lateral true hermaphrodites do occur -- having an ovary and Müllerian-
duct derivatives on one side, and a testis and Wolffian-duct derivatives on the other -- such a vertical midline split is confined
strictly to the "innards." There is no left-right asymmetry in
their external sexual development. Their circulating testosterone
levels uniformly determine the extent of masculine manifestation;
e.g., beard growth, penis size, etc. While their circulating
estradiol levels control the extent of postpubertal feminine manifestation; e.g., breast fullness, hip roundness, etc. In mammals,
XX and XY cells are equally responsive to testosterone and estradiol. Thus, depiction of the androgyne as only a figment of wildly
unrealistic imagination illustrates that, in truth, there is total
hormonal dependence of the mammalian secondary sex-determining
mechanism. Furthermore, even with regard to the primary (gonadal)
sex-determining mechanism, XX and XY gonadal cells are not irreversibly committed to their respective organogenetic destinies.
Accordingly, XX// XY mosaic or chimaeric gonads seldom develop into
ovotestes. Instead, they most often organize testes, or, occasionally, ovaries.

By contrast, androgynes, there known as gynandromorphs, do
occur among those insects in which a sex-determining mechanism
based on male heterogamety operates (and where XO is male). A nondisjunctional event occurring in an early cleavage division of the

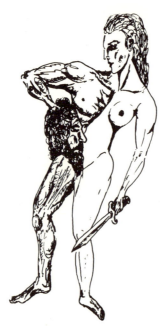

FIGURE 1. My own version of androgyny. The drawings and paintings
    in existence include one attributed to Pliny the Elder (62—
    113 A.D.).

XX zygote produces an XX// XO mosaic. One half of the body, populated by XX cells, manifests the feminine phenotype, whereas the
other half, populated by XO cells, assumes the appearance of a
male. In insects, sexual type resides within each individual cell
as its intrinsic, irreversible property. Even the sexual behav-
iours of an insect appear to be determined by the sex-chromosome
constitution of neurons in relevant regions (Whiting 1932; Hotta
and Benzer 1976).

     In this paper, I shall examine hormonal mechanisms with
regard to both the primary (gonadal) and secondary (extragonadal)
sex-determining mechanisms of mammals, which enables XX// XY mosaic
or chimaeric individuals to develop either as males or as females,
each one more or less normal.

DEVELOPMENTAL STRATEGY OF COMPETITIVE DISPLACEMENTS

AND THE FATE OF XX// XY GONADS

No biological system can be error free, and embryonic organogenesis is no exception. Natural selection must have included, as
part of the mammalian embryonic plan, various accommodations to
either negate or minimize the effects of these mishaps. Accidental
mix-ups between differently committed cells are bound to occur at
territorial boundaries during the process of organogenesis. What
if the diverticulum of a primitive gut destined to be liver, acci-
dentally incorporated a number of stray cells that had already made
an initial commitment to be intestinal cells? Purely autonomous
organogenesis by irreversibly committed individual cells would have
produced an island of intestinal structure in the midst of liver.
The very fact that such a mosaic organ is seldom, if ever, seen
indicates the existence of a developmental strategy that avoids the
formation of mosaic organs. The study of the fate of XX// XY mosaic
or chimaeric gonads has revealed the nature of this developmental
strategy and has shown it to be based on the principle of competitive displacements.

Random fusions of two blastocysts should be producing XX ↔ XY
sex-chromosome chimaeras 50% of the time. Were XX and XY gonadal
cells to follow their own inherent organogenetic dictates, the
overall sex ratio of chimeric mice should be 1:1:2 for XX ↔ XX
females, XY ↔ XY males, and XX ↔ XY true hermaphrodites, respectively. The fact is that true hermaphrodites seldom occur among
chimeric mice. My literature survey revealed that of 550 chimeras
described, only eight were hermaphrodites: an incidence of 1.4%.
A curious dichotomy in reported sex ratios cannot, however, be ig-
nored. When the data reported by Tarkowski, McLaren, and their
respective colleagues were combined, I found the sex distribution
to be 9 females (16.7%), 41 males (75.9%), and 4 true hermaphrodites (7.4%). In sharp contrast, the combined data reported by
Mintz and Gardner gave a nearly one-to-one sex ratio; 200 females,
192 males, and only 4 true hermaphrodites. The above discrepancy
is mainly due to a difference in strain combinations used.* The
first group, of Tarkowski and McLaren, used two genetically very
similar or compatible strains for their blastocyst aggregations.
For example, Tarkowski regularly used two congenic strains that
differed from each other only with regard to T6 marker chromosomes
and a coat color gene. The second group, of Mintz and Gardner, on
the other hand, customarily used genetically distant strain combinations. Whitten (1975), among others, has pointed out that in
strain combinations such as B10 ↔ BALB, one cell line being more
vigorous tends to outgrow the other, thus producing so-called

_____

* See also Mullen & Whitten (1971), J. exp. Zool. 178: 165-176 (ed.)

unbalanced chimeras. Under these circumstances, it is not surprising that XX ↔ XY chimeras always develop the sex of the dominant cell line. For example, if the cells of strain A tend to outgrow the cells of strain B, XX(A) ↔ XY(B) chimaeras would develop as females, whereas XX(B) ↔ XY(A) chimaeras would develop as males, thus leading to an overall sex ratio of 1:1 among chimaeras of the A ↔ B strain combination. Inasmuch as naturally occurring XO// XY or XX// XY heterosexual mosaics usually develop from the XY zygote, the XO or XX cell line, being a derivative, is genetically identical to the ancestral XY line except for the absence of the Y. It follows than that the finding of the first group of chimeras is more relevant than that of the second group to our understanding of the fate of naturally occurring heterosexually mosaic gonads. It appears that heterosexual gonads made of a nearly one-to-one mixture of XX and XY cells most often organize testes, less often ovaries, and rather infrequently ovotestes. Here I should point out that, as far as the laboratory mouse is concerned, a majority of true hermaphrodites (66.9%) belong to the type that has a testis on one side and an ovary on the other, whereas the type having a pair of ovotestes is the rarest (5.2%), as summarized by Whitten (1975).* In man, however, the situation is somewhat different: the type having a testis or an ovary on one side and an ovotestis on the other appears to be most common (Polani 1970).

I have proposed the XY-to-XX transfer of H-Y antigen as the reason for testicular differentiation of XX// XY mosaic or chimeric gonads. By saturating the plasma membrane sites of neighbouring XX cells with disseminated H-Y antigen, XY cells manage to entice XX cells in the same gonad to cooperate in the act of testicular organization (Ohno 1976). An ample amount of H-Y antigen found in exceptionally virilized testis-like fetal bovine freemartin gonads that were essentially made of XX cells confirmed the postulated transfer of H-Y antigen to XX gonadal cells (Ohno, Christian, Wachtel, and Koo 1976). However, in the case of bovine freemartinism, there exists an uncertainty as to the source of gonadal H-Y antigen (Ohno 1978). For this reason, we felt the need to study chimeric mice whose testes were roughly a one-to-one mixture of XX and XY cells. While such testes are less likely to be found among XX ↔ XY chimeric males of genetically distant strain combinations, such combinations nevertheless enable us to exploit allelic differences at H-2 and at certain enzyme loci as tools to assess XX : XY ratios of various cell types.

Accordingly, we have chosen the BALB/c ↔ C3H combination. All chimeric males produced in the laboratory of Dr. J. Melnyk of this institution were progeny tested by mating them to *albino* BALB/c females. XX primordial germ cells in the testicular environment

---

* See also paper by Beamer *et al.*, these Proceedings.

are incapable of undergoing neonatal differentiation to become
definitive spermatogonia. Accordingly, they become extinct at
that stage. For this reason, XX ↔ XY chimeric males of our strain
combination, if they were fertile, sired only either all *agouti*
or all *albino* progeny when mated to *albino* BALB/c females. Needless to say, *agouti* progeny were derived from a C3H-XY germ line,
and *albino* progeny from a BALB/c-XY germ line. Of several XX ↔
XY chimeric males, so identified by the progeny test, most revealed
a great preponderance of XY cells in all parts of their bodies as
expected. They were of little use.

Fortunately, one XX(BALB/c) ↔ XY(C3H) male, while producing
39 *agouti* (18 males and 21 females) and no *albino* progeny, demonstrated more white than colored patches in his coat. Subsequent
analysis indeed revealed the presence of 50% or more BALB/c(XX)
cells in every somatic type examined. The XX : XY ratios in his
spleen and tail epidermal cells were determined by cytotoxicity
tests using anti-H-2^d antibody directed against BALB/c(XX) cells,
and anti-H-2^k antibody directed against C3H(XY) cells. Testicular
cells were first fractionated into germ cells and somatic elements
by successive treatments with collagenase and then trypsin in two
concentrations. While germ cells, comprising 90% of more of the
total, were exclusively of the C3H(XY) line, as expected from the
progeny test, the starch-gel electrophoretic study of glucosephosphate isomerase revealed the XX : XY ratio among Sertoli and Leydig
cells to be 1 : 1. H-Y absorption tests performed on the various
cell types revealed no evidence of the XY-to-XX transfer of H-Y
antigen among spleen and epidermal cells. This negative finding
is relevant in interpreting the H-Y antigen expression reported
on essentially XX cell populations of peripheral blood leukocytes
and cultured fibroblasts of one human XX male who actually was an
XX//XXY mosaic (Wachtel, Koo, Breg, Thaler *et al*. 1976). It may
be that the XY-to-XX transfer of H-Y antigen among extragonadal
somatic elements can occur only if the two cell lines involved are
MHC (major histocompatibility) compatible. This is almost certainly the case with naturally occurring human sex-chromosome mosaics,
as already noted.

The situation found in the testicular Sertoli and Leydig cells
of this balanced XX(BALB/c) ↔ XY(C3H) chimeric male mouse was very
different from that found in his spleen and epidermal cells. In
spite of the fact that half of these testicular cells were
XX(BALB/c), the H-Y antibody absorption capacity shown by them
actually surpassed that of normal males of either parental strain.
Thus, the reason that XX gonadal cells in a mosaic or chimeric
gonad are often enticed to participate in testicular organogenesis
can now be attributed to the XY-to-XX transfer of H-Y antigen. A
more detailed description of this most informative XX ↔ XY chimeric male mouse has been given elsewhere (Ohno, Ciccarese, Nagai,

and Wachtel 1978). Because of the neonatal elimination of XX germ
cells from the XX ↔ XY testis, we were unable to witness the XY-
to-XX transfer of H-Y on germ cells of this sexually mature
XX(BALB/c) ↔ XY(C3H) male. Were we to have studied him at the
fetal stage, I am reasonably certain that H-Y antigen would have
also been found on the plasma membrane of XX primordial germ cells.
It is worth remembering that differentiation from primordial germ
cells to much smaller definitive spermatogonia invariably occurs
neonatally (Roosen-Runge 1964).

     Although less frequent than XX ↔ XY males, XX ↔ XY chimeric
female mice have also been identified. When fertile, they may ovu-
late XY oocytes (Evans, Ford, and Lyon 1977). It would appear that
the reverse competitive displacement of testis-organizing H-Y antigen with a yet-to-be-identified ovary-organizing antigen can occur
on the plasma membrane of XY gonadal cells. However, the absence
of H-Y antigen on the plasma membrane of XY ovarian cells, germline
and soma alike this time, is technically hard, if not impossible,
to prove by H-Y antibody absorption tests. Mouse ovaries are simply too small to supply the large number of cells (40 to 80 x 10^6)
required for proof of the absence of H-Y antibody absorption capacity. Nevertheless, it may be recalled that, in the absence of H-Y
antigen, XY gonadal cells of fertile XY wood-lemming females readily organized a functional ovary (Fredga, Gropp, Winking, and
Frank 1976; Wachtel, Koo, Ohno, Gropp *et al.* 1976). Furthermore,
in *in vitro* reaggregation experiments, testicular Sertoli cells
lysostripped of their H-Y antigen behaved as though they were now
ovarian follicular cells (Ohno, Nagai, and Ciccarese 1978; Zenzes,
Wolf, Gunther, and Engel 1978), as schematically shown in Figure 2.

     The study on the XX(BALB/c) ↔ XY(C3H) chimeric mouse testes
indeed provided strong supportive evidence for the notion that competitive displacements of one organogenesis-directing antigen with
another on the plasma membrane of engaged cells is the developmental strategy that mammals employ to avoid the formation of mosaic
organs (Fig. 3). The reason that an XX ↔ XY gonad shows a far
greater tendency to develop as a testis than as an ovary is rather
self evident. Both, nature's experiment witnessed in the wood
lemming, and *in vitro* reaggregation experiments performed on newborn mouse and rat testicular cells, have shown that XY gonadal
cells, too, have the inherent inclination to organize an ovary,
and that it is the H-Y antigen that prevents this inclination from
manifesting itself. Thus, it is likely that the production of a
yet-to-be-identified ovary-organizing antigen is constitutive in
both sexes. It follows, then, that during the process of normal
testicular organogenesis, XY gonadal cells have the need to dis-
place their own ovary-organizing plasma membrane antigen with disseminated H-Y antigen. Quite obviously, this physiological need
to disseminate testis-organizing H-Y antigen during the normal

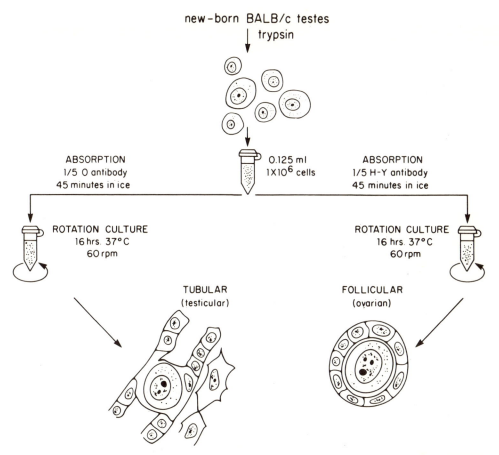

FIGURE 2. Moscona-type *in vitro* reaggregation experiment performed
on dissociated XY gonadal cells from newborn BALB/c mouse testis. These cells, lysostripped of H-Y antigen, reorganized
in vitro to yield ovarian follicle-like aggregates (right);
whereas the same cells, allowed to retain H-Y antigen, readily reorganized seminiferous tubule-like aggregates.

course of testicular organogenesis give XY gonadal cells a decisive
advantage over XX gonadal cells when the two confront each other
in the XX// XY mosaic or chimeric gonad.

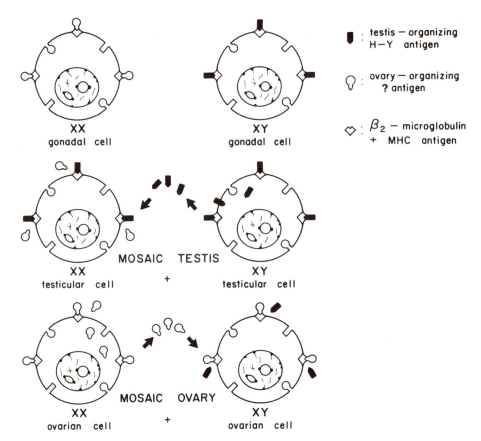

FIGURE 3. The developmental strategy of competitive displacements
            that avoids the formation of ovotestes by XX∥XY mosaic or
            chimeric gonads is schematically illustrated. Most often,
            testis-organizing H-Y antigen disseminated by XY gonadal
            cells, manages to dislodge a yet-to-be-defined ovary-organiz-
            ing antigen from the plasma membrane of neighbouring XX
            gonadal cells and to occupy the vacated sites (middle row).
            In this manner, XY gonadal cells entice XX gonadal cells to
            engage in testicular organogenesis. The XY to XX transfer of
            H-Y antigen has actually been observed among Sertoli and Ley-
            dig cells of XX(BALB)∥XY(C3H) chimeric mouse testes (Ohno,
            Ciccarese, Nagai, and Wachtel 1978).

            Less often, testis-organizing H-Y antigen on the plasma mem-
            brane of XY gonadal cells is dislodged and replaced by an
            ovary-organizing antigen disseminated by neighbouring XX go-
            nadal cells (bottom row). In this rare event, XX∥XY gonads
            develop as functional ovaries. The developmental strategy of
            competitive displacements is made operative only because these

SEX-CHROMOSOME CONSTITUTIONS ARE IRRELEVANT TO SECONDARY

SEX DETERMINATION

At the time of embryonic development, when the fate of the gonads is about to be determined, mammalian embryos of both sexes are equipped with a pair of parallel ducts on each side which open into the cloaca: the Wolffian (mesonephric) duct system and the Müllerian (paramesonephric) duct system. Subsequent development of Müllerian ducts into Fallopian tubes, uterus, and vagina, and of the urogenital sinus and external genitalia into vaginal vestibule, clitoris, and labia minora and majora, are intrinsically programmed developmental processes that require no inducer. Complete regression of the Wolffian ducts is also an intrinsic process, and its prevention requires active intervention. Indeed, the basic mammalian embryonic plan is inherently feminine with regard to secondary sex determination as well. Accordingly, male embryos castrated at an appropriately early stage follow the intrinsic developmental pathway outlined and acquire feminine secondary sex characters (Jost 1947a). Immediately following castration of male embryos, if they are continuously exposed to exogenously supplied testosterone by daily treatments of their mother, not only these castrated males but also their sisters acquire male secondary sexual features. Wolffian ducts develop into epididymides, ducti deferentia, seminal vesicles, and ejaculatory ducts; while the urogenital sinus and external genitalia are masculinized to form prostates, scrotum, and penis (Jost 1947b). In this manner, it has been established that the survival and differentiation of Wolffian ducts, and the masculinization of the urogenital sinus and external genitalia, are entirely androgen-dependent developmental processes, and that XX and XY cells are equally responsive to androgen.

The above testosterone treatment, however, does not cause the regression of Müllerian ducts -- either in castrated males or in intact females. Quite obviously, the fetal testis secretes another factor that has the single function of causing regression of the Müllerian ducts. This factor has now been identified as the anti-Müllerian hormone, which is thought to be a rather large peptide synthesized by testicular Sertoli cells (Josso, Picard, and Tran 1977).

In rodents, but not in man, testosterone-induced masculine differentiation includes severance of the connection between the

---

two opposing organogenesis-directing antigens utilize an identical set of plasma-membrane anchorage sites. I have assigned this anchorage function to β_2-microglobulin-H-2 or HLA antigen dimers (Ohno 1977).

nipple and underlying mammary glands. As a result, male nipples become far less conspicuous than female ones (Raynaud 1947).

FETAL SYNTHESIS OF TESTOSTERONE, AND THE TWO MEANS

OF ITS DELIVERY TO TARGETS

Inasmuch as the mammalian embryonic plan is inherently feminine, the fetal testis has to function as an endocrine organ almost immediately following completion of its organogenesis; and it has to keep playing this role for a considerable period, until the forced regression of Müllerian ducts, as well as the induced masculine development of the urogenital sinus and external genitalia, have been completed. While the extremely short gestation period of laboratory mice and rats hinders the identification of this period of intense endocrine activity by the fetal testis, such a period is readily definable in larger mammalian species with long gestation periods, such as man. The newly-emerged human testis of gestational day 56 already contains over 4 ng testosterone/mg tissue, the intratesticular testosterone concentration reaching a peak of 5 ng on day 84. The circulating testosterone level reaches its peak of 3.0 ng/ml on about day 112, returning to the characteristically low level of less than 0.5 ng/ml roughly on day 168 (Reyes, Boroditsky, Winter, and Faiman 1974). Indeed, for a period of nearly two months, starting from day 84, circulating testosterone levels of male fetuses approach the low normal testosterone level of adult human males. It is no coincidence that this period of nearly two months corresponds to that during which the urogenital sinus and external genitalia remain amenable to testosterone-induced masculine differentiation. On the other hand, the androgen-sensitive period of Wolffian ducts, during which testosterone can prevent their regression by inducing masculine differentiation, is considerably shorter and occurs earlier, coinciding with the peak in intratesticular testosterone concentration (day 84). We have proposed that the masculine development of Wolffian ducts of male fetuses is not due to circulating testosterone, but is due exclusively to testosterone secreted directly from the adjacent testis into the lumen and the immediate surroundings of the Wolffian duct (Ohno, Dofuku, and Tettenborn 1971). As already noted, human true lateral hermaphrodites characteristically show Wolffian duct development on the side that has the testis, and Müllerian duct development on the side that has the ovary. It would appear that the anti-Müllerian hormone produced by the fetal testis also acts by this direct route.

EVEN *TFM/+*; *SXR/+* MALE MICE DO NOT BECOME ANDROGYNES

The X-linked testicular feminization (*Tfm*) mutation of the mouse (Lyon and Hawkes 1970), apparently by specifying a defective nuclear-cytosol androgen receptor, renders all the target-cell types of affected individuals totally nonresponsive to androgen (Ohno 1976). Furthermore, being X linked, the *Tfm* locus is subject to the X-inactivation process (Lyon 1961). Hence, the body of *Tfm/+* heterozygotes consists of androgen-responsive wild-type (*+*) cells and nonresponsive mutant (*Tfm*) cells. An autosomal dominant gene, *Sxr* (Cattanach, Pollard, and Hawkes 1971), can give testes -- and therefore a source of androgen -- to these *Tfm/+* heterozygotes. My last hope of creating androgynes rested on these sex-reversed *Tfm/+ Sxr/+* male mice. Indeed, we often obtained a beautiful vertical midline split with regard to *Blo/+* coat color (Fig. 4), *Blo* being coupled with *Tfm* on the same X. Even these animals, however, have shown the all-or-none phenomenon of their nipple development. Most often, all five pairs of nipples were conspicuously feminine in type. Occasionally, however, we did observe all male-type nipples (Drews, Blecher, Owen, and Ohno 1974). Of several hundred male mice of the above genotype that we have examined, not a single individual has been observed that has a complete vertical split with regard to nipple development. Needless to say, all the extragonadal male reproductive organs were subnormal to varying degrees in these *Tfm/+; Sxr/+* males. However, two peculiarities were noted: (1) the inconspicuousness of left-right asymmetries; (2) the absence of independence in clonal composition of different organs -- i.e., if epididymides were extremely underdeveloped, so were seminal vesicles, etc. (Drews *et al.* 1974). In short, androgynes were not observed among *Tfm/+; Sxr/+* male mice. The reason became rather obvious. Fetal testosterone induction of Wolffian-duct and urogenital-sinus derivatives is due to the androgen responsiveness of underlying mesenchymal cells. Accordingly, the clonal compositions of epithelial elements are totally irrelevant.

THE FETAL TARGETS OF TESTOSTERONE ARE MESENCHYMAL CELLS

The important role that the underlying mesenchyme plays in organogenesis has long been emphasized by Grobstein (1967). The testosterone dependence of masculine differentiation of the mouse urogenital sinus has been explored by Cunha (1973). A fetal heterotypic recombinant made of 12th-day snout dermis mesenchyme and 15th-day urogenital sinus epithelium, when grown in the anterior eye chamber of adult males, produced epithelial keratinization, suggesting that, in the absence of androgen-responsive mesenchyme, the urogenital-sinus epithelium differentiated as an ordinary epidermis. In sharp contrast, the recombinant, composed of 16th-day

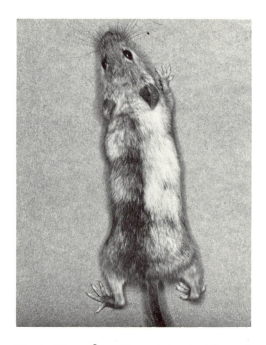

FIGURE 4. *Tfm + Blo/+ Ta +* ♀. The right half of her body was
entirely *Blo* hemizygous. As judged by the expression of the
coat-color gene *Blo*, which was in coupling with *Tfm* on the
same X chromosome, her right half was effectively *Tfm*-mono-
clonal, whereas the left half was roughly a 1 : 1 mixture of
the *+* and *Tfm* clones. Yet, when this type was found among
sex-reversed *Tfm + Blo/+ Ta +; Sxr/+* males, no left-right
asymmetry was noted with regard to nipple formation, male
genital ducts, gland development, and androgen sensitivity of
the kidney.

seminal vesicle mesenchyme and 12th-day snout skin epithelium produced single and branched epithelial tubules, suggesting that the
androgen-responsive mesenchyme was able to entice ordinary skin
epidermal cells to differentiate as though they were seminal-vesi-
cle epithelial cells. By combining the technique of heteroplastic
recombinations with that of organ culture in the presence of androgens, Kratochwil and Schwartz (1976) proved that mesenchymal cells
are entirely responsible for the testosterone-induced severance of
the connection between the nipple and the underlying mammary gland.
The combination of *Tfm*/Y epidermal cells of the nipple-forming area
with *+*/Y or *+*/*+* mesenchymal cells of the corresponding area responded to androgens and yielded an inconspicuous masculine nipple.

However, the converse combination proved totally androgen resistant
and proceeded to develop the conspicuous feminine nipple and underlying mammary glands.

The notion of fetal masculine differentiation being determined
by mesenchymal androgen responsiveness found further support in an
observation made on sex-reversed *Tfm/+; Sxr/+* mosaic males. One of
the more striking findings was that the androgen-nonresponsive *Tfm*
cells of the Wolffian ducts, which should have perished during
early fetal development, were actually found in good numbers among
epididymal epithelial cells of these mosaic males (Drews *et al.*
1974). This was obviously due to metabolic cooperation with neighbouring androgen-responsive (+) cells. The fact that as many as
500 *Tfm*-type epithelial cells may constitute a local clone effectively ruled out the possibility of the metabolic help coming from
adjacent +-type epithelial cells for the simple reason of distance.
It had to be a sufficient number of +-type fibroblasts in the underlying mesenchyme that were sustaining the survival of the *Tfm*-type
epithelial cells. Subsequently, Drews and Drews (1975) indeed
showed that in response to administered androgens, these *Tfm*-type
epithelial cells of the epididymis divided as often as did the
adjacent +-type epithelial cells, and that this was the sole reason
for their persistence to early adulthood in spite of continuous
death among them. Figure 5 illustrates this point. There remains
little doubt that mitotic stimuli to epithelial cells of the
Wolffian duct and most likely also of the urogenital sinus, so

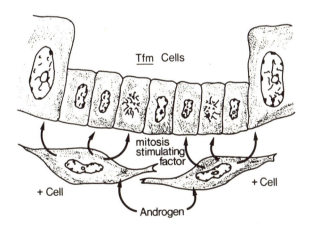

FIGURE 5.   Schematic illustration of the metabolic cooperation
       between androgen-responsive +-mesenchymal cells and androgen-
       nonresponsive *Tfm*-epithelial cells observed in the epididy-
       mides of sex-reversed *Tfm/+; Sxr/+* males.

essential to the fetal masculine differentiation of these structures, are supplied by androgen-responsive mesenchymal cells.   It
would appear that, as far as mesenchymal cells are concerned, there
occurs no left-right asymmetry in clonal compositions with regard
to +-cells and *Tfm*-cells.

CONCLUSIONS

1)   In mammals, in contrast to insects, the sex-chromosome
constitution of extragonadal cells is totally irrelevant to their
sexual development.   This is because, XX and XY cells are equally
responsive to the masculinizing influence of testosterone, as the
testosterone-induced masculine differentiation is mediated through
underlying mesenchymal cells and not through epithelial elements
of the fetal target organs.   Even *Tfm/+; Sxr/+* male mice failed to
demonstrate the left-right asymmetry in sexual development.   Androgynes do not exist in mammals.

2)   Even with regard to the primary (gonadal) sex-determining
mechanism, the fate of XX// XY mosaic gonads tends to be determined
collectively by a hormone-like function of testis-organizing H-Y
antigen disseminated by XY gonadal cells, and able to entice
neighbouring XX gonadal cells to differentiate into testicular Sertoli and Leydig cells.

REFERENCES

Cattanach, B. M., C. E. Pollard and S. G. Hawkes.   1971.   Sex-
reversed mice: XX and XO males.   Cytogenetics 10: 318-327.

Cunha, R.   1972.   Tissue interactions between epithelium and mesenchyme of urogenital and integumental origin.   Anat. Rec. 172: 529-
542.

Drews, U., S. R. Blecher, D. A. Owen and S. Ohno.   1974.   Genetically directed preferential X-activation seen in mice.   Cell 1:
3-8.

Drews, U. and U. Drews.   1975.   Metabolic cooperation between *Tfm*
and wild-type cells in mosaic mice after induction of DNA synthesis.   Cell 6: 475-479.

Evans, E. P., C. E. Ford and M. F. Lyon.   1977.   Direct evidence
of the capacity of XY germ cells in the mouse to become an oöcyte.
Nature 267: 430-431.

Fredga, K., A. Gropp, H. Winking and F. Frank. 1976. Fertile XX-
and XY-type females in the wood lemming (*Myopus schisticolor*).
Nature <u>261</u>: 255-257.

Grobstein, C. 1967. Mechanism of organogenetic tissue interaction. Nat. Cancer Inst. Monogr. <u>26</u>: 279-299.

Hotta, Y. and S. Benzer. 1976. Courtship in *Drosophila* mosaics
and sex-specific foci for sequential behavior pattern. Proc. Nat.
Acad. Sci. USA <u>73</u>: 4154-4158.

Josso, N., J. Y. Picard and D. Tran. 1977. The anti-Müllerian
hormone. In (R. J. Blandau and D. Bergsma, eds.) Morphogenesis
and Malformation of the Genital System, National Foundation Original Article Series, Vol. 8, pp. 59-84. Alan R. Liss, Inc., New
York.

Jost, A. 1947a. Sur les effets de la castration précoce de l'embryon mâle de lapin. C. R. Soc. Biol. (Paris) <u>141</u>: 126-219.

Jost, A. 1947b. Action de la testostérone sur l'embryon male
castré de lapin. C. R. Soc. Biol. (Paris) <u>141</u>: 275-276.

Kratochwil, K. and P. Schwartz. 1976. Tissue interaction in androgen response of embryonic mammary rudiment of mouse: Identification of target tissue for testosterone. Proc. Nat. Acad. Sci.
USA <u>173</u>: 4041-4044.

Lyon, M. F. 1961. Gene action in the X-chromosome of the mouse
(*Mus musculus L.*). Nature <u>190</u>: 372-373.

Lyon, M. F. and S. G. Hawkes. 1970. An X-linked gene for testicular feminization of the mouse. Nature <u>227</u>: 1217-1219.

Ohno, S. 1976. Major regulatory genes for mammalian sexual
development. Cell <u>7</u>: 315-321.

Ohno, S. 1977. The original function of MHC antigens as the general plasma membrane anchorage sites of organogenesis-directing
proteins. Immunol. Rev. <u>33</u>: 59-69.

Ohno, S. 1978. <u>Major sex determining genes</u>. Springer-Verlag,
Berlin-Heidelberg-New York.

Ohno, S., R. Dofuku and U. Tettenborn. 1971. More about X-linked
testicular feminization of the mouse as a noninducible (i^S) mutation of a regulatory locus: 5α-androstan-3α-17β-diol as the true
inducer of kidney alcohol dehydrogenase and β-glucuronidase.
Clin. Genet. <u>2</u>: 128-140.

Ohno, S., L. C. Christian, S. S. Wachtel and G. C. Koo. 1976. Hormone-like role of H-Y antigen in bovine freemartin gonad. Nature 261: 597–598.

Ohno, S., Y. Nagai and S. Ciccarese. 1978. Testicular cells lysostripped of H-Y antigen organize ovarian follicle-like appearance. Cytogenet. Cell Genet. 20: 351–364.

Ohno, S., S. Ciccarese, Y. Nagai and S. S. Wachtel. 1978. H-Y antigen in testes of XX (BALB)/XY (C3H) chimaeric male mouse. Arch. Androl. 1: 103–109.

Polani, P. E. 1970. Hormonal and clinical aspects of hermaphroditism and the testicular feminization syndrome in man. Phil. Trans. Roy. Soc. Lond. B 259: 187–204.

Rayaud, A. 1947. Effet des injections d'hormones sexuelles á la souris gravide, sur le développment des ébauches de la glande mammaire des embryons. I. Action des substances androgénes. Ann. Endocrinol. 8: 248–253.

Reyes, F. I., R. C. Boroditsky, J. S. D. Winter and C. Faiman. 1974. Studies on human sexual development. II. Fetal and maternal serum gonadotropin and sex steroid concentrations. J. Clin. Endocrinol. Metab. 38: 612–617.

Roosen-Runge, E. C. 1964. Primordial germ cells and the spermatogonia. In: Congenital Malformation, p. 32, International Medical Congress, New York.

Wachtel, S. S., G. C. Koo, W. R. Breg, H. T. Thaler, G. M. Dillarad, I. M. Rosenthal, H. Dosik, P. S. Gerald, P. Saenger, M. New, E. Lieber and O. J. Miller. 1976. Serological detection of a Y-linked gene in XX males and XX true hermaphrodites. New England J. Med. 295: 750–754.

Wachtel, S. S., G. C. Koo, S. Ohno, A. Gropp, V. G. Del, R. Tantravahi, D. A. Miller and O. J. Miller. 1976. H-Y antigen and the origin of XY female wood lemmings (Myopus schisticolor). Nature 264: 638–639.

Whiting, P. W. 1932. Reproductive reactions of sex mosaics of a parasitic wasp, Habrobracon inglandis. J. Comp. Psychol. 14: 345–346.

Whitten, W. K. 1975. Chromosomal basis for hermaphroditism in mice. In The Developmental Biology of Reproduction, 33rd Symp. of the Society for Developmental Biology. Academic Press, New York.

Zenzes, M. T., U. Wolf, E. Günther and W. Engel. 1978. Studies on the function of H-Y antigen: Dissociation and reorganization experiments on rat gonadal tissue. Cytogenet. Cell Genet. 20: 365-372.

CELL INTERACTIONS IN THE SEX ORGANS OF SEX REVERSED MICE HETERO-ZYGOUS FOR TESTICULAR FEMINIZATION

Ulrich Drews

Anatomisches Institut der Universität Tübingen,
D-7400 Tübingen, West Germany

ORIGIN OF THE MOSAIC MICE

The X-linked mutation for testicular feminization (*Tfm*) described by Lyon and Hawkes (1970) causes androgen insensitivity of the testosterone target cells. The molecular basis of the phenotype is a defect of the androgen receptor protein (Attardi and Ohno, 1974; Gehring and Tomkins, 1974). Due to random X inactivation, XX mice heterozygous for *Tfm* are mosaics with respect to androgen sensitivity. They can be converted to males by the autosomal dominant mutation for "sex reversal" (*Sxr*) described by Cattanach, Pollard, and Hawkes (1971). By imitating the Y-chromosome, *Sxr* induces formation of testes in XX embryos. The testosterone produced by the embryonic testes in turn induces formation of male sex organs. In sex-reversed embryos heterozygous for *Tfm*, testosterone encounters a mixed population of androgen-insensitive and androgen-sensitive cells. In the androgen-insensitive cells the X chromosome bearing *Tfm* is active. The *Tfm* cells express the defective receptor protein and therefore are constitutively bound to form female organs. In the androgen-sensitive cells the wild-type X is active. The wild-type cells therefore express an intact androgen receptor protein. They respond to testosterone and are bound to form male sex organs. Depending on the quantitative representation of the two cell types, mice with an intersexual genital tract develop (Drews et al., 1974; Drews, 1975a). They range from males with hypospadia and minor asymmetries of prostate lobes and vesicular glands to heavily feminized animals with a sinus vagina and only rudimentary male sex organs. As in other sex-reversed XX males, the testes are devoid of germ cells. The Leydig-cell function is however not impaired.

183

GENERAL EXPRESSION OF THE MOSAIC CONDITION

Although, due to variation in the X-inactivation pattern, each
of the mosaic animals is unique, a general principle is nevertheless discernible. Figure 1 shows schematically the intersexual
genital tract in animals with a high contribution of *Tfm* cells.
Figure 4 gives an example of such a genital tract dissected out
from the animal as seen in dorsal view. As indicated in Figure 1,
three levels of expression of the mosaic can be distinguished.
Before dealing with more detailed aspects, the three levels will be
briefly characterized.

At the upper level, the Wolffian and the Müllerian ducts are
originally present. During embryonic life the Müllerian duct
regresses. Under the action of testosterone the Wolffian duct is

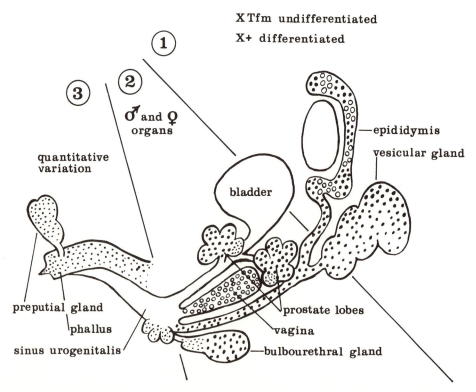

FIGURE 1.   Schematic representation of the three levels along the
     genital tract with different expressions of the mosaic
     (Drews, 1975a).

transformed into epididymis, deferent duct, and vesicular gland.
In the epididymis the original mosaic of *Tfm* and wild-type cells
is preserved and is still directly visible in the adult animal.
The *Tfm* cells form patches of undifferentiated epithelium between
regularly differentiated, high columnar wild-type cells (Fig. 2).
The presence of *Tfm* cells in the epididymis is a constant finding
in all mosaic animals, although the absolute amount varies with the
degree of feminization and decreases with age. Deferent ducts and
vesicular glands usually contain no *Tfm* cells. An originally high
contribution of *Tfm* cells is indicated by short ducts and small
irregular size of the vesicular glands (Fig. 4).

The middle level (Fig. 1) comprises the derivatives of the
urogenital sinus. In the male the indifferent urogenital sinus
forms the urethra, with prostate lobes and bulbo-urethral glands.
In the female it forms urethra and vagina. In the mosaics with
high contribution of *Tfm* cells, a mixture of male and female
organs develops. The male organs are represented by small and
distorted prostate lobes and relatively well developed bulbo-
urethral glands. In a number of cases they contain contributions
of indifferent urethral gland lobules formed by *Tfm* cells (see
"mixed glands" below). The female organ is a blindly ending sinus
vagina which keeps the deferent ducts from opening into the urethra
at their regular site below the bladder (Figs. 1, 4, and 5). Instead, the ducts run down behind the vagina to the diverticulum of
the bulbus penis where they finally join the urethra together with
the vagina.

The lowest level is represented by the external genitals.
Here, the indifferent state is normally transformed into the male
phenotype by growth of the phallus and closure of the sinus to a
penile urethra, or into the female phenotype by development of a
separate vaginal outlet. In the mosaics a range of intersexual
external genitals is produced solely by variations in phallus size
and extent of hypospadia. The final outcome is always symmetrical
and appears quite orderly, but is, of course, nonfunctional for
reproduction.

DETAILED FEATURES OF MOSAICISM

Epididymal mosaic

During development of the Wolffian duct into an epididymis,
testosterone induces cellular differentiation in the wild-type
cells. As in the normal male, they form epididymal epithelial
cells with definite excretory and resorptive functions. By contrast the *Tfm* cells remain undifferentiated (Drews and Alonso-
Lozano, 1974). However, although the *Tfm* cells cannot respond to

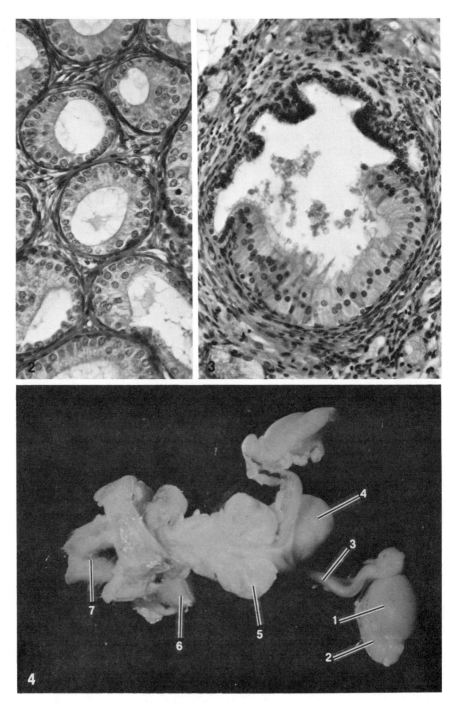

FIGURES 2, 3&4

←*FIGURE 2.* Mosaic of *Tfm* and wild-type cells in the epididymal duct.

←*FIGURE 3.* Patch of undifferentiated *Tfm* cells in the deferent
        duct. Note the irregular structure of connective tissue
        beneath *Tfm* cells. (Drews and Dieterich 1978).

←*FIGURE 4.* Whole genital tract dissected out from a mosaic animal.
        Dorsal view, 8 x. Constituent parts indicated by numbers, as
        follows: 1, testis; 2, epididymis; 3, deferent duct; 4,
        bladder; 5, vesicular gland; 6, bulbo-urethral gland; 7,
        phallus with broad opening of urogenital sinus.

testosterone, they survive in the mosaic environment. This is primarily not what one would expect, since in the *Tfm*/Y mouse the
Wolffian ducts regress as in the female.

We conclude that for induction of differentiation the intact
androgen protein is required in the respective cell. On the other
hand, the trophic effect of testosterone is mediated from the wild-
type cells to the *Tfm* cells. In line with this notion, we have been
able to demonstrate that in the epididymis of juvenile mosaic mice
the stimulus for DNA-synthesis is mediated from the wild-type to the
Tfm cells. After a single dose of testosterone, followed by [3]H-
thymidine, the labeling index went up in both cell types to the
same extent (Drews and Drews, 1975).

The following observations indicate, however, that mediation
of the trophic effect of testosterone is far from being perfect:
the mosaic epididymis is smaller than the epididymis of sex-reversed
males without *Tfm*; there are fewer *Tfm* cells than expected from
random X-inactivation; in the deferent duct, usually no *Tfm* cells
are present, the case shown in Fig. 3 being a rare exception. We
therefore studied cell death in the mosaic epididymis in more detail
(Drews and Dieterich 1978). It turned out that, in the adult
animal, a steady loss of *Tfm* cells takes place. Cell death is,
however, not restricted to the *Tfm* cell population but is also
enhanced in wild-type cells and in the connective tissue. If adult
mosaic mice are castrated or injected by cyproterone acetate, the
epididymis reacts not only by involution as in the sex reversed
controls, but also by massive necroses in the epithelium and in the
underlying connective tissue. Again, both *Tfm* and wild-type sections are involved. Two or three weeks after castration the necro-
tic lesions have disappeared. At their sites, abnormal sprouts and
outpocketings of the epididymal duct are left behind. Close inspection shows that the necroses in the mosaic are accompanied by pre-
existing or newly arising disorganized sections in the wall layers
of the epididymal duct.

We conclude from these observations that the trophic effect of
testosterone is mediated by the connective tissue component. In

line with this assumption is the observation that preservation or
loss of *Tfm* cells in the Wolffian duct are correlated with the
duct's definitive structural organisation in the adult. In the
convoluted epididymal duct, intermingling and exchange of cells
between the wall layers of *Tfm* and wild-type sections is possible,
allowing the *Tfm* cells in the epithelium to survive, but also ren-
dering the wild-type cells sensitive to necrosis. By contrast,
in the straight deferent duct, secondary contacts between adjacent
duct sections are not formed. The *Tfm* cells usually die off. If,
as shown in Fig. 3, a remaining *Tfm* section is encountered in a
young animal, the defective structure of the wall underneath the
Tfm cells is particularly evident when compared with the structure
in the epididymis (Fig. 2).

During destruction of the mammary gland anlagen of the male
mouse embryo by testosterone, the mesenchyme plays a comparable
mediating role. By *in vitro* recombination of epithelial buds and
respective mesenchyme from *Tfm* and wild-type mammary gland anlagen
Kratochwil and Schwartz (1976) and we (Drews and Drews, 1977)
demonstrated that testosterone acts via the mesenchyme. We were
motivated for these experiments by the observation that in our sex-
reversed *Tfm* heterozygotes all ten nipples were always present.
The presence of some *Tfm* cells must therefore suffice to neutralize
the destructive influence of testosterone on the whole mammary
gland anlage.

Mixed glands

In the epithelium of the embryonic urogenital sinus, testosterone normally induces the outgrowth of prostate lobes and bulbo-
urethral glands. In the adult male, these glands produce secre-
tions which, together with the content of the vesicular glands,
form the vaginal plug after copulation. They are homologous to
the small urethral glands in the submucous coat of the male and
female urethra. In the mosaic mice, the male glands sometimes also
contain some lobules of indifferent urethral glands. An example is
the prostate lobe shown in Fig. 5. Obviously, these urethral gland
lobules are formed by *Tfm* cells being unable to differentiate into
prostate epithelium. They must have joined the wild-type cells
which, under the regimen of testosterone, formed the outgrowth of
the respective prostate bud during fetal life. The *Tfm* moiety in
turn influences the shape and location of the whole prostate lobe.
The mixed prostate lobe has no stalk and is broadly fixed to the
wall of urethra and vagina. In the bulbo-urethral gland we encountered one mixed gland, the proximal rectangular half of which was
made up from urethral glands only. On the other hand, several
bulbo-urethral glands were observed from which polypous tissue
masses were expelled, presumably representing *Tfm* cells (Drews,

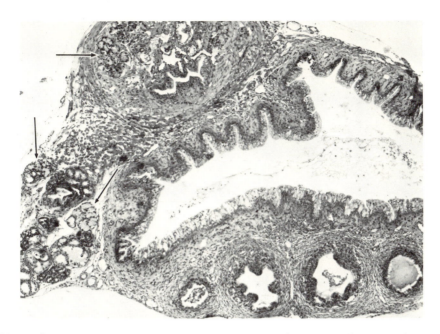

FIGURE 5. Cross section through urogenital tract of a mosaic mouse.
Broad vagina between urethra and Wolffian ducts, accompanied
laterally by the excretory ducts of the vesicular glands.
Urethral glands (arrow) in front of the urethra and in a mixed
prostate lobe. 63 x (Drews, 1975a).

1975a). It follows from these observations that the stimulus for
the outgrowth of testosterone-dependent glands can be mediated from
the wild-type to the *Tfm* cells. The final mixed gland is a unique
compromise between the morphogenetic properties of the male and the
indifferent urethral gland component.

Formation of the sinus vagina

The lower part of the vagina stems from the urogenital sinus
and is present in *Tfm*/Y animals. In the male its formation is prevented by testosterone. In heavily feminized mosaic animals, a
sinus vagina is also formed. However, instead of opening to the
outer surface, it joins the urethra together with the deferent ducts
at the level of the penile bulb (compare Figs. 1, 4, and 5). The
course of the deferent ducts behind the vagina is, on first glance,
hard to explain. It is, however, also known in the human female
where remnants of the Wolffian ducts may be present as Gartner's
ducts or cysts in a similar position. Ectopic ureters also often

take a similar course. The malformations are better understood if the normal morphogenetic processes involved in the formation of the vagina are considered.

Morphogenetic processes can be visualized by means of the histochemical cholinesterase reaction. In earlier studies we have shown that, in general, morphogenetic movements in the embryo are marked by cholinesterase activity (Drews, 1975b). Fig. 6 shows a sagittal cryostat section through a *Tfm*/Y embryo stained for cholinesterase. Intense enzyme activity is present in mesenchymal cells at the dorsal wall of the urogenital sinus where separation of the vaginal anlage is under way. In horizontal sections, the cholinesterase activity extends laterally around the vaginal anlage and is also present in the epithelial cells at the level where vagina and urethra separate. In the indifferent stage of the genital tract, the mesenchymal cholinesterase activity is located immediately beneath the junction of Wolffian and Müllerian ducts with the sinus. In the case of male development, the active mesenchyme

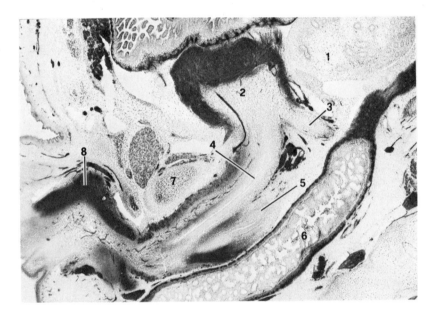

FIGURE 6. Sagittal cryostat section through *Tfm*/Y embryo on day 17 of pregnancy. Histochemical cholinesterase reaction after Karnovsky and Roots. Note cholinesterase activity in the mesenchyme of the urogenital sinus during formation of the vagina. Key to numbers: 1, testis; 2, bladder; 3, ureter; 4, urethra; 5, vagina; 6, rectum; 7, symphysis; 8, corpus cavernosum penis (intense activity).

forms a cap into which the buds of the vesicular glands grow out.
In female and *Tfm*/Y embryos, it moves down at the dorsal and lateral
wall of the sinus while the vagina is formed concomitantly. Going
back to the mosaics, we assume that after the wild-type cells in
the mesenchyme have initiated vesicular-gland formation, leftover
Tfm cells start with the demarcation of the vagina. Thereby the
process of demarcation and elongation also involves Wolffian ducts
and vesicular glands. The ducts of the vesicular glands may then
be separated from the Wolffian ducts as in the case shown in Fig.
5. In some of our mosaics, the separation of the Wolffian ducts
and their elongation to the penile bulb had occurred even without
formation of a vagina. For initiation of the male or female alternative of mesenchymal behavior, a critical number of wild-type
or *Tfm* cells is presumably required.

CONCLUSIONS

The effect of testosterone as embryonic inducer and trophic
hormone of the male sex organs depends on an intact cytoplasmic
receptor protein. If the hormone encounters a mixture of cells,
some with intact and some with defective receptor proteins, its
action is primarily restricted to cells with intact receptor. As
shown in the mosaics, this is in particular true for cellular differentiation of the epididymal epithelial cells, and of the secre-
tory cells in the vesicular glands, the prostate, and the bulbo-
urethral glands. On the other hand, the detailed analysis of
mosaics has shown that other effects such as stimulation of proliferation, induction of morphogenetic processes, and the trophic
effects of the hormone can be mediated from the wild-type to the
defective *Tfm* cells. The cellular interactions inferred from these
observations work only over very short distances. Epitheliomesen-
chymal interactions have been proved to be involved. Communication
through gap junctions or local hormones, such as chalones, are other
possible mechanisms.

The efficiency of regulation by cellular interactions is particularly evident in the expression of the mosaic in the external
genitals. At this level of the genital tract, no difference in
terms of cellular differentiation exists between male and female.
All actions of testosterone belong to the category of mediated
effects. By cellular interactions, the random mosaic is transformed into orderly anatomical structures representing a quantitative variation between male and female phenotype. Varying amounts
of *Tfm* cells therefore affect male development in the same way as
does lack of testosterone or administration of antiandrogens during
the sensitive period of development, as described by Neumann et al.,
1970.

It is known that the subunits of the cytoplasmic receptor protein finally function as regulatory proteins on the chromatin. In this respect the *Tfm* cells in the mosaic cannot be supplemented by the wild-type cells. In analogy, one may infer that the malignancy of teratocarcinoma cells which can be cured by passage through embryonic development, is not due to a structural defect of a regulatory protein but to a defect in one of the communicable functions (see Illmensee, this volume).

The work presented was supported by the Deutsche Forschungsgemeinschaft (SFB 87 and SFB 88).

REFERENCES

Attardi, B. and S. Ohno. 1974. Cytosol androgen receptor from kidney of normal and testicular feminized (Tfm) mice. Cell 2: 205-212.

Cattanach, B. M., C. E. Pollard and S. G. Hawkes. 1971. Sex-reversed mice: XX and XO males. Cytogenetics 10: 318-337.

Drews, U. 1975a. Direct and mediated effects of testosterone: The development of intersexes in sex reversed mosaic mice, heterozygous for testicular feminization. Anat. Embryol. 146: 325-340.

Drews, U. 1975b. Cholinesterase in embryonic development. Progr. Histochem. Cytochem. Vol. 7, No. 3. Stuttgart: Gustav Fischer Verlag.

Drews, U. and V. Alonso-Lozano. 1974. X-inactivation pattern in the epididymis of sex reversed mice heterozygous for testicular feminization. J. Embryol. exp. Morph. 32: 217-225.

Drews, U., St. R. Blecher, D. A. Owen and S. Ohno. 1974. Genetically directed preferential X-activation seen in mice. Cell 1: 3-8.

Drews, U. and H. J. Dieterich. 1978. Cell death in the mosaic epididymis of sex reversed mice, heterozygous for testicular feminization. Anat. Embryol. 152: 193-203.

Drews, U. and U. Drews. 1975. Metabolic cooperation between Tfm and wild-type cells in mosaic mice after induction of DNA synthesis. Cell 6: 475-479.

Drews, U. and U. Drews. 1977. Regression of mouse mammary gland
anlagen in recombinants of Tfm and wild-type tissues: testosterone
acts via the mesenchyme. Cell 10: 401-404.

Gehring, U. and G. M. Tomkins. 1974. Characterization of a hormone receptor defect in the androgen-insensitivity mutant. Cell 3:
59-64.

Illmensee, Karl. 1978. Reversion of malignancy and normalized
differentiation of teratocarcinoma cells in chimeric mice. In,
Genetic Mosaics and Chimeras in Mammals, Liane B. Russell, Ed.
Plenum Press, New York and London.

Kratochwil, K. and P. Schwartz. 1976. Tissue interaction in androgen response of embryonic mammary rudiment of mouse: identification of target tissue for testosterone. Proc. Nat. Acad. Sci.
USA 73: 4041-4044.

Lyon, M. F. and S. G. Hawkes. 1970. X-linked gene for testicular
feminization in the mouse. Nature 227: 1217-1219.

Neumann, F., R. von Berswordt-Wallrabe, W. Elger, H. Steinbeck,
J. D. Hahn and M. Kramer. 1970. Aspects of androgen-dependent
events as studied by antiandrogens. Recent Progr. Horm. Res. 26:
337.

SPONTANEOUS SEX MOSAICISM IN BALB/cWt MICE

W. G. Beamer, W. K. Whitten and E. M. Eicher

The Jackson Laboratory, Bar Harbor, Maine 04609

HISTORICAL PERSPECTIVES

The spontaneous appearance of an individual with somatic and gonadal characters typical of both sexes is rather rare, but not unknown, among men and mice. Such individuals have been labeled intersexes, hermaphrodites, or gynandromorphs, depending upon the investigator's emphasis. In the following discussion of BALB/cWt strain mice, we have adopted the term hermaphrodite because of its general usage vis-a-vis phenotypic morphology. However, we do not wish to imply that connotations associated with intersex or gynandromorph are unacceptable.

In 1956, Hollander, Gowan, and Stadler published their observations on 25 adult hermaphrodites in BALB/cGw mice. The hermaphrodites, derived from both control and experimental populations in an X-irradiation experiment, appeared with an overall incidence of approximately 0.3%. The authors suggested that, while the variety of reproductive-tract elements found within hermaphrodites represented hormonal control problems, the composition of the gonads themselves reflected chromosome differences. Nearly two decades later, Whitten (1975) reported observations on approximately 100 hermaphrodites in the inbred strain BALB/cSnGnSnRrDgWt (hereafter BALB/cWt) mice maintained by him at the Jackson Laboratory. Additional characteristics of this colony were low numbers of weaned male offspring (often as low as 38% of the total weaned), and some indications for the presence of XO females within the colony. Results of chromosome counts in suitably prepared bone-marrow cells of adult hermaphrodites implied chromosomal mosaicism. From the available data, Whitten hypothesized that nondisjunctional events were responsible for the generation of BALB/cWt hermaphrodites.

195

Hollander *et al.* (1956) suggested that BALB/c mice might be unique with respect to hermaphroditism. Support for that idea was derived from unpublished cases (cited in Hollander *et al.*) of Dr. M. C. Green's of two hermaphrodites in the BALB/cSnGn, the progenitor stock of the BALB/cWt subline. Further evidence comes from the discovery, among approximately 4000 young BALB/cJ males, of two hermaphrodites that were subsequently confirmed, histologically, by Dr. L. C. Stevens (personal communication). Finally, although no hermaphrodites have been found to date in the BALB/cBy subline, a significant depression in number of males was found during studies of 14–15 day fetal gonads (370 ♀♀, 291 ♂♂, χ^2 = 9.44). It is possible to reconstruct the chronological history of and relationships among at least 18 sublines of BALB/c mice. The four sublines referred to above can be traced to the original Bagg albino strain inbred by McDowell (Staats 1972), as demonstrated by Bailey (1978). Thus, it would seem that there indeed may be something unique about BALB/c sublines and disturbances in sex differentiation.

BALB/cWt MICE

Before delving into our studies of hermaphroditism in BALB/cWt mice, the reader is directed to the basic features of the subline that are presented in Table 1. During the time period of July 1976 to March 1977, 201 14–17 day pregnant BALB/cWt females were killed

TABLE 1. Sex distribution of offspring in BALB/cWt mice

	♀♀	♂♂	♂♀/♀♂
Fetuses,*	814	582	43
14–17 days	(56.6)[†]	(40.4)	(3.0)
			P < 0.01
Weanlings,	1919	1377	14
21–28 days	(58.0)	(41.6)	(0.4)

*243 resorptions were found in the fetal examinations.

[†]Numbers in parentheses are percentages of total offspring.

by cervical dislocation and the fetuses removed for further study.
Fetal gonads were dissected out, placed in a drop of phosphate-
buffered saline, and the gonadal sex identification made under 25x
with a dissection microscope. A total of 1439 live fetuses and
243 resorbing embryos were recorded. The number of male fetuses
represented 40.4% of the total live fetuses examined — significantly less than the expected proportion of 50% males (χ^2 = 52.5,
p <.01). The resorptions averaged 1.21/litter. Forty-three offspring (3.0% of total live fetuses) were identified

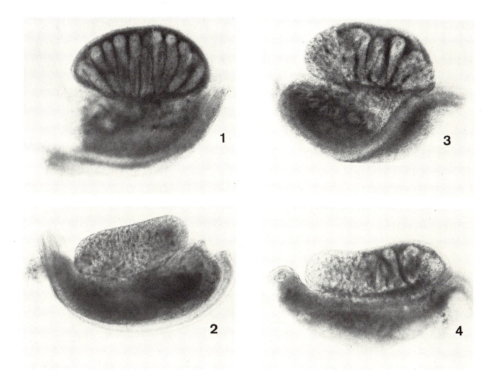

FIGURES 1-4. Photomicrographs of gonads from 15-day fetal BALB/cWt
    mice.
    1. Normal testis with 10 seminiferous tubules. Note promi-
    nent, dark testicular capsule.
    2. Normal ovary. Gonad is granular in appearance, smaller
    in size, and without a prominent capsule.
    3. Ovotestis with all or portions of four seminiferous
    tubules equatorially located and ovarian tissue at both gon-
    adal poles. Note absence of capsule over ovarian region.
    4. Ovotestis with all or portions of 3 tubules equatorially
    located, ovarian tissue at the cranial pole, and a disorgan-
    ized tubule at the caudal pole.

as hermaphrodites by the presence of both male and female gonadal tissue within the same fetus (see Fig. 1—4). Colony weanling data revealed a comparable picture with respect to a deficiency of males, but the proportion of hermaphrodites was significantly less (χ^2 = 19.1, p <.01). We presume that a majority of the hermaphrodites are not identified at weaning because they have developed as phenotypically normal males or females and thus are overlooked. Although exact records on losses between birth and weaning were not kept, our impressions are that the number of missing offspring was not substantial.

In Table 2, we have summarized the gonadal classification from 108 F_1 and inbred BALB/cWt fetal hermaphrodites identified during the studies reported herein. The classification was made from hand drawings and photographs of the fresh specimens. We were impressed with the apparent ovotesticular organization. Ovarian tissue was most often located at the cranial pole or at both

TABLE 2. Classification of gonads in 108 fetal BALB/cWt hermaphrodites

Classification	Right gonad	Left gonad
Ovotestis		
Cranial pole only ovarian	44	31
Both poles ovarian	43	38
Caudal pole only ovarian	4	3
Equatorial zone ovarian	3	3
Normal gonad		
Ovary	5	12
Testis	5	12
Unclassified	4	9

Laterality	No. of mice
Lateral — Ovary, testis	2
Unilateral — Normal gonad, ovotestis	29
Bilateral — Ovotestis	68
One or both gonads unclassifiable	9

poles. The testicular tubules were almost always located in the
equatorial, or equatorial and caudal regions of the gonads. Ovarian tissue appeared in the equatorial region or caudal pole in
fewer than 7% of ovotestes. There was no significant tendency for
either left or right gonad to be either wholly ovarian or testicular in composition. Finally, the most frequent class of hermaphrodites observed was that of bilateral ovotestes.

The nonrandom organization of the ovotestes is intriguing.
We have considered such ideas as differential rates of migration
into the gonad of germ cells according to sex-chromosome composition to explain the ovotesticular organization. Alternatively,
those cells elaborating H-Y antigen for organizing testicular tubules may become functional in the center of the gonad first, and
at the poles slightly later. Such a time differential may allow
the rete to surround and separate individual germ cells (creating
ovary) and thus may prevent later-appearing H-Y antigen from
organizing tubules. Clearly, additional investigations are required to provide the explanation for the ovotestis organization.

The excess proportion of female offspring in BALB/cWt mice
could conceivably arise by (1) selective prenatal death of male
embryos, (2) generation of XO females from XY embryos following
loss of Y chromosomal material, or (3) the presence of unsuspected
XO females within the mating colony, which produce excess female
offspring. Selective prenatal death of male embryos is very difficult to evaluate. However, if one were to assume that all of the
observed 243 resorbing embryos were male and to add them to the 582
live male fetuses of Table 1, there would be no disparity in sex
distribution of the 14—17 day fetuses. This tidy conclusion becomes partly compromised by the results from genetic analysis of
the BALB/cWt females. Randomly selected BALB/cWt females were
mated to males hemizygous for the X-linked dominant gene, tabby
(Ta). Eleven of 63 BALB/cWt females (17%) produced Ta/O female
offspring. These data clearly show that the BALB/cWt colony contains XO females that in all probability arise both from XO dams
and from new generation via loss of Y chromosomal material from XY
embryos. This dual source seems essential, since the sex distribution of offspring in the BALB/cWt colony has remained the same
for over a decade.

                              GENETIC STUDIES

The consistently high incidence of hermaphroditism in BALB/cWt
allowed us to initiate genetic studies directed at understanding
this phenomenon. Whitten (1975) previously reported that matings
between SJL/Wt female and BALB/cWt male mice produced hermaphrodite
offspring, but the reciprocal matings did not. Hermaphrodites have

TABLE 3. Fetal sex distribution of F_1 offspring from BALB/cWt females mated to either BALB/cWt or SJL/Wt males consomic for the reciprocal Y chromosomes

	Gonad classification		
Genotype of sire	♀♀	♂♂	⚥⚥
C.SJL/Wt-Y N8	283 (53.2)*	249 (46.8)	0
SJL.C/Wt-Y N8	285 (53.3)	245 (46.0)	3[†] (0.6)

* % of total offspring

[†] In addition, 2 ♂♂ were identified in SJL.C/Wt N8

not been found in SJL/Wt inbred mice. Following the hint of male-related inheritance, we began the construction of consomic BALB/cWt and SJL/Wt mouse stocks with reciprocally exchanged Y chromosomes. Males from the eighth backcross generation of each strain were mated to BALB/cWt females and the 15-day-old fetal gonads examined as described earlier. The data in Table 3 show that the BALB/cWt strain males carrying the SJL/Wt Y chromosome (C.SJL/Wt-Y) did not sire F_1 hermaphrodites among more than 500 offspring, whereas the SJL/Wt strain males carrying the BALB/cWt Y chromosome (SJL.C/Wt-Y) sired three hermaphrodites. In addition, two SJL.C/Wt-Y N8 hermaphrodites were found, strengthening the suggestive evidence that the BALB/cWt Y chromosome is uniquely involved with the generation of hermaphroditism. Backcrossing of these incipient congenic lines to the appropriate inbred strains is continuing with the objective of more definitive studies when greater portions of the genomes have been made homozygous.

Since an embryo results from paternal and maternal genome interaction, we have studied the maternal genetic contribution to the potential for hermaphroditism. Outcrossing of BALB/cWt males to females from several different strains was carried out in search of F_1 combinations that would not yield fetal hermaphrodites. The results summarized in Table 4 make three points. First, there is a diverse range of inbred strains that permit the expression of hermaphroditism in F_1 offspring sired by BALB/cWt males. Second, the disturbed male sex ratio (% males) is not invariably associated with hermaphroditism. Third, the incidence of F_1 hermaphroditism

TABLE 4. Sex ratio and incidence of gonadal hermaphroditism in 14—15 day fetal offspring from hybrid matings with BALB/cWt males

Strain of dam	No. of fetuses	Sex ratio (% ♂♂)	No. of ♀♀	% ♀♀
A/HeJ	815	49	10	1.2
C3H/HeJ	650	47	0	0
C3HeB/FeJ	594	48	1	0.2
C57BL/6J	720	45*	0	0
C57BL/10Wt	627	50	0	0
SJL/Wt	552	41[†]	14	2.5
SWR/J	532	49	4	0.8

* Significantly different from 50.0 at .05 level.

[†] Significantly different from 50.0 at .01 level.

is variable but may be separable into two classes — relatively high (F_1's with strains A/HeJ, SJL/Wt, SWR/J), and low or non-detectable (F_1's with strains C3H/HeJ, C3HeB/FeJ, C57BL/6J, C57BL/10Wt). Such data lend credence to the idea of maternal factors associated with the expression of hermaphroditism, but do not distinguish between such diverse features as maternal environment or maternal genome contributed to oocytes.

The search for an explanation of the maternal influence was extended to females of the inbred strains C57BL/6By, BALB/cBy, and their 7 Recombinant Inbred (RI) strains (Bailey 1971). These RI strains, resulting from sister-brother matings derived from F_1 mice that originated from BALB/cBy x C57BL/6By crosses, represent unique recombinations of the original genomes. If the progenitor strains differ by a measurable characteristic, analyses of the RI strains for that characteristic can provide genetic evidence for single or multiple gene inheritance and, if the character is governed by a single gene, about the chromosomal location of that gene. The data collected, as of the date of this conference, although not complete, are presented in Table 5. The two progenitor strains,

TABLE 5. Sex ratio and hermaphrodite incidence in F_1 fetal offspring from BALB/cWt males mated to females of strains C57BL/6By,
BALB/cBy, and their 7 recombinant inbred (RI) strains

	Total	No. ♂♂	Sex ratio (% ♂♂)	No. ♀♀	Resorptions average (no. dams)
Progenitor strain					
C57BL/6By	595	297	50*	0	0.41 (74)
BALB/cBy	592	246	42[†]	14	1.35 (83)
RI strains					
CXBD	462	237	51*	3	0.56 (70)
CXBE	577	272	47*	5	0.46 (69)
CXBG	503	238	47*	2	0.78 (50)
CXBH	535	142	26	17	1.25 (61)
CXBI	400	156	39[†]	13	2.15 (99)
CXBJ	512	227	44[†]	5	1.23 (60)
CXBK	612	265	43[†]	1	0.81 (67)

* Values not significantly different from each other.

[†] Values not significantly different from each other but are so
from 50.0%.

when mated to BALB/cWt males, differed markedly with respect to
offspring sex ratio, expression of hermaphroditism, and average
number of embryonic resorptions per dam. The C57BL/6By females
produced normal numbers of fetal males, no hermaphrodites, and low
embryonic loss. On the other hand, the BALB/cBy females produced
a significant deficiency of fetal males, 14 hermaphrodites, and
an increase in embryonic loss. Since examination of offspring
from (BALB/cBy x C57BL/6By)F_1 females mated to BALB/cWt males has
yet to be completed, it is premature to speculate about recessive
or dominant characters. Nevertheless, the two progenitor strains
differed with respect to the tabulated phenomena, thus justifying
the use of RI strains for genetic analyses.

One can begin to appreciate the analytical complexity of the hermaphroditism phenomenon by inspecting the data from the RI strains in Table 5. For instance, the sex ratio of offspring from the seven RI strains mated to BALB/cWt males was found to be distributed into three classes: a normal sex ratio (strains CXBD, CXBE, and CXBG) similar to the parental C57BL/6By mice; a significant reduction in sex ratio (strains CXBI, CXBJ, and CXBK) similar to the parental BALB/cBy mice; and a very marked reduction in sex ratio (strain CXBH) that is clearly different from either progenitor strain. Again, it appears that a decline in sex ratio is not necessarily associated with hermaphroditism since all RI strains produce hermaphrodites. On the other hand, there is a consistently higher mean embryonic loss in those strains with a deficient male sex ratio than in those with a normal sex ratio. Since lowered viability has been demonstrated for XO females (Morris 1968), the failed embryos could be XO's that begin development as XY embryos. However, we now suspect there are XO females within the BALB/cBy strain (15-day fetal male sex ratio is 43%) and potentially within one or more RI strains. Thus, it is essential to know that dams mated to BALB/cWt males are XX females before attempting to evaluate the offspring sex ratios.

The actual incidence of hermaphroditism shown in the data of Table 5 appears to vary considerably. However, one could conclude that there may be a pattern of "low" incidence (strains CXBD, CXBE, CXBG, CSBJ, and CXBK) similar to the C57BL/6By data and "high" incidence (strains CXBH and CXBI) similar to the BALB/cBy. In a purely speculative vein, there may exist a low but significant tendency in most inbred strains for F_1 hermaphroditism if the BALB/cWt Y chromosome is present. The low incidence of hermaphroditism could then be markedly enhanced by a hypothetical gene, or genes, present in strains such as BALB/cWt, SJL/Wt, A/HeJ, and in BALB/cBy plus the RI strains CXBH and CXBI. Before experimentally pursuing ideas from such speculation on maternal genes enhancing hermaphrodite incidence, it will be prudent to develop the evidence regarding the effects of the maternal environment itself, as opposed to the genetic contribution to the embryo.

CHROMOSOME ANALYSES

The fundamental issue of hermaphrodite chromosome constitutions was approached by studying liver metaphases of BALB/cWt fetal hermaphrodites, along with those of normal male and female littermates. We anticipated that the hermaphrodites would be sex-chromosome mosaics, and since the entire fetal liver was utilized to obtain the metaphase chromosomes, the karyotype probably represented proliferating liver parenchyma, hemopoietic cells (extra hepatic in origin?), and perhaps other types of cells as well. Similarly, tissue of the fetal gonad also is derived from several sources, i.e., gonadal blastema from the genital ridge, gonadal rete from the mesonephros, coelomic epithelium of the gut cavity, and primordial germ cells from the embryonic yolk sac. Although we would not argue that the liver-chromosome data applied to any one population of cells within the liver or gonad, it is reasonable to assume that such data are indicative of the cell populations comprising the gonads or fetus in general.

A substantial number of BALB/cWt x BALB/cWt matings was made, and eventually 15 litters of gestational age 14—15 days were identified that contained one to two fetal hermaphrodites each, as determined by gonadal examination. The hermaphrodite gonads were photographed and fixed for subsequent histological analyses. The livers of the hermaphrodites and of nearby gonadally normal male and female littermates were separately processed by the technique of Eicher and Washburn (1978) for mitotic metaphase nuclei. Well spread, Giemsa-banded chromosomes were identified by low-power microscopic examination, and the number of chromosomes per metaphase was counted at 1000x. Table 6 contains a sample of the metaphase classes encountered in liver metaphase preparations. Two of the three hermaphrodites were XO/XY mosaics, while the third was XO/XY/XYY. Only cells bearing two X chromosomes were found in the gonadally normal female controls. The gonadally normal male

TABLE 6. Examples of karyotype data from 14—15 day BALB/cWt fetal liver preparations

Fetal no. and classification	(n)	XX		XO		XY		XYY	
		40	39	39	38	40	39	41	40
656.9 ⚥	(50)	0	0	33	3	12	2	0	0
656.8 ♀	(14)	13	1	0	0	0	0	0	0
656.10 ♂	(23)	0	0	0	0	23	0	0	0
1828.1 ⚥	(140)	0	0	110	0	30	0	0	0
1828.10 ⚥	(194)	0	0	99	0	64	4	25	2
1828.2 ♀	(63)	59	4	0	0	0	0	0	0
1828.6 ♂	(26)	0	0	13	1	12	0	0	0

controls were different from each other: the first contained only
XY cells, and the second contained both XO and XY cells.

The examples in Table 6 were quite typical, as may be inferred
from the summarized data of Table 7. Twenty fetal hermaphrodites
were found whose combined gonadal proportion of ovarian tissue
varied from approximately 5% to 95%, with a mean of 35%. Ten of
the twenty hermaphrodites were XO/XY mosaics, while the remaining
were XO/XY/XYY. The overall ratio of XO:XY cells was approximately
2:1, with the XYY clone in the minority at 6% of the total cells
counted. Fourteen of 15 female controls were XX; one female had
two of 29 cells that were 39 XO. The male controls were found to
fall into two groups: those with a normal cellular complement of
XY chromosomes, and those with both XO and XY or with XO, XY, and
XYY cells. In the mosaic male controls, the ratio of XO:XY cells
was approximately 1:2; essentially the reverse of the ratio found
in the hermaphrodites. The XYY clone was very small and present
in only two mosaic males.

Data on liver chromosomes of six F_1 fetal hermaphrodites were
gathered with the specific purpose of verifying the sex-chromosomal
mosaicism previously found in BALB/cWt fetuses. The data, summarized in Table 8, reveal the expected chromosome mosaicism, the relative paucity of XYY bearing clones, and the larger proportion of
the XO cells.

TABLE 7. Summary of gonad classification and sex-chromosome karyotypes in livers from 14–15 day BALB/cWt fetal mice

Classification	Mean % ovarian tissue	Total metaphases analyzed			
		XX	XO	XY	XYY
Hermaphrodites n = 20	35 (5–95)	1	1150	599	107
Females normal n = 14	100	398	0	0	0
mosaic (?) n = 1	100	27	2	0	0
Males normal n = 8	0	0	0	224	0
mosaic n = 7	0	0	113	211	3

TABLE 8. Summary of sex-chromosome karyotypes in livers from 14—15 day fetal F_1 offspring produced by matings with BALB/cWt males

Dam genotype	% Ovarian tissue	Karyotype			
		XX	XO	XY	XYY
A/HeJ	15	0	33	26	0
BALB/cByJ	15	0	51	21	0
SJL/Wt	10	0	36	13	1
SJL/Wt	10	0	74	23	1
SJL/Wt	5	0	23	54	0
SWR/J	35	0	23	12	8

The karyotype data for the 20 BALB/cWt hermaphrodites, summarized in Table 7, support the hypothesis that these unique mice arise from male embryos by nondisjunction of the Y chromosome. Since the XYY clone is considerably less frequent than either the XO or XY clones, there also appears to be a substantial probability for loss of Y chromosomal material associated with the nondisjunctional event(s). The proportion of female cells (XO) to male cells (XY and XYY) in the hermaphrodites demonstrates that the differentiation of gonads in the direction of ovaries is likely to occur when the number of XO cells exceeds XY and XYY cells. If the number of XO cells is less than that of XY and XYY cells, a gonadally normal, but sex-chromosomally mosaic male usually results. Although there were not spectacular numbers of metaphases to count in the male controls ($\bar{X} \pm SEM = 37 \pm 7$), about half of these animals possessed some female cells. This, of course, implies that at least half the BALB/cWt males are mosaics. This mosaicism could be even more extensive if, by chance, we simply did not recover XO clones from every "normal" male liver. It is worth noting that no XX/XY mosaic males or hermaphrodites were found, thus excluding from consideration for BALB/cWt mice the hypothesis of Mintz (1971) that spontaneous hermaphroditism results from aggregation of separate embryos following early shedding of zonas.

If one excludes reports on chimeric hermaphrodite mice, there are few papers on true hermaphrodite mice with accompanying chromosome data. Lyon (1969) reported on a sterile phenotypically

normal male that on dissection proved to be a true hermaphrodite.
Corneal mitoses were prepared and found to be XO and XY. Beechey
and Searle (1975) similarly found a true hermaphrodite mouse to
possess XO/XY mosaicism in corneal mitotic preparations. Sparse
as the literature is, the findings are compatible with those reported herein for BALB/cWt mice.

Of course, the cytogenetic data from true hermaphrodite human
beings are more complex, with major karyotype classes of 46 XX, 46
XY, and mixed sex chromosome constitutions. Both Jacobs (1969)
and Polani (1970) reported that the finding of 45 XO/46 XY mosaicism
among true hermaphrodites was not uncommon. Thus, the BALB/cWt
mouse, as a model of chromosomal nondisjunction associated with a
high frequency of true hermaphroditism, has relevance to a significant portion of human true hermaphroditism.

MECHANISMS OF MOSAICISM

Spirited discussion among the authors has centered on the timing, the mechanism(s), and the number of occurrences associated with
the aberrant cytogenetic events that yield the BALB/cWt mosaicism.
Whitten (1975) suggested that the first cleavage of the zygote was
most likely to be affected and to yield nondisjoined Y chromosomes
in the two-celled embryo (XO/XYY). The XYY clone would be unstable
and Y chromosome loss would occur progressively with time. An
alternative hypothesis is that there is a high probability of nondisjunction in several of the early cleavage divisions, and that
each nondisjunction has associated with it a high probability for
loss of Y-chromosomal material. A third hypothesis is that there
is very late replication of the Y, associated with subsequent loss
of Y-chromosomal material. Although, at present, there are no data
to eliminate these or other hypotheses, we believe that the high
frequency of mosaicism in BALB/cWt mice presents the opportunity to
study cytogenetic and genetic processes associated with chromosomal
nondisjunction and with developmental events resulting in intersex
individuals.

The authors wish to express their appreciation and thanks to
S. C. Carter, A. M. Cleary, L. J. Maltais, and L. L. Washburn for
their dedicated technical assistance in conducting these studies.
This work was supported by NIH grant numbers AM-17947, HD-04083,
and GM-20919.

The Jackson Laboratory is fully accredited by the American
Association for Accreditation of Laboratory Animal Care (AAALAC).

REFERENCES

Bailey, D. W. 1971. Recombinant-inbred strains: an aid to finding identity, linkage, and function of histocompatibility and other genes. Transplantation 11: 325-327.

Bailey, D. W. 1978. Sources of subline divergence and their relative importance for sublines of six major inbred strains of mice. Workshop on the Origins of Inbred Mice, held in Washington, D.C., February 1978. Ed. H. C. Morse, III.

Beechey, R. and A. Searle. 1975. Report of a hermaphrodite mosaic mouse. Private communication, Mouse News Letter 53: 31.

Eicher, E. M. and L. L. Washburn. 1978. Assignment of genes to regions of mouse chromosomes. Proc. Nat. Acad. Sci. 75: 946-950.

Hollander, W. F., J. W. Gowen and J. Stadler. 1956. A study of 25 gynandromorphic mice of the Bagg albino strain. Anat. Rec. 124: 223-239.

Jacobs, P. A. 1969. The chromosome basis of some types of intersexuality in man. J. Reprod. Fert. suppl. 7: 73-78.

Lyon, M. F. 1969. A true hermaphrodite mouse presumed to be an XO/XY mosaic. Cytogenetics 8: 327-331.

Mintz, B. 1971. Control of embryo implantation and survival. Adv. Biosci. 6: 317-340.

Morris, T. 1968. The XO and OY chromosome constitutions in the mouse. Genet. Res. 12: 125-137.

Polani, P. E. 1970. Hormonal and clinical aspects of hermaphroditism and the testicular feminizing syndrome in man. Phil. Trans. Roy. Soc. Lond. B 259: 187-204.

Staats, J. 1972. Standardized nomenclature for inbred strains of mice: fifth listing. Cancer Res. 32: 1609-1646.

Whitten, W. K. 1975. Chromosomal basis for hermaphroditism in mice. In 33rd Symp. Developmental Biology of Reproduction. Academic Press, New York.

EVIDENCE FROM MUTABLE GENES CONCERNING THE ORIGIN OF THE GERM LINE

A. G. Searle

Medical Research Council Radiobiology Unit, Harwell,
Didcot, Oxon. OX11 ORD, England

In recent years, studies on aggregation and injection chimaeras and on the genetic mosaics that result from X-chromosomal
inactivation have done a great deal to elucidate what goes on in
the early stages of mammalian development. Other kinds of genetic
mosaic, namely those arising through forward and reverse mutation
at particular loci, can also provide useful information. This is
particularly so because the initial mutational event in these
mosaics can occur at different stages in development, from the
first cleavage division on, and can therefore provide us with a
sort of running commentary on developmental processes; whereas the
initiating events with respect to X-chromosome inactivation and
the formation of chimeras are limited to very early stages in
embryogenesis. Another point which may be of importance is that
there would seem to be much less chance of preferential proliferation of one of the clonal components of such a mosaic than in most
chimeras. In these mosaics, the genetic difference between the
clones normally involves two viable alleles at a single locus controlling some aspect of coat colour. In chimeras, however, there
are usually many genetic differences between the components.

The potential value of these genetic mosaics was fully appre-
ciated by L. B. Russell (1964) when she wrote that their study
"constitutes a perfect meeting place for the fields of genetics
and developmental biology providing, as it does, interrelated information on mutability, cell lineage (including the special problems of cell lineage of the germ line) and the effect of genotype
on part of the organism versus the whole." In pioneer studies on
mosaicism in mammals, Russell (1964) analysed a series of coat-
colour mosaics which had arisen by forward mutation (probably all
spontaneously) in specific-locus experiments on mice (W. L. Russell

209

1951). In one group, both the coat and the gonads were involved, in another this was probably the case, while in a third group the gonad was mosaic but the coat not so, because the mutation was to a recessive condition in a homozygous wild type animal. Russell observed that, on average, about 50% of the gonad was affected and deduced that the initiating event was either mutation in one strand of a double-stranded gametic chromosome or at the first cleavage division. From the broadness of the observed distribution she also deduced that if the gonad primordium was set aside as a random assortment of n cells then n must be very small, "perhaps around 5". However, some of the progeny ratios differed significantly from expectation on this hypothesis, which suggested either that n was not constant, or that the idea of random assortment did not hold.

UNSTABLE GENES

Russell's specific-locus series is the only large group of mosaics that has been studied in mammals in which the mutations have been in normal stable genes. However, two unstable genes, which revert spontaneously to wild type, have also been worked on. These are $pearl$ (pe), a gene which dilutes coat colour, and $pink-eye\ unstable$ (p^{un}), in which the melanocytes produce very little eumelanin pigmentation and in which the eye loses virtually all its pigmentation.

Pearl

Russell and Major (1956) and Russell (1964) studied somatic reversions of pearl and concluded that these occurred either very early in embryonic life (probably at the first cleavage division) or fairly late (in 10-day embryos), with few if any at intermediate stages. All six examples of early reversion, with a high propor-tion (up to 100%) of the coat affected, showed gonadal involvement, although in two this was very slight and may actually have been the result of an independent mutation. In three of the remaining four, nearly half the progeny were wild type, which suggested that the germinal tissue was entirely +/pe. If these embryos were indeed a mixture of 50% +/pe and 50% pe/pe cells, then these breeding re-sults suggest that the primordial germ cells in mice are derived from a very small initial population.

Pink-eyed unstable: Previous work

The p^{un} allele of $pink-eyed\ dilution$ (p) in the mouse was first described by Wolfe (1963) with the symbol p'. It occurred

in the C57BL/6J inbred strain and was noteworthy for the sporadic
production, in the homozygote, of mice with mosaic coat-colour
patterns, in which some of the pigmentation had reverted from the
very pale pp phenotype on eumelanin to wild type (black on the
C57BL background). Eye colour was affected in a similar way, and
some mosaics produced wild-type progeny as well as pink-eyed dilute
ones, which showed that the gonads could also be mosaic.

Melvold (1971) reported that the proportion of coat affected
in mosaic p^{un} homozygotes tended to follow a bimodal distribution,
since it was generally either very small or quite large, with few
intermediate cases. He pointed out the striking similarity to the
distribution of pe reversions and concluded that the same embryonic
stages (2-cell and 10-day) as postulated by Russell seemed to be
involved. On this basis, Melvold calculated reversion rates at
the 2-cell and 10-day embryonic stages and concluded that the rate
was significantly lower at 10 days. He assumed that 200 melanoblasts were present at 10 days, on the basis of work by L. B.
Russell and Major (1957). He also reported that the reversion
rate was higher if the parents were heterozygous for p^{un} or were
somatically mosaic. The effect of heterozygosity suggested to him
that intragenic recombinational events might be involved in the
reversion phenomenon and that the choice of mosaic mice might result in selection for unstable alleles. However, genetic background per se also seems to affect the p^{un} reversion rate, since
Melvold (1972) found that this rate was much lower in p/p^{un} mice
on a hybrid 129/Re x C57BL/6 background than on an inbred C57BL/6
background.

Present studies with p^{un}

Our interest in p^{un} was stimulated by the search for a good
method of studying somatic mutation at the cellular level, since
the known high reversion rate would make it easier to develop a
suitable technique (Searle 1977). Besides keeping p^{un} on a *non-
agouti* background, we have also placed it on *non-agouti dilute
(a/a d/d)* and on *non-agouti piebald (a/a s/s)*. *Dilute* was used to
clump the revertant epidermal melanocytes (Markert and Silvers
1956) and thus make them more visible; while it was thought that
the presence of piebald might make the individual pigment areas
(Schaible and Gowen 1960; Mintz 1967) show up more clearly. This
has indeed proved to be the case (Fig. 1a, b, c). The externally
visible mosaics arising in our p^{un} breeding colony have been
recorded (with outline drawings showing the extent of the revertant
areas), and the most striking have been photographed. Some examples are given in Figure 1, to show the appearance of high-grade
mosaics (with gonadal involvement) in the presence and absence of
piebald, as well as of intermediate mosaics in which only one or

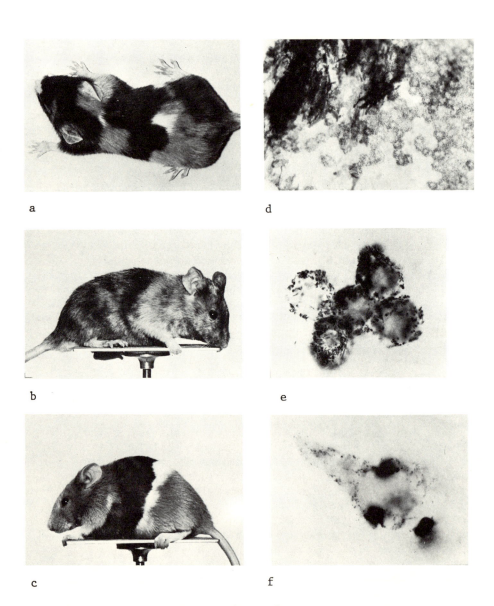

a

b

c

d

e

f

Figure 1

FIGURE 1.   Phenotypic effects of *pink-eyed unstable* (p^{un})
      (a)   High-grade coat-colour mosaic, homozygous for piebald (s).
      On this genetic background, the revertant (black) regions
      become more clearly defined, so that the individual pigment
      areas are revealed.
      (b)   High-grade mosaic without piebald.
      (c)   Intermediate-grade piebald mosaic, with only one pigment
      area affected.
      (d)   RPE and choroid of high-grade mosaic, showing revertant
      retinal and dendritic (choroidal) melanocytes.
      (e)   Small clone of revertant retinal melanocytes in retinal
      pigment epithelium (RPE).
      (f)   Hair follicle from mount of epidermis of young homozygote
      for dilute (d) and p^{un}, showing revertant melanocytes, clumped
      because of the effect of d.

two pigment areas are affected.   The proportion of the mosaic coat
which had the revertant phenotype was roughly estimated by eye and
by measurements of the size of revertant patches.

      Intermediate and high-grade mosaics, as well as some low-grade
ones, were mated to p^{un}/p^{un} or p/p stocks to check on gonadal involvement, which we have found only in high-grade mosaics.   Uni-
lateral testicular biopsies were performed on two male high-grade
mosaics, so that numbers of revertant and pink-eyed offspring could
be compared when both testes were present and when only one was
functional.

      Eyes of mosaic and non-mosaic p^{un}/p^{un} mice were fixed in 10%
formalin and cleared in benzyl alcohol, so that revertant retinal
melanocytes could be seen (Searle 1977) in the retinal pigment epithelium (RPE) as well as epidermal melanocytes in the choroid.
After removal of the lens and the sensory part of the retina, parts
of the RPE with adjacent choroid were mounted in Euparal for microscopic examination.   Areas of the epidermis of 2–3 day p^{un}/p^{un} mice
were also fixed, cleared, and mounted for microscopic study, because at this stage the epidermal melanocytes can be seen clearly
in the developing hair follicles.

Results

      In the non-mosaic p^{un} homozygotes, small clones of fully pig-
mented (and therefore revertant) melanocytes could be seen in both
the RPE and the epidermis.   Those in the RPE were clearest, since
they stood out against the almost completely pigment-free background (Fig. 1d) while there was still some residual background
pigment in the epidermis.   In the high-grade mosaics, large patches

of revertant retinal melanocytes (Fig. 1e), usually containing several hundred cells, could be seen extending from the iris region down towards the optic nerve. They were partially obscured by other large patches of choroidal melanocytes, immediately distinguishable by their prominent dendritic processes (Fig. 1e), except that in some eyes from piebald mice no choroidal pigment was found.

With the help of a Wild dissecting microscope, clones of revertant melanocytes were counted in the cleared eyes of five adult $a/a;p^{un}/p^{un}$ mice (three were also s/s; and the two others, d/d). It was interesting to note that the number of clones seemed higher in the s/s mice than in d/d, which supports Melvold's (1971, 1972) report of an influence of genetic background. The overall picture is shown in Table 1. The number of retinal melanocytes per eye was estimated from the number spanning a microscope field of known diameter, and from the average diameter of an adult mouse eye, with allowance made for the cornea and iris. This estimate (Table 1) is lower than that used previously (Searle 1977), in which the iris was included; but it is double the estimate of 4.2×10^4 for the RPE of adult mosaic mice, made by West (1976).

Table 1 shows that as the clone size increases the clone number decreases, as would be expected if the reversion rate per cell division was constant. Theoretically, one would expect a clone-size distribution close to the following, if synchrony of division is assumed: 16 of size 1, 8 of size 2, 4 of size 4, 2 of size 8, 1 of size 16. The observed distribution does not differ very markedly from this expected one. From these data, therefore, we can tentatively estimate the reversion rate per cell division to be about $16/4.4 \times 10^5 = 3.6 \times 10^{-5}$.

Similar clones of revertant dendritic melanocytes can be seen in the mounted epidermis of 2—3 day old p^{un} mice. The actual size of the clone can only be determined in *dilute* mice, in which the nucleopetal melanocytes are distinct (Fig. 1f). From these results it is clear that reversions also occur at stages later than day 10 of embryonic life, but are not visible to the naked eye.

TABLE 1. Distribution of clones of revertant melanocytes in ten RPE's of five non-mosaic p^{un}/p^{un} mice

	Number of clones of different sizes										Total revertants
	1	2	3	4	5	6	7	8	9	Total	
	13	10	3	4	1	2	0	0	1	34	84

Estimated no. melanocytes per eye = 8.8×10^4.
Thus reversion frequency = 10^{-4}.

TABLE 2. Frequency of high-grade mosaicism of coat in non-mosaic p^{un}/p^{un} intercross progeny

Series	No. > 30% dark	Total
Melvold (1971)	3	1618
Searle	3	1787

Frequency = 1.8×10^{-3}

It is interesting to contrast these frequencies for the latest cell divisions with those for the earliest cell divisions shown in Table 2. The three mosaics in Melvold's series were all estimated to have more than 60% of the coat affected, as was one in our series. The overall frequency of these high-grade mosaics is clearly higher than the reversion frequency during the final cell divisions. The pattern of pigmentation found in these high-grade mosaics (Fig. 1a, b) is very similar to that found in chimeras (as pointed out by Mintz 1974), and the individual pigment areas can be clearly seen in piebald mice. In our series, apart from one mosaic with about 15% of the coat affected, the rest of the recorded mosaicism (20 mice) involved 5% or less of the coat. No special effort was made to record all the very low-grade mosaics in our series.

For four of the higher-grade mosaics, the proportion of the coat affected was compared with the proportion of the RPE affected and thus showing normal pigmentation. The latter was rather

TABLE 3. Comparison of the extent of coat and retinal pigmentation in four p^{un}/p^{un} mosaics

Mating PUN/	Estimated percent reversion	
	Coat	RPE
123	70	60
57	45	45
124*	15	0
163*	15	30

*Gonads not affected

difficult to estimate in some eyes, where the revertant choroidal pigmentation tended to obscure the RPE. However, as Table 3 shows, there is fairly close correspondence between the two. This suggests a fairly late separation of the lineages leading to neural crest (and thus to epidermal melanocytes) and to optic cup (from which retinal melanocytes are derived).

Gonadal involvement

Analysis of gonosomal mosaics with respect to the amount of the coat and the gonads affected can help to throw light on the separation of the germ-line lineage. Table 4 is based partly on our own breeding records for individual p^{un} mosaics, but mainly on much additional information kindly supplied by Dr. Roger Melvold and Professor H. Glenn Wolfe. It should be remembered that even if 100% of the diploid germ cells have reverted from p^{un}/p^{un} to $+/p^{un}$ the mosaic concerned will still be expected to have 50% p^{un} progeny on crossing to p^{un}/p^{un}. Thus the percent $+/p^{un}$ in the gonads is obtained by doubling the percentage of offspring which are revertant, i.e. $+/p^{un}$. With the highest-grade mosaics (over 60% dark), the numbers of individuals at each end of the distribution (i.e., with all p^{un}/p^{un} or all $+/p^{un}$ germ cells) are of particular interest. It can be seen that, even if we discount the two entries based on rather few progeny, we are still left with a proportion of one quarter of the mosaics being at the extremes. The estimated percentages of $+/p^{un}$ germ cells in these three mosaics were 0, 95, and 118. With decreasing amounts of coat affected, the proportion of mosaics with gonadal involvement also decreases, as expected. It is interesting to note that in one mating, in which both parents were recorded as having less than 1% of the coat affected, three out of 14 offspring had a completely black coat (Melvold 1977). Apart from this exceptional mating, the least

TABLE 4. Gonadal involvement in different grades of p^{un}/p^{un} mosaics

Percent coat dark	Percent $+/p^{un}$ in gonads						Total analysed
	0	-20	-40	-60	-80	-100	
Over 60	2*	0	2	3	4	3†	14
30–60	3	0	1	2	1	0	7
Below 30	44	2	1	2	0	0	49

*1 based on 6 progeny only
†1 based on 11 progeny

amount of coat which was dark in the most affected parent of more
than one revertant offspring (actually 3/16) was estimated as 7.3%
(Melvold 1977). Those parents having only one black offspring were
discounted as this might have been the result of germinal mutation.

Only two black offspring were found in 3407 progeny from inter-
crosses of non-mosaic p^{un} homozygotes (Table 5). These were presumably the result of reversions in the germ line which could have
occurred either in a maternal or paternal germ cell. An alternative explanation would be that these were really high-grade mosaics
in which the lineage leading to coat pigmentation had by chance
started with only $+/p^{un}$ cells. Melvold (1977) found that three out
of twelve completely black offspring from high-grade mosaics bred
as if they had mosaicism of the germ line with respect to p^{un}.
However, neither of the two black offspring from Table 5 were progeny tested, so this point must remain in doubt.

Two mosaic males were allowed to mate with a number of p^{un}/p^{un}
or p/p females both before and after removal of the left testis.
As Table 6 shows, results were very different for the two mice.

TABLE 5.   Revertant offspring from p^{un}/p^{un} matings without coat-
colour mosaicism

Series	Phenotype		
	+	p^{un}	Total
Melvold (1971)	1	1618	1619
Searle	1	1787	1788

Reversion frequency = 2.9×10^{-4} per gamete

TABLE 6.   Progeny of high-grade mosaic p^{un} males before and after
removal of left testis

Mating PUN/		No. offspring with phenotype		Percent $+/p^{un}$ germ-cells	χ^2
		+	p^{un}		
57	Before	31	89	52	6.0
	After	15	16	97	
180	Before	27	48	72	<0.1
	After	34	61	72	

In the first one, there was a significant difference in the frequency of wild-type offspring before and after the operation; while
in the second one, the frequencies were remarkably alike. The
second male produced a high-grade mosaic among its progeny. A number of the wild-type offspring are being tested to see if they
really are mosaic.

DISCUSSION

Reversion frequency

Before considering the relevance of these results to the origin of the germ line, it seems desirable to consider when these
reversions take place. From her work on *pe* L. B. Russell (1964)
concluded that they "can occur either very early or moderately late
in embryonic development". The very early ones seemed to be at
the first cleavage division, while the late visible ones seemed to
have arisen on about the tenth day of embryonic life. The reversion frequency seemed about an order of magnitude higher in the
first cleavage stage than in 10-day embryos. Melvold (1971) also
reported that in p^{un} the reversion rate at the 2-cell stage was
significantly higher than at the 10-day stage by a factor of about
4. Thus the same embryonic stages seemed to be involved in this
reversion.

We have found small revertant clones of melanocytes in both
the epidermis and the RPE of postnatal p^{un} homozygotes, which shows
that reversion occurs at very late stages also. Therefore it seems
worthwhile to consider whether the p^{un} reversion frequency per cell
division could really be essentially the same from conception
throughout life, with the apparent peaks and troughs being the
result of what goes on in development. Recent studies have shown
that the embryo proper develops from part of the inner cell mass
(ICM) of the blastocyst, which is the product of the first six cell
divisions (Graham 1971). The ICM also goes to form the extraembryonic membranes. The number of ICM cells that contribute to
the embryo proper seems to be quite small. Mintz (1974) suggested
that it might be only 3, while Gardner's (1968) findings, that when
2—5 cells injected into blastocysts did lead to chimerism (in less
than 20% of cases) they made a substantial contribution to the
phenotype, also indicated that the number was low.

Let us assume that the embryo proper does indeed stem from
three ICM cells. If, in a p^{un} homozygote, one or more of these
three is the product of $p^{un} \rightarrow +$ reversion, then the initial lineage
of embryonic cells will be at least one-third $+/p^{un}$, and the resultant mouse would have quite a high probability of being a high-
grade mosaic with respect to coat colour. Any revertant cell in

the ICM might have arisen from reversion at any of the previous six cleavage divisions, not only the first. If the reversion rate per cell division is uniform and low, with the value r, then after six cleavage divisions the chance that a particular ICM cell contains a p^{un} reversion is about 6r. The chance that one or more out of a group of three cells is a revertant is theoretically about three times this, although much would depend on the extent of mixing. If r is approximately 3.6×10^{-5}, as estimated from clones in the RPE, then the frequency of these lineages with one-third or more revertant cells would thus be about 6.5×10^{-4}, one-third the frequency of high-grade mosaicism (Table 2). The discrepancy might be fully explained if there was another "bottleneck" some generations later in the lineage leading to neural-crest-derived melanocytes. This possibility is supported by Melvold's (1977) finding that three out of twelve completely black progeny of p^{un} mosaics bred as if they were mosaics. This suggests that the chance of picking n all-revertant cells out of a mixed lineage is quite high, presumably because n is small. On the other hand, if the bottleneck was too narrow, one would not expect the sort of reasonably close correspondence between the extent of coat and of germ-line mosaicism which is found.

If the high proportion of high-grade mosaics means that they can arise by reversion at any one of quite a large number of cell divisions, because of "bottlenecks," then the low proportion of intermediate-grade mosaics would imply that they are likely to arise at relatively few divisions. The fact that in neither of the two found in our colony (each with about 15% of the coat affected) was the germ line involved, while the germ line was usually involved in higher-grade mosaics, suggests that the reversions occurred shortly after separation of the ectodermal lineage leading to melanocytes from the others. In fact, from their appearance, they seem to arise just when the separate pigment areas are being established, i.e., on or before the 8th day of embryonic life according to Mintz (1967). If Mintz is correct in thinking that there are 34 separate pigment areas, 16 of which are on the tail, then about half the revertants at this time should merely have a small dark patch on the tail, which would probably not be counted as a coat mosaic and certainly not as an intermediate-grade one. This may also help to account for the sparseness of intermediate-grade mosaics.

With p^{un} reversion at successive stages of proliferation of melanoblasts within a particular pigment area, one would expect the appearance of dark patches of successively smaller size on the coat. Clearly a fairly large number of cell divisions would be concerned. Russell and Major (1957) estimated that the extremes of the range of spot size they found after irradiation of $10\frac{1}{4}$-day embryos were separated by six cell divisions. The range coming within the small but visible category of p^{un} revertants would be larger than this and would probably encompass at least ten cell divisions. Melvold's (1971) finding that the frequency of these small spots was nevertheless significantly lower than that of high-grade mosaics is another indication that, on the hypothesis of a constant reversion rate per cell division, it would have to be possible to generate high-grade coat mosaics over a large number of cell divisions. This would also seem to confirm the need for a bottleneck in the melanocyte lineage as well as that postulated in the ICM after six cell divisions.

It can be concluded, perhaps, that the idea of a constant reversion rate per cell division is not completely untenable but that much further work is needed before it can be tested properly. One particularly important subject for investigation is the relationship between the extent of reversion in mosaics as estimated from inspection of the coat and the actual proportion of all dendritic melanocytes which have the $+$ rather than the p^{un}. Cattanach and Isaacson (1967) found that scoring the coats of mosaic female mice heterozygous for Cattanach's translocation overestimated the true level of variegation for albinism by about 10—15%.

Germ-line initiation

No large clusters of wild-type progeny were found in matings of externally non-mosaic mice, in line with the general belief that the germ line is not separated off precociously but comes from the same population of totipotent cells as the rest of the embryo. One small cluster was found in a mating involving very low-grade mosaicism. This may have been the result of reversion shortly after separation of the germ line, leading to a fairly large clone of revertant germ cells. The actual reversion frequency in the germ line (Table 5) seems lower than would be expected on the basis of a constant reversion frequency per cell division. In fact, it remains possible that reversions do not occur in germ cells, since we cannot be certain that these two apparent germ-line reversions were not really mosaic.

The finding that about one quarter of all high-grade mosaics with respect to the coat appeared to have germ cells that were either all $+/p^{un}$ or all p^{un}/p^{un} (see Table 4 and text) supports the belief that the germ line is initiated from a very small number of embryonic cells. If the basic cell population was a random mixture of half p^{un} and half revertant cells, then, if a group of three cells was separated off, one would expect one quarter of the resultant organs to be all $+$ or all p^{un}. The actual situation is much more complex, of course, but our results do not seem to contradict L. B. Russell's (1964) estimate of "perhaps around 5" or Mintz's (1974) estimate of approximately 2—9 primordial germ cells.

The experiments on mosaic males, in which breeding results are
compared before and after removal of one testis, throw some light
on the time of separation of the germ-cell primordia going to right
and left genital ridges. The significant difference between pre-
and postoperative results found in one of the two males suggests
that the lateral separation occurs soon after the segregation of
the germ line itself, when the number of primordial germ cells is
still small. In fact, the results for the first males could be
explained if there were only two precursor cells, one of $+/p^{un}$
genotype going to the right testis and one of p^{un}/p^{un} genotype going to the left. However, the result for the second male would
seem to require a minimum of eight precursor cells, six $+/p^{un}$ and
two p^{un}/p^{un}.

Conclusions

The uncertainties involved in the present approach are obvious.
It is impossible to know the actual degree of p-locus mosaicism in
the totipotent embryonic cells of any individual; one can only infer
it from the extent of mosaicism in some derivatives. Moreover, the
actual expectations after separation of lineages will depend on the
extent of cell mixing (McLaren 1972; Lewis, Summerbell, and Wolpert
1972). Although this is thought to be more pronounced after the
ICM stage, at a time when cell lineages are being formed, yet it
remains a factor of great uncertainty. However, our results seem
to be in line with others which suggest that primordial germ cells
are first separated off as a very small group, with an early decision on which ones are destined for the right and left sides.
There is evidence that the lineage from which melanoblasts are
derived also originates as a small group of cells. However, the
most intriguing and pressing problems arising out of this work concern the actual pattern of reversions with respect to developmental processes. If indeed they are equally likely at any cell division, .as postulated here, then the observed frequency and appearance
of different grades of mosaicism can help to elucidate these early
developmental processes.

SUMMARY

Mosaics arising from somatic mutation at coat-colour loci can
throw light on what happens in early development. Mutable recessive
alleles at the *pearl* (*pe*) and *pink-eyed unstable* (p^{un}) loci of mice,
which revert to wild type, have proved especially useful. With both
genes, coat-colour mosaics tend either to be high-grade (mainly
affecting the germ line also) or low-grade (namely, a small spot
in a particular pigment area), with few intermediates. This has
led to the suggestion that reversion tends to occur predominantly

at the first cleavage division or at the 10-day stage. Work with p^{un} has now shown that small clones of revertant melanocytes can be found in the retinal pigment epithelium (RPE) as well as in the developing hair follicles of 2—3 day mice. The distribution of those in the RPE corresponds to expectation if the reversion rate per cell division is constant during the last stages in RPE formation. This has led to the hypothesis that there is a constant reversion rate per cell division in these mutable genes, with the peaks and troughs in frequency of different grades of mosaic being a consequence of developmental processes. If so, high-grade mosaics must arise at any one of a large number of early cell divisions, rather than at just the first. This only seems possible if the embryo proper develops from a small proportion of the inner cell mass of the blastocyst (favoured also by evidence from some other workers), and if there is also a later "bottleneck" in the lineage leading to melanocyte formation.

Analysis of different grades of p^{un} mosaic with respect to the distributional pattern of germ-line involvement suggests that the initial number of primordial germ cells at the time of their separation is very small, in line with previous estimates. The proportions of p^{un} and wild type offspring from two high-grade male mosaics were compared before and after removal of the left testis. In one, the difference was significant. This suggested an early separation of the primordial germ cells destined for each genital ridge, when numbers are still small.

I am particularly grateful to Dr. Roger Melvold and Professor H. Glenn Wolfe for kindly allowing me to use their extensive breeding data on the p^{un} mutation, without which a detailed analysis would not have been possible. I am also indebted to Dr. Bruce Cattanach for kindly performing the testicular biopsies, and to Mr. David Papworth for statistical advice. I am grateful to Messrs. Colin Beechey and Gordon Wilkins for the photography, and to Mr. Roland Quinney for looking after the mice.

REFERENCES

Cattanach, B. M. and J. H. Isaacson. 1967. Controlling elements in the mouse X chromosome. Genetics 57: 331-346.

Gardner, R. L. 1968. Mouse chimaeras obtained by the injection of cells into the blastocyst. Nature 220: 596-597.

Graham, C. F. 1971. The design of the mouse blastocyst. Symp. Soc. exp. Biol. 25: 371-378.

Lewis, J. H., D. Summerbell and L. Wolpert. 1972. Chimaeras and cell lineage in development. Nature 239: 276-279.

Markert, C. L. and W. K. Silvers. 1956. The effects of genotype and cell environment on melanoblast differentiation in the house mouse. Genetics 41: 429-450.

McLaren, A. 1972. Numerology of development. Nature 239: 274-276.

Melvold, R. W. 1971. Spontaneous somatic reversion in mice: effects of parental genotype on stability at the p-locus. Mutation Res. 12: 171-174.

Melvold, R. W. 1972. Factors affecting the spontaneous somatic reversion of pink-eyed unstable in the mouse. Unpublished Ms.

Melvold, R. W. 1977. Personal communication.

Mintz, B. 1967. Gene control of mammalian pigmentary differentiation. I. Clonal origin of melanocytes. Proc. Nat. Acad. Sci., Wash. 58: 344-351.

Mintz, B. 1974. Gene control of mammalian differentiation. Ann. Rev. Genet. 8: 411-470.

Russell, L. B. 1964. Genetic and functional mosaicism in the mouse. In Role of Chromosomes in Development, pp. 153-181. (Michael Locke, Ed.) Academic Press, New York.

Russell, L. B. and M. H. Major. 1956. A high rate of somatic reversion in the mouse. Genetics 41: 658 (Abstr.).

Russell, L. B. and M. H. Major. 1957. Radiation-induced presumed somatic mutations in the house mouse. Genetics 42: 161-175.

Russell, W. L. 1951. X-ray-induced mutations in mice. Cold Spring Harbour Symp. Quant. Biol. 16: 327-336.

Schaible, R. H. and J. W. Gowen. 1960. Delimitation of coat pigment areas in mosaic and piebald mice. Rec. Genet. Soc. Amer. 29: 92.

Searle, A. G. 1977. The use of pigment loci for detecting reverse mutations in somatic cells of mice. Arch. Toxicol. 38: 105-108.

West, J. D. 1976. Clonal development of the retinal epithelium in mouse chimaeras and X-inactivation mosaics. J. Embryol. exp. Morph. 35: 445-461.

Wolfe, H. G. 1963. Two unusual mutations affecting pigmentation in the mouse. <u>In</u> Genetics Today, Vol. 1, p. 251. (S. J. Geerts, Ed.) Pergamon Press, New York.

X Chromosome Inactivation and Depression

BIMODAL DISTRIBUTION OF α-GALACTOSIDASE ACTIVITIES IN MOUSE EMBRYOS

V. M. Chapman, J. D. West[*], and D. A. Adler

Roswell Park Memorial Institute, 666 Elm Street,
Buffalo, New York 14263

It is widely accepted that only one of two X chromosomes present in the somatic cells of female mammals is active (Lyon 1961). This results in a similar dosage relationship between functional X chromosomes and autosomes in females and males. This compensation occurs early in development between the 2-cell stage (Hoppe and Whitten 1972) and the time of implantation of the embryo into the uterus (Gardner and Lyon 1971). An important issue concerning X-chromosome differentiation is the functional state of X chromosomes during early embryogenesis, before irreversible dosage compensation occurs. That is, does X-chromosome differentiation involve a process of X-chromosome inactivation or X-chromosome activation? Choosing between these alternatives is important for understanding a number of features of X-chromosome differentiation, including:

(1) the derivation of molecular and genetic models of this process, and

(2) the determination of the timing of this differentiation.

In the latter instance, activation and inactivation events may pose entirely different conditions for using biochemical variants of X-linked genes for studying the developmental timing of the event.

Two X-chromosome-linked gene products, hypoxanthine phosphoribosyl transferase (HPRT) and α-galactosidase, show marked increases in enzyme activity during the preimplantation period. Three

---

* Present address: Department of Zoology, Oxford University,
  Oxford, United Kingdom

separate laboratories working with HPRT in early embryos have
arrived at the conclusion that a dosage difference exists between
male and female embryos for this enzyme during preimplantation
development (Monk 1978a, b; Kratzer and Gartler 1978; and Epstein,
Travis, Tucker, and Smith 1978). These findings suggest that both
X chromosomes are functioning in females before X chromosome differentiation occurs.

Similar studies have been conducted in our laboratory, using
the enzyme α-galactosidase (Adler, West, and Chapman 1977). In
this instance, α-galactosidase activity levels showed a more pronounced increase than HPRT during the preimplantation stages. Furthermore, the distributions of single embryo α-galactosidase activities were consistent with a dosage difference between males and
females, but specific tests were not performed to ascertain whether
the distributions of α-galactosidase activities differ significantly
from normal. We have reexamined the results of the α-galactosidase
experiments using probit analysis techniques to test whether the
distributions are bimodal. Where a distribution significantly
differs from normal, we have estimated the mean and standard deviation of component sub-populations using probability graph paper, or
probit analysis. The 66 h (morula stage) sample significantly differed from normal. Using probit analysis, we determined that
morula-stage embryos were bimodally distributed and that the modes
differed in specific activity by a factor of 1.7. A similar analysis technique has been previously reported for glucose-6-phosphate-
dehydrogenase activities in rabbit and mouse embryos (Brinster
1970).

α-GALACTOSIDASE ACTIVITY LEVELS IN PREIMPLANTATION EMBRYOS

Preimplantation mouse embryos of the strain C3H/HeHa were collected at each cleavage stage from artificially inseminated females.
The age of the embryos in hours post insemination, and the corresponding cell number, are shown in Table 1. α-Galactosidase activity was assayed in single embryos, using the fluorogenic substrate
4-methyl-umbelliferyl-α-D-galactoside in a microassay procedure
previously described for β-glucuronidase (Wudl and Chapman 1976).
The mean α-galactosidase activity per embryo increased 300-fold
(from 10^{-14} to 3×10^{-12} mol product hr^{-1} embryo^{-1} @ 37°C) between
the two-cell stage and the blastocyst stage (Fig. 1). Good agree-
ment between the results of the single-embryo microassay and the
standard test-tube assay procedure that uses pooled embryo samples
was observed. The increased α-galactosidase per embryo also represents a substantial increase in activity per cell up to the morula
stage (66 hr) (Table 1). After that time, the rate of increase in
α-galactosidase activity per embryo is coincident with the increase
in cell number.

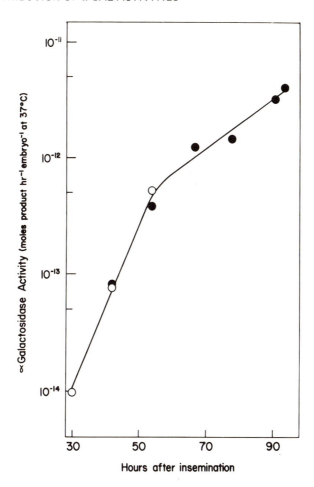

FIGURE 1.   Increase in mean α-galactosidase activity during preim-
    plantation development of C3H/HeHa mouse embryos.   Enzyme
    activity is expressed as moles of product per hr per embryo
    at 37°C.   Results from both the microassay (o) and test-tube
    assay (●) are shown.   Time 0 is the time of artificial in-
    semination (West, Frels, Papaioannou, Karr, and Chapman 1977).
    [Reprinted, by permission, from Adler et al. (1977), Nature
    267: 838–839.]

    Other lysosomal acid hydrolases, β-galactosidase and β-glucu-
ronidase, show similar but slightly delayed increases in activity
during the preimplantation stages (Wudl and Chapman 1976; Chapman,
Adler, Labarca, and Wudl 1975; Esworthy, personal communication).
In the case of β-glucuronidase, it has been possible to use genetic
variation of the glucuronidase locus (Gus) to determine that the

TABLE 1. Mean cell number and mean α-galactosidase activity per cell during preimplantation development

Age[*]	Mean cell no.[†]	Mean α-galactosidase activity per cell[‡] (fmol hr^{-1} at 37°C)	χ^2 for normal distribution[§]	
30	2	5	8.564	12df.
42	4	21	28.922	20df.
54	8	48	17.692	17df.
66	17.3 ± 0.9	72	30.270	13df.[**]
78	30.1 ± 2.0	49	26.684	14df.[††]
90	60.5 ± 4.0	57	25.808	9df.[††]

[*] h. after artificial insemination.

[†] Cell numbers at 30, 42, and 54 h are by direct count using a dissecting microscope. Cell numbers at 66, 78, and 90 h were determined using the air-drying method of Tarkowski (1966).

[‡] Mean α-galactosidase activity was determined by microassays of 2-cell embryos and test-tube assays of older embryos. (From Fig. 1).

[§] χ^2 for normal distribution of data in Fig. 2. Degrees of freedom (df) are derived from the number of classes in a distribution minus the number of parameters estimated (mean and standard deviation) plus 1.

[**]Probability that the distribution is normal < 0.5%.

[††]Probability that the distribution is normal < 5.0%.

paternally derived allele, is expressed in early cleavage, possibly by the two- to four-cell stage (Chapman, West, and Adler 1977). Thus, we conclude that autosomally inherited genes are expressed in early cleavage stages. However, we cannot unequivocally demonstrate that the paternally derived X chromosome is functional during the increase in α-galactosidase. If both X chromosomes of female embryos are active during the early increase in α-galactosidase activity, we would predict that a dosage difference should

exist between male and female embryos. As a consequence, the distribution of α-galactosidase activities of embryos would be expected to be bimodal before X-chromosome inactivation occurs, and
would become unimodal afterwards.

The distributions of single embryo α-galactosidase activities
are shown in Figure 2 for six stages of preimplantation development. Bimodal distributions were previously observed at the 54 h
(8-cell) and 66 h (morula) stages (Chapman, West, and Adler 1977),
but in this experiment the distributions are not clearly bimodal.
To test whether these distributions are bimodal we initially tested
whether they significantly differed from normal. An expected normal
frequency distribution for each of the times sampled was derived
using the mean and standard deviations of those samples. The estimated frequency distributions were compared with those observed in
each of the samples, using a χ^2 analysis (Table 1). The distributions at 30, 42, and 54 h did not differ significantly from normal.
However, the distribution at 66 h differed from normal at the 0.5%
level of significance. Significant differences from normal at the
5% level occurred at the 78 and 90 h stages of development.

To determine whether the samples were composed of a mixture of
subpopulations, the cumulative percentages within a distribution
are plotted on Hagan's probability graph paper (Harding 1949; Cassie
1954). If a bimodal distribution is compounded of two distributions
that are normally distributed, it will give a curve which is the
result of two straight lines. These lines can be determined, and
the positions and slopes of these lines can be used to derive estimates of the means and standard deviations of the component subpopulations. Because the comparable area under the normal curve of
a subpopulation is approximately double that observed in the mixed
population, the position of the line estimating one subpopulation
mean is derived by multiplying the low end of the mixed distribution by a factor of about 2. The second subpopulation is estimated
by multiplying the high end by the reciprocal.

The probit analysis of each of the time periods sampled is
shown in Figure 3. Only the 66-hour sample has a distribution
that significantly differs from normal and a curve that indicates
bimodality. The 42 h sample shows a curve that is suggestive of
a bimodal distribution. However, the variability within this sample was too large (CV = 62.3%) to detect bimodality resulting from
a 2-fold difference in component subpopulation means. The 78 h
and 90 h distributions differ significantly from normal, but there
is no clear indication of bimodality either in the histograms or
the probit analysis.

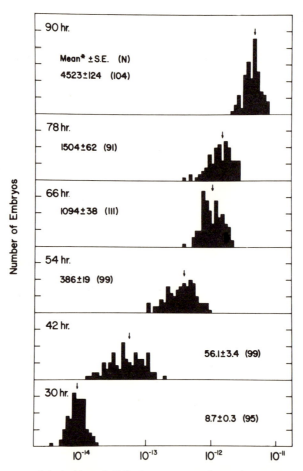

∝Galactosidase Activity (moles product hr⁻¹embryo⁻¹ at 25°C)

FIGURE 2. Distributions of single-embryo α-galactosidase activities
at six sampling times after artificial insemination. Individual embryos were assayed at 25°C using the microassay. The
number of embryos in each activity class is indicated by the
vertical scale marked in intervals of five embryos. The mean
activity for each distribution is indicated with an arrow.
From top to bottom: 90 h mean α-galactosidase activity (±
s.e.) 4,523 ± 124 fmol product/hr/embryo at 25°C (n=104);
78 h, 1,504 ± 62 (n-91); 66 h, 1,094 ± 38 (n=111); 54 h, 386
± 19 (n=99); 42 h, 56.1 ± 3.4 (n=99); 30 h, 8.7 ± 0.3 (n=95).
[Reprinted, by permission, from Adler _et al._ (1977), Nature
267: 838-839.]

The compound frequency distribution of a 50:50 mixture of estimated subpopulations was compared with the observed distribution at 66 hours (Fig. 4). The observed distribution does not differ significantly from the predicted compound mixture (χ^2 = 10.572 with 10 df. P = 0.50). The estimated mean values of the subpopulations are 77.6 x 10^{-14} and 135.0 x 10^{-14} moles hr^{-1} embryo^{-1}. This 1.7-fold difference is close to the expected female vs. male dosage difference of two-fold.

DISCUSSION

The observation of bimodality for α-galactosidase activity at the morula stage, taken by itself, provides only circumstantial evidence for a dosage difference between male and female embryos at this stage. However, it is consistent with the findings in HPRT expression presented in the accompanying papers (Kratzer and Gartler 1978; Monk 1978b; Epstein et al. 1978). Furthermore, distributions of embryo activities for the autosomal gene product, β-glucuronidase, do not show clear evidence of bimodality at any of the preimplantation stages (Wudl and Chapman 1976; Wudl and Sherman 1976). Taken together, these findings strongly indicate that both X chromosomes are functional in females before an X chromosome becomes irreversibly inactive. In other words, the process of dosage compensation appears to be one of inactivation of active X chromosomes, rather than activation of X chromosomes that have been inactive during cleavage.

Several features of X inactivation remain unresolved. The timing of inactivation, and whether it occurs in all cells at the same time, are issues that have received considerable attention. The lack of bimodality in the 78 h and 90 h samples may be consistent with X inactivation occurring in at least some of the cells at this stage of development (Takagi 1974), but could also be explained by developmental variability among embryos.

The disappearance of a dosage difference between males and females will also depend upon the relative rates of synthesis of α-galactosidase after X inactivation occurs. It will also depend upon the turnover of the previously synthesized message and enzyme protein. Without some knowledge of these parameters, it may be premature to use the loss of bimodality of α-galactosidase or other X-linked enzymes as an indication of the timing of X-chromosome inactivation.

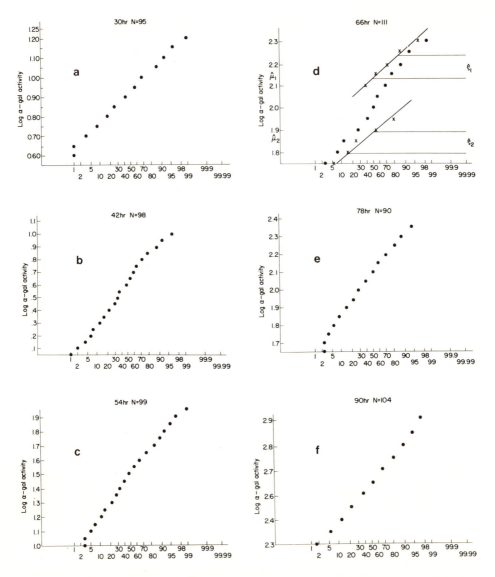

FIGURE 3. Probability graph plots of the distributions in Figure 2. The percentage points of the distribution are shown on the bottom of each figure and the $\log_{10}$ of α-galactosidase activity on the vertical axis. The 30 h time is the log of fmol/hr/embryo. The other times are the log of 10^{-14} moles/hr/embryo. For the 66 h sample the points marked (x) and heavy lines estimate the distributions of the component subpopulations. The intervals $\hat{\sigma}_1$ and $\hat{\sigma}_2$ estimate the standard deviations of the subpopulations while $\hat{\mu}_1$ and $\hat{\mu}_2$ are the estimates of the subpopulation means.

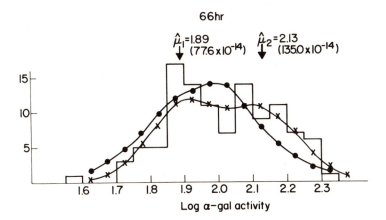

FIGURE 4. Histogram distribution of individual-embryo α-galactosidase (α-gal) activities at 66 h. The number of embryos in
each class is indicated by the scale on the left. The expected normal distribution estimated from the mean and standard
deviation of the observed population is indicated by (●).
The estimated compounded distribution of two subpopulations
derived from the probit analysis is indicated by (x). The
estimated means of the component subpopulations is indicated
by $\hat{\mu}_1$ and $\hat{\mu}_2$.

SUMMARY

The distribution of α-galactosidase activities in single preimplantation embryos significantly differs from normal at the
morula and early blastocyst stages. A probit analysis of activity
distributions at the morula stage clearly indicates that the distribution is bimodal. A bimodal distribution of α-galactosidase
is consistent with a dosage difference between male and female
embryos, suggesting that both X chromosomes are functional in
females during early development. We conclude from our data, and
from the similar findings for HPRT, that X-chromosome differentiation in mammals involves inactivation of an active X chromosome.

Supported by grant from the National Institutes of Health
HD08768-3 and GM24125-01.

REFERENCES

Adler, D. A., J. D. West and V. M. Chapman. 1977. Expression of
α-galactosidase in preimplantation mouse embryos: indications for
X-chromosome inactivation. Nature 267: 838-839.

Brinster, R. L. 1970. Glucose-6-phosphate dehydrogenase activity
in the early rabbit and mouse embryo. Biochem. Genet. 4: 669-696.

Cassie, R. M. 1954. Some uses of probability paper in the analysis of size frequency distributions. Aust. J. Marine and Fresh
Water Res. 5: 513-522.

Chapman, V. M., J. D. West and D. A. Adler. 1977. Genetics of
early mammalian embryogenesis. In, Concepts in early mammalian
development, M. I. Sherman, Ed. M.I.T. Press, pp. 95-126.
Observer Excerpta Medica, North-Holland, Assoc. Scientific
Publishers, New York.

Chapman, V. M., J. D. West and D. A. Adler. 1977. Genetics of
early mammalian embryogenesis. Concepts in early mammalian development. M. I. Sherman, Ed. M.I.T. Press, pp. 95-126.

Epstein, C. J., B. Travis, G. Tucker and S. Smith. 1978. The
direct demonstration of an X-chromosome dosage effect prior to
inactivation. In, Genetic Mosaics and Chimeras in Mammals, Liane
B. Russell, Ed. Plenum Press, New York and London.

Esworthy, R. S. personal communication.

Gardner, R. L. and M. F. Lyon. 1971. X-chromosome inactivation studied by injection of a single cell into the mouse blastocyst. Nature (Lond.) 231: 385-386.

Harding, J. P. 1949. The use of probability paper for the graphical analysis of polymodal frequency distributions. J. Marine Biol. Assoc. 28: 141-153.

Hoppe, P. C. and W. K. Whitten. 1972. Does X chromosome inactivation occur during mitosis of first cleavage. Nature (Lond.) 239: 520.

Kratzer, P. and S. M. Gartler. 1978. HGPRT expression in early mouse development. In, Genetic Mosaics and Chimeras in Mammals, Liane B. Russell, Ed. Plenum Press, New York and London.

Lyon, M. F. 1961. Gene action in the X-chromosome of the mouse (*Mus musculus*). Nature (Lond.) 190: 372-373.

Monk, M. 1978*a*. Biochemical studies on mammalian X-chromosome activity. In, Development in Mammals. Vol. 3, M. H. Johnson, Ed. North-Holland Publ. Co., Amsterdam.

Monk, M. 1978*b*. Biochemical studies on X-chromosome activity in preimplantation mouse embryos. In, Genetic Mosaics and Chimeras in Mammals. Liane B. Russell, Ed. Plenum Press, New York and London.

Takagi, N. 1974. Differentiation of X chromosomes in early female mouse embryos. Exp. Cell Res. 86: 127.

Tarkowski, A. K. 1966. An air-drying method for chromosome preparations from mouse eggs. Cytogenetics 5: 394-400.

West, J. D., W. I. Frels, V. E. Papaioannou, J. Karr and V. M. Chapman. 1977. Development of interspecific hybrids of *Mus*. J. Emb. Exp. Morph. 41: 233-243.

Wudl, L. R. and V. Chapman. 1976. The expression of β-glucuronidase during preimplantation development of mouse embryos. Develop. Biol. 48: 104-109.

Wudl, L. R. and M. I. Sherman. 1976. *In vitro* studies of mouse embryos bearing mutations at the T locus t^{w5} and t^{12}. Cell 9: 523-532.

BIOCHEMICAL STUDIES ON X-CHROMOSOME ACTIVITY IN PREIMPLANTATION MOUSE EMBRYOS

Marilyn Monk

MRC Mammalian Development Unit, Wolfson House, (University College London), London NW1, 2HE, England

During early development of female (XX) eutherian mammals, one or the other of the X chromosomes is rendered inactive in all, or most, of the cells of the embryo. This differentiation of the X chromosomes is irreversible, and the adult female is a mosaic with respect to clones of cells with either the maternally-derived or paternally-derived X chromosome inactive. The timing of X-chromosome differentiation has been a subject of considerable interest. Cytogenetic evidence suggests that it occurs around the time of implantation, or at the late blastocyst stage (e.g., see Takagi 1974; Mukherjee 1976). However, other genetic evidence (Gardner and Lyon 1971) suggests that both X chromosomes are active at this stage, at least in the inner cell mass cells of the blastocyst. The subject of X-chromosome inactivation has been extensively reviewed (e.g., see Lyon 1968, 1972, 1974; Eicher 1970; Gartler and Andina 1976; and Monk 1978).

It has been generally assumed that both X chromosomes are active in very early development, and that one or the other is *inactivated* at random in embryo precursor cells. However, there has to date been no direct evidence that this is so. Consequently this work was undertaken in an attempt to answer the following questions:

(1) Are both X chromosomes active in early female XX embryos?

(2) If both X chromosomes *are* active, when does X-chromosome inactivation take place?

(3) Does X-chromosome differentiation occur in all tissues of the
     embryo at the same time, or is the event perhaps linked in
     some way to cellular differentiation?

The work presented here strongly suggests that both X chromosomes
are active in XX preimplantation embryos, but that inactivation
occurs in the majority of the cells by the blastocyst stage.
Preliminary data indicating that both X chromosomes are active in
the inner cell mass (ICM) cells of XX blastocysts supports the
hypothesis (Monk 1978) that X-chromosome differentiation is linked
in some way to cellular differentiation and occurs in cells as
they "depart" from the multipotent "stem line." The evidence is
presented below.

    Biochemical analysis of X-chromosome function in early em-
bryos ideally requires distinguishable variant forms of an X-
linked enzyme on the two X chromosomes, a microassay sensitive
enough to measure them in individual embryos, and the absence of
a high concentration of that enzyme in the maternal cytoplasm of
the egg (which would mask the embryo-coded contributions). In
the absence of a suitable system for variant forms of an X-linked
enzyme (but see Chapman and Shows 1976) it remained possible to
look at gene-dosage effects (see Epstein 1969, 1972) for two enzymes satisfying the other criteria, namely, α-galactosidase
(Adler, West, and Chapman 1977; Chapman, West, and Adler 1978)
and hypoxanthine phosphoribosyl transferase (HPRT, E.C.2.4.2.8;
Monk and Kathuria 1977; Monk 1978; Monk and Harper 1978; Kratzer
and Gartler 1978). The idea is that if both X chromosomes are
active in early female embryos, and if the level of an X-linked
enzyme is proportional to gene dosage, then embryos with two X
chromosomes (XX) should show twice the activity of the enzyme as
do embryos with one X chromosome (XY or XO). If the assay for
the X-linked enzyme can be developed to sufficient sensitivity to
allow assays of individual embryos, half of which we expect to be
XX and half XY, then the distribution of activities should be
bimodal with a twofold separation of the modes.

    The assay system used is based on that reported by McBurney
and Adamson (1976), and details and controls justifying its validity are described in Monk and Kathuria (1977) and Monk and Harper
(1978). The activities of two enzymes, HPRT (X-linked) and APRT
(adenine phosphoribosyl transferase, E.C.2.4.2.7, on chromosome
8 [Kozak, Nichols and Ruddle 1975]), are measured in extracts of
individual embryos in the same reaction mix. The phosphorylated
products of the substrates for HPRT and APRT, ^{3}H guanine and [14]C
adenine respectively, are precipitated by lanthanum chloride, the
precipitates collected on filters and counted. The activities of
HPRT and APRT in each embryo extract may be evaluated. The

expression of the results as a ratio, HPRT:APRT, for each embryo
eliminates sampling errors.

Figure 1 shows distributions of activities of HPRT, APRT, and
HPRT:APRT ratios in extracts of large numbers of individual 9- to
16-cell morulae, blastocysts, and inner cell masses isolated from
blastocysts. In morulae (Fig. 1a) the distributions of HPRT
activities and HPRT:APRT ratios are bimodal, with a twofold
separation of the modes. The distribution of the autosomally
coded APRT activities is unimodal. These results strongly suggest
that both X chromosomes are active in XX morulae (Monk 1978; Monk
and Harper 1978). Such a situation was previously tentatively
claimed for the distribution of α-galactosidase activities in
single morulae by Adler *et al.* (1977) and Chapman *et al.* (1978).
The conclusion that both X chromosomes are active in XX morulae
rests on the plausible assumption that the two modes represent
male (XY) and female (XX) embryos. Epstein, Travis, Tucker, and
Smith (1978) have performed analyses for karyotype and HPRT activity in twin blastocysts grown from earlier divided embryos, and
have shown that twins of XX karyotype have higher HPRT activity
than do those of XY karyotype.

Monk and Kathuria (1977) reported that a two-fold separation
of XX and XY embryos with respect to HPRT activities could not be
seen for 8-cell embryos and for blastocysts. They concluded that
some form of dosage compensation was operating at these developmental stages. The apparently unimodal distributions for HPRT and
APRT activities and HPRT:APRT ratios in individual blastocysts are
shown in Figure 1b. There is possibly, however, an indication of
two populations of embryos with an approximately 1.5-fold separation of modes at the 8-cell and the blastocyst stages when the data
are reexamined at the level of single litters (data not shown, but
see Monk and Harper 1978; Kratzer and Gartler 1978). What form of
dosage compensation could be operating at these stages that might
prevent a two-fold difference between XX and XY embryos?

Let us consider first the 8-cell embryos. Monk and Harper
(1978) assayed HPRT, APRT, and HPRT:APRT ratios in embryos derived
from XX and XO mothers. Because both X chromosomes are active
during oogenesis, XX-derived embryos begin development with twice
the HPRT activity as do XO-derived embryos. We showed that, although there is a considerable increase in HPRT activity by the
8-cell stage, XX-derived 8-cell embryos still show approximately
twice as much HPRT activity as do XO-derived 8-cell embryos. APRT
activities in the two groups of embryos remain similar, while also
rising with advancing development. We concluded that there is a
significant maternal contribution of HPRT activity at the 8-cell
stage. This would explain why the two-fold separation of XX and
XY populations is not seen. Moreover, since there was an

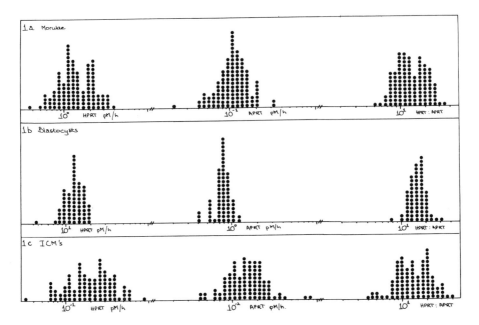

FIGURE 1. HPRT and APRT activities and HPRT:APRT ratios in ex-
    tracts of individual morulae (1a), blastocysts (1b) and inner
    cell masses (ICM, 1c).
    Morulae and blastocysts were isolated from the oviducts and
    uteri of superovulated MF1 females on the third and fourth
    day of pregnancy, respectively (at 74 hours and 94 hours post
    HCG injection). Inner cell masses were isolated from blasto-
    cysts by the method of Solter and Knowles (1975). Each
    figure contains the pooled results of two experiments.
    Details of the methods of embryo isolation, preparation of
    extracts, and enzyme assays are given in Monk and Harper
    (1978). Data similar to those shown in Figures 1a and 1b
    have previously been presented in Monk and Harper (1978) and
    Monk and Kathuria (1977), respectively.

approximate ten-fold increase in HPRT activity by the 8-cell stage, we suggested that these data may represent the first evidence in mammalian embryos of active maternal messenger RNA. Other interpretations, such as an earlier onset of activity of the HPRT gene on the maternally-inherited X chromosome, were also considered.

As for the situation in blastocysts, it is well established that these consist of two discrete tissues, trophectoderm and inner cell mass (ICM). Is it possible that X inactivation has occurred in the trophectoderm, which constitutes the majority of cells of the blastocyst, but not in the ICM? My results for HPRT, APRT, and HPRT:APRT ratios in extracts of individual inner cell masses isolated microsurgically (Solter and Knowles 1975) are shown in Figure 1c. The results are highly suggestive that both X chromosomes are active in ICMs of the presumptive XX blastocysts, and therefore that inactivation has occurred only in the differentiated trophectoderm at this stage. This conclusion is consistent with the genetic evidence of Gardner and Lyon (1971) suggesting that both X chromosomes are potentially active in inner cell mass

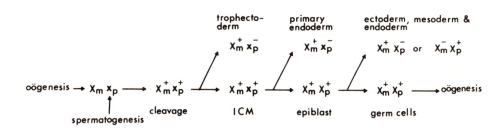

FIGURE 2. An interpretation of X-chromosome differentiation (Monk 1978).

X-chromosome differentiation is depicted as occurring at different times in different lineages of cells as they depart from the multipotent embryonic stem line (m = maternal, p = paternal, + = active, − = inactive). This differentiation shows: (a) a preferential recall that the paternal X chromosome was previously inactive (during spermatogenesis), (b) a later loss of this recall in embryo precursor cells (epiblast), and (c) the maintenance of two active X chromosomes through early development and throughout the germ line. Evidence concerning the preferential inactivation of the paternal X chromosome in cells differentiating early in development is given in Takagi and Sasaki (1975), West, Frels, Chapman, and Papaioannou (1977), and West, Papaioannou, Frels, and Chapman (1978). It is reviewed by Monk (1978).

cells. It also provides support for the hypothesis (Fig. 2; and Monk 1978) that X-chromosome differentiation occurs at different times in different cell lineages, and is associated with the departure, or differentiation, of cells from the "stem line." Further predictions of the hypothesis presented in Figure 2 are currently under test.

REFERENCES

Adler, D. A., J. D. West and V. M. Chapman. 1977. Expression of α-galactosidase in preimplantation mouse embryos. Nature 267: 838-839.

Chapman, V. M. and T. B. Shows. 1976. Somatic cell genetic evidence for the X-chromosome linkage of glucose-6-phosphate dehydrogenase, phosphoglycerate kinase and hypoxanthine-phospho-ribosyl transferase. Nature 259: 665-667.

Chapman, V. M., J. D. West and D. A. Adler. 1978. Bimodal distribution of α-galactosidase activities in mouse embryos. In Genetic Mosaics and Chimeras in Mammals, Liane B. Russell, Ed., Plenum Press, New York and London.

Eicher, E. M. 1970. X autosome translocations in the mouse: total inactivation versus partial inactivation of the X chromosome. Adv. Genet. 15: 175-259.

Epstein, C. J. 1969. Mammalian oocytes: X chromosome activity. Science 163: 1078-1079.

Epstein, C. J. 1972. Expression of the mammalian X chromosome before and after fertilisation. Science 175: 1467-1468.

Epstein, C. J., B. Travis, G. Tucker and S. Smith. 1978. The direct demonstration of an X-chromosome dosage effect prior to inactivation. In Genetic Mosaics and Chimeras in Mammals, Liane B. Russell, Ed., Plenum Press, New York and London.

Gardner, R. L. and M. Lyon. 1971. X chromosome inactivation studied by injection of a single cell into the mouse blastocyst. Nature 231: 385-386.

Gartler, S. M. and R. J. Andina. 1976. Mammalian X-chromosome inactivation. Adv. in Human Genet. 7: 99-140.

Kozak, C., E. Nichols and F. H. Ruddle. 1975. Gene linkage analysis by somatic cell hydridisation: assignment of adenine phosphoribosyltransferase to chromosome 8 and α-galactosidase to the X chromosome. Somatic Cell Genet. 1: 371-382.

Kratzer, P. G. and Gartler, S. M. 1978. HGPRT expression in early mouse development. In Genetic Mosaics and Chimeras in Mammals, Liane B. Russell, Ed., Plenum Press, New York and London.

Lyon, M. F. 1968. Chromosomal and subchromosomal inactivation. Ann. Rev. Genet. 2: 31–52.

Lyon, M. F. 1972. X-chromosome inactivation and developmental patterns in mammals. Biol. Rev. 47: 1–35.

Lyon, M. F. 1974. Mechanisms and evolutionary origins of variable X-chromosome activity in mammals. Proc. Roy. Soc. Lond. B. 187: 243–268.

McBurney, M. W. and E. D. Adamson. 1976. Studies on the activity of the X chromosome in female teratocarcinoma cells in culture. Cell 9: 57–70.

Monk, M. 1978. Biochemical studies on mammalian X-chromosome activity. In Development in Mammals III, M. H. Johnson, Ed., North Holland Publishing Company, Amsterdam.

Monk, M. and M. Harper. 1978. X-chromosome activity in preimplantation mouse embryos from XX and XO mothers. J. exp. Embryo. Morph. 46: 53–64.

Monk, M. and H. Kathuria. 1977. Dosage compensation for an X-linked gene in preimplantation mouse embryos. Nature Lond. 270: 599–601.

Mukherjee, A. B. 1976. Cell cycle analysis and X-chromosome inactivation in the developing mouse. Proc. Nat. Acad. Sci. USA 73: 1608–1611.

Solter, D. and B. A. Knowles. 1975. Immunosurgery of mouse blastocyst. Proc. Nat. Acad. Sci. USA 72: 5099–5102.

Takagi, N. 1974. Differentiation of X chromosomes in early female mouse embryos. Exp. Cell Res. 86: 127–135.

Takagi, N. and M. Sasaki. 1975. Preferential inactivation of the paternally derived X chromosome in the extraembryonic membranes of the mouse. Nature 256: 640–642.

West, J. D., W. I. Frels, V. M. Chapman and V. E. Papaioannou. 1978. Preferential expression of the maternally derived X chromosome in the mouse yolk sac. Cell 12: 873–882.

West, J. D., V. E. Papaioannou, W. I. Frels and V. M. Chapman. 1978. Preferential expression of the maternally derived X chromosome in extraembryonic tissues of the mouse. In Genetic Mosaics and Chimeras in Mammals, Liane B. Russell, Ed., Plenum Press, New York and London.

HYPOXANTHINE GUANINE PHOSPHORIBOSYL TRANSFERASE EXPRESSION IN

EARLY MOUSE DEVELOPMENT

Paul G. Kratzer and Stanley M. Gartler

Departments of Genetics and Medicine, University of
Washington, Seattle, Washington 98195

Dosage compensation for X-linked genes occurs by the process
of X-chromosome inactivation (XCI) in mammalian somatic cells
(Lyon 1972). The inactivation of one X chromosome in females takes
place early in development, although the exact time is unknown.
One method of ascertaining the time of XCI is to determine the
activity of the X chromosome at different stages of development as
measured by the activity of an X-coded enzyme. Prior to XCI, and
in the absence of other dosage compensating mechanisms, the activity for an embryonically expressed X-coded enzyme should be twice
as high in female embryos with two X chromosomes, as in male embryos
with one X chromosome. The distribution of enzyme activities for
single embryos from a litter would have two equal-sized peaks that
are separated by a factor of two. The convergence of the two peaks
into one would indicate that XCI had occurred.

This approach has been applied to two X-coded enzymes: α-
galactosidase (Adler, West, and Chapman 1977; Chapman, West, and
Adler 1978), and hypoxanthine guanine phosphoribosyl transferase
(HGPRT) (Monk and Kathuria 1977; Monk 1978a, b; Kratzer and Gartler
1978). The results of these studies indicate that early preimplantation embryos (8-cell and morula) lack dosage compensation. In
this report, we extend the work on HGPRT to earlier and later stages
of development and to dissected blastocysts.

247

MATERIALS AND METHODS

Embryo preparation

Mouse embryos and oocytes were obtained from superovulated (BALBxS1)F_1 hybrid females mated to S1 males (Eklund and Bradford 1977). Methods for obtaining 2-cell to blastocyst stages are given in Kratzer and Gartler (1978). Unfertilized eggs were collected from the ampulla 15 hours after the injection of human chorionic gonadotropic (HCG) and freed from cumulus cells by brief exposure to hyaluronidase. Sections of embryonic ectoderm covered by proximal embryonic endoderm were sliced off day-6 and day-7 egg cylinders for assay.

Inner cell masses (ICM) were isolated from very late blastocysts by immunosurgery (Solter and Knowles 1975). The sequence of incubations in antisera and complement effectively removes the outside cells of the embryo. In two cases, the trophectoderm was torn with needles, exposing the primitive endoderm to the action of immunosurgery.

Embryonic specimens for assay were washed in rinsing solution and frozen on dry ice in a small volume of rinsing solution plus bovine serum albumin (Kratzer and Gartler 1978).

Enzyme assays

HGPRT assays as described by Kratzer and Gartler (1978) were carried out using ^{14}C-hypoxanthine as substrate and thin-layer chromatography to isolate the product.

Lactate dehydrogenase (LDH) was assayed either on whole extracts, or in the case of double (HGPRT and LDH) assays, on part of the HGPRT incubation mixture before freezing to stop the reaction. The LDH assay was carried out at 37° in 2 ml of Tris, pH 8.6, 100 mM; NAD, 100 µM; and sodium lactate, 50 mM. Fluorescence measurements were linear for 24 hours when the activity was low.

RESULTS AND DISCUSSION

HGPRT activity increases continuously from the egg through development, with two exceptions (Fig. 1). A drop in activity first occurs at compaction, where after increasing 17-fold from the egg to the 8-cell stage, there is a 10% decrease in activity. Other enzymes are known to decrease in activity at this stage (Epstein 1975). The second drop, constituting a 40% decrease, occurs just before implantation. The cause or causes of these

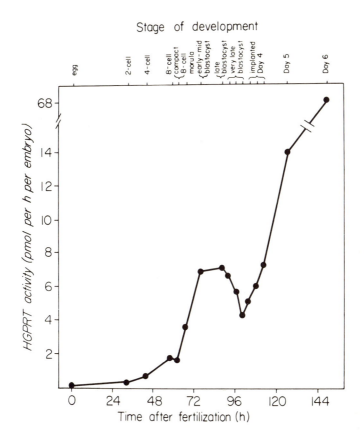

FIGURE 1. HGPRT activity is plotted versus developmental stage and hours after fertilization. Fertilization is assumed to occur between 13 and 17 hours after the HCG injection, since this is the interval following ovulation, but before checking for vaginal plugs. Blastocysts were substaged as follows: early-mid blastocysts are cavitating, late blastocysts have expanded, and very late blastocysts have hatched from the zona pellucida.

decreases in enzyme activity during early development are not apparent at this time. However, it is of interest that both decreases occur during periods of morphogenetic reorganization in the early embryo (compaction, when differences appear between inside and outside cells [Johnson, Handyside, and Braude 1977]; and changes occurring just prior to implantation).

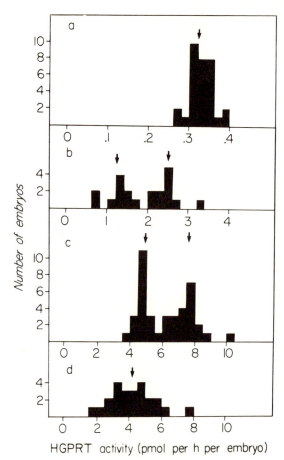

FIGURE 2. Distributions of HGPRT activity in single embryos from
    litters at four different developmental stages: (a) 2-cell,
    litter no. 317; (b) 8-cell, litter no. 294; (c) late blasto-
    cyst, litter no. 278; and (d) very late blastocyst, litter
    no. 280. Arrows indicate the means of the distributions,
    which are plotted on different scales in the various parts
    of the figure.

    The presence or absence of dosage compensation will be re-
vealed by the shape of the distribution of HGPRT activity per embryo
at stages in which the embryonic gene is active. For HGPRT, the
early increase in activity may be maternally derived, but by day 3
it is embryonically coded (Epstein 1972). At the 2-cell stage,
the distributions are definitely unimodal (Fig. 2, Table 1). At

the 4-cell stage, there is some hint of bimodality, in which new
synthesis is added to the 2-cell level; however, the distributions
are not significantly bimodal (P>.1). By the 8-cell stage, clear
bimodality (P<.001) is present, where the peaks have equal proportions, and the upper mean has twice the value of the lower mean.
The bimodality does not result from developmental heterogeneity
among littermates, since LDH, an autosomally coded enzyme shows
little tendency toward bimodality (P>.1) at any stage (Table 2).
The simplest explanation for the bimodality is that both X chromosomes are active in female embryos. It has recently been reported
that, in early blastocysts, female embryos do have twice as much
HGPRT activity as male embryos (Epstein, Smith, Travis, and Tucker
1978; Epstein, Travis, Tucker, and Smith 1978).

In later preimplantation stages, the distributions of HGPRT
activity differ from those at the 8-cell stage in two respects.
First, between the 8-cell and late-blastocyst stages, the bimodality of the distributions is only marginally significant (.05<P<.1).
The lower chi-square values might result from increased variability
in enzyme activity between embryos. The coefficient of variation
is 36, 22, and 20% for compact 8-cell, morula, and early-mid blastocysts, respectively, compared to 17 and 11% for 8-cell and late
blastocysts. Both of the stages (8-cell and late blastocyst) which
are highly significantly bimodal (P<.001) occur when enzyme activity
is changing least rapidly, and both stages are followed by a decrease in enzyme activity. Theoretically, the faster the enzyme
activity is changing, the more variable should be the embryos'
activities. Second, the ratio of the upper mean to the lower mean
decreases from 2 : 1 to 1.5 : 1 to unimodality. The decrease begins between the morula (ratios: 1.78, 2.13, 2.24) and early-mid
blastocysts (ratios: 1.04, 1.65, 1.66, 1.76) and continues through
the late blastocysts (ratios: 1.41, 1.55, 1.58). The distributions
are unimodal for very late blastocyts, and for ratios of HGPRT/LDH
activity for day-5 and day-6 embryos (Table 3).

Convergence of the two peaks is expected as a consequence of
XCI, since female embryos would no longer have twice as many active
X chromosomes as male embryos, yet would have twice as much activity
from enzyme synthesized before XCI. As enzyme and mRNA turnover
proceeds, the peaks should merge together. The time of XCI estimated from the initiation of convergence thus does not depend upon
the half-life of either the mRNA or the enzyme, since these parameters will only affect the rate of convergence. The initiation
of convergence does depend on the interval between the decision to
inactivate an X chromosome, and the enzymatic expression of this
inactivation. Despite the uncertainty in when the decision to
inactivate an X chromosome is made, the appearance of XCI occurs
before blastulation.

TABLE 1. Distribution of HGPRT activities per embryo

Stage	Litter no.	No. of embryos	χ^2	Coef. of variation	Peak means[§]		Ratio($\frac{upper}{lower}$)	Peak proportions	
					Lower	Upper		Lower	Upper
2-cell	317	32	.00	8.5	.32	.33	1.03	.51	.49
	328	30	3.33	5.7	.40	.48	1.19	.70	.30
	330	29	.00	13.5	.39	.41	1.05	.70	.30
			Sum 3.33*						
4-cell	322	40	4.90	12.3	.58	.86	1.49	.73	.27
	326	28	2.25	13.1	.74	1.07	1.44	.56	.44
	329	22	1.58	13.8	.52	.73	1.41	.60	.40
			Sum 8.73*						
8-cell	264	18	5.06	17.3	1.29	2.68	2.07	.72	.28
	291	25	11.76	15.6	1.06	2.20	2.08	.58	.42
	294	21	7.58	17.3	1.23	2.50	2.04	.52	.48
			Sum 24.40‡						
Compact 8-cell	292	15	1.39	34.5	1.14	2.22	1.95	.66	.34
	295	15	2.40	38.5	1.46	2.33	1.60	.53	.47
			Sum 3.79*						
Morula	267	16	6.59	18.5	1.75	3.93	2.24	.37	.63
	274	24	3.85	18.5	3.43	6.11	1.78	.66	.34
	288	28	.56	29.4	2.89	6.16	2.13	.72	.28
			Sum 11.00†						

Early-mid blastocyst	262	13	.95	16.2	6.13	10.19	1.66	.63	.37
	271	32	6.12	17.5	4.46	7.83	1.76	.53	.47
	275	30	7.51	20.2	6.06	10.00	1.65	.47	.53
	287	16	.00	24.0	5.76	5.97	1.04	.63	.37
			Sum 14.58[†]						
Late blastocyst	277	49	13.96	10.9	5.63	7.96	1.41	.53	.47
	278	40	12.42	12.8	4.89	7.59	1.55	.53	.47
	293	21	14.44	9.0	6.45	10.20	1.58	.56	.44
			Sum 40.82[‡]						
Very late blastocyst	276	16	2.18	15.7	5.61	8.84	1.58	.67	.33
	280	24	.06	33.5	3.95	6.64	1.68	.91	.09
	289	28	.31	22.2	4.40	7.00	1.59	.67	.33
	290	15	3.61	10.0	5.18	6.96	1.35	.48	.52
			Sum 6.16[*]						

[*] $P>.10$ [†] $.05<P<.10$ [‡] $P<.001.$

[§] Mean HGPRT activities are expressed as pmol per hour per embryo.

TABLE 2. Distribution of LDH activity per embryo

Stage	Litter no.	No. of embryos	χ^2	Peak means[†]		Ratio($\frac{upper}{lower}$)	Peak proportions	
				Lower	Upper		Lower	Upper
8-cell	83	16	5.74	18.0	22.0	1.22	.64	.36
	99	31	0	20.2	21.0	1.04	.26	.74
	100	11	3.53	15.7	23.5	1.50	.73	.27
			Sum 9.57*					
Early-mid blastocyst	66	17	5.61	7.41	10.49	1.42	.59	.41
	90	13	0	9.52	10.72	1.13	.43	.57
	91	22	0	11.55	12.30	1.06	.48	.52
			Sum 5.61*					
Late blastocyst	73	10	0	8.67	8.98	1.04	.51	.49
	104	15	7.68	6.62	10.79	1.63	.68	.32
			Sum 7.68*					

* P > .10

† Mean LDH activities are expressed as nmoles per hour per embryo

The estimate of the time of XCI obtained here by measurement of enzyme activities agrees with the cytological estimations based on the detection of sex chromatin (DeMars 1967), prophase hetero-pycnosis (Takagi 1974), and replication asynchrony (Takagi 1974). On the other hand, later estimates are obtained by the genetic approaches of blastocyst injection (Gardner and Lyon 1971) and analyzing the extent of variegation in females heterozygous for an X-coded marker (Nesbitt 1971; Deol and Whitten 1972). This dis-crepancy is not surprising, since the genetic approaches necessar-ily look at XCI in the ICM derivatives, while the cytological and enzymatic observations can additionally look at XCI in the tro-phectoderm, which makes up most of the preimplantation blastocyst (McLaren 1976). Since the trophectoderm cells outnumber the ICM cells, one would expect enzyme measurements to reflect primarily the activity of the trophectoderm cells. Therefore, our enzyme approach probably estimates the time of XCI in the trophectoderm, while XCI in the ICM may occur at a later time.

To test the hypothesis that XCI occurs earlier in the trophec-toderm than in the ICM, immunosurgically isolated ICMs from very late blastocysts were assayed. Preliminary results are presented in Table 3. The ICMs in these isolations have about 25% of the embryo's activity, roughly corresponding to the proportion of ICM cells in the embryo. ICMs from embryos, in which the trophecto-derm had been torn, presumably facilitating lysis of the primitive endoderm during immunosurgery, had slightly lower activities than ICMs from intact blastocysts. The distributions from embryos with torn trophectoderms are significantly bimodal (P<.001), and the ratios (1.75, 1.80) are higher than those in whole very late blas-tocysts. In ICMs from intact blastocysts, the distributions are marginally significant (.05<P<.1), and the ratios are lower (1.58, 1.58). Sections of day-6 and day-7 egg cylinders containing mainly embryonic ectoderm plus proximal embryonic endoderm show no bimo-dality (P>.1). These preliminary results suggest that XCI does occur earlier in the trophectoderm than in the ICM, and that, within the ICM, XCI may occur earlier in the primitive endoderm than in the embryonic ectoderm. This difference in time of XCI would add to the differences in randomness (West, Frels, Chapman, and Papaioannou 1977; West, Papaioannou, Frels, and Chapman 1978) and replication patterns (Takagi and Sasaki 1975; Takagi 1978) of XCI noted between ectoderm-derived and non-ectoderm-derived tissues.

SUMMARY

Early preimplantation embryos show no dosage compensation, as evidenced by bimodal distribution for HGPRT activity. Before blas-tulation, the two peaks in the distributions begin to converge, signifying XCI. Preliminary results suggest that XCI occurs ear-lier in the trophectoderm, than in the ICM.

TABLE 3. Distribution of ratios for HGPRT/LDH activities per embryo

| | HGPRT activity | | | HGPRT/LDH ratios | | | | |
| | No. of embryos | Mean* | χ² | Peak means** Upper | Peak means** Lower | Ratio(upper/lower) | Peak proportions Upper | Peak proportions Lower |
Litter no.								
ICMs from intact very late blastocysts								
310	14	1.34	2.28	2.59	4.09	1.58	.71	.29
305	17	1.15	5.90	1.48	2.34	1.58	.52	.48
			Sum 8.18‡					
ICMs from very late blastocysts with torn trophectoderm								
312	7	1.41	5.38	2.17	3.80	1.75	.57	.43
319	11	.68	13.62	1.35	2.43	1.80	.38	.62
			Sum 19.00§					
Implanted embryos - whole								
day 5 - 279	24		.89	.49	.67	1.35	.47	.53
day 6 - 114	16		4.82	1.04	1.35	1.30	.51	.49
day 6 - 313	23		.39	1.39	1.70	1.22	.57	.43
			Sum 6.10†					

Implanted embryos - slice of
ectoderm plus endoderm

day 6 - 321	13	2.76	.75	.97	1.29	.40	.60
day 7 - 315	15	2.26	.97	1.19	1.23	.52	.48
		Sum 5.02[†]					

* Mean HGPRT activities are expressed as pmol per hour per embryo.

† P>.10   ‡ .05<P<.10   § P<.001

** Means for HGPRT/LDH ratios are expressed as pmol per nmol

We are grateful to Dr. Eric Bradford for the Sl strain of mice, Dr. Jon Gallant for advice on chromatography, Dr. Jurg Ott for statistical help, and Bill Frels for helpful discussion. This work was supported by NIG grants GM15253-11 and GM670727. S.M.G. is a recipient of an NIH Research Career Award.

REFERENCES

Adler, D. A., J. D. West, and V. M. Chapman. 1977. Expression of α-galactosidase in preimplantation mouse embryos. Nature, Lond. 267: 838-839.

Chapman, V. M., J. D. West, and D. A. Adler. 1978. Bimodal distribution of α-galactosidase activities in mouse embryos. In, Genetic Mosaics and Chimeras in Mammals, Liane B. Russell, Ed. Plenum Press, New York and London.

DeMars, R. 1967. The single-active X: functional differentiation at the chromosome level. Nat. Cancer Inst. Monogr. 26: 327-351.

Deol, M. S. and W. K. Whitten. 1972. X-chromosome inactivation: does it occur at the same time in all cells of the embryo? Nature New Biol. 240: 277-279.

Eklund, J. and G. E. Bradford. 1977. Genetic analysis of a strain of mice plateaued for litter size. Genetics 85: 529-542.

Epstein, C. J. 1972. Expression of the mammalian X chromosome before and after fertilization. Science 175: 1467-1468.

Epstein, C. J. 1975. Gene expression and macromolecular synthesis during preimplantation embryonic development. Biol. Reprod. 12: 82-105.

Epstein, C. J., S. Smith, B. Travis, and G. Tucker. 1978. Both X chromosomes function prior to X-chromosome inactivation in female mouse embryos. Nature, Lond., in press.

Epstein, C. J., B. Travis, G. Tucker, and S. Smith. 1978. The direct demonstration of an X-chromosome dosage effect. In, Genetic Mosaics and Chimeras in Mammals, Liane B. Russell, Ed. Plenum Press, New York and London.

Gardner, R. L. and M. F. Lyon. 1971. X-chromosome inactivation studied by injection of a single cell into the mouse blastocyst. Nature 231: 385-386.

Johnson, M. H., A. H. Handyside, and P. R. Braude. 1977. Control mechanisms in early mammalian development. In, Development in Mammals, Volume 2. M. H. Johnson, Ed.

Kratzer, P. G. and S. M. Gartler. 1978. HGPRT activity changes in preimplantation mouse embryos. Nature, Lond., in press.

Lyon, M. F. 1972. X-chromosome inactivation and developmental patterns in mammals. Biol. Rev. 47: 1-35.

McLaren, A. 1976. Growth from fertilization to birth in the mouse. In, Embryogenesis in Mammals (CIBA Found. Symp. 40 New Series), Elsevier, Amsterdam, pp. 47-51.

Monk, M. 1978a. Biochemical studies on mammalian X-chromosome activity. In, Development in Mammals, Volume 3. M. H. Johnson, Ed.

Monk, M. 1978b. Biochemical studies on X-chromosome activity in preimplantation mouse embryos. In, Genetic Mosaics and Chimeras in Mammals, Liane B. Russell, Ed. Plenum Press, New York and London.

Monk, M. and H. Kathuria. 1977. Dosage compensation for an X-linked gene in preimplantation mouse embryos. Nature, Lond. 270: 599-601.

Nesbitt, M. N. 1971. X-chromosome inactivation mosaicism in the mouse. Develop. Biol. 26: 252-263.

Solter, D. and B. B. Knowles. 1975. Immunosurgery of mouse blastocyst. Proc. Natl. Acad. Sci. USA 72: 5099-5102.

Takagi, N. 1974. Differentiation of X chromosomes in early female mouse embryos. Exp. Cell Res. 86: 127-135.

Takagi, N. 1978. Preferential inactivation of the paternally derived X chromosome in mice. In, Genetic Mosaics and Chimeras in Mammals, Liane B. Russell, Ed. Plenum Press, New York and London.

Takagi, N. and M. Sasaki. 1975. Preferential inactivation of the paternally derived X chromosome in the extraembryonic membranes of the mouse. Nature, Lond. 256: 640-642.

West, J. D., V. E. Papaioannou, W. I. Frels, and V. M. Chapman. 1978. Preferential expression of the maternally derived X chromosome in extraembryonic tissues of the mouse. In, Genetic Mosaics and Chimeras in Mammals, Liane B. Russell, Ed. Plenum Press, New York and London.

West, J. D., W. I. Frels, V. M. Chapman, and V. E. Papaioannou.
1977. Preferential expression of the maternally derived X chromosome in the mouse yolk sac. Cell 12: 873–882.

THE DIRECT DEMONSTRATION OF AN X-CHROMOSOME DOSAGE EFFECT PRIOR

TO INACTIVATION

Charles J. Epstein, Bruce Travis, Georgianne Tucker,
and Sandra Smith

Departments of Pediatrics and of Biochemistry and Biophysics, University of California, San Francisco,
California 94143

When the X-linked enzyme, hypoxanthine guanine phosphoribosyltransferase (HGPRT), was found to increase significantly in activity
during the morula stage of preimplantation mouse embryonic development (Epstein 1970), it was obvious that this enzyme would be a
useful marker for studying the control of X-chromosome expression.
This conviction was strengthened by the finding that, while still
present at the 2-cell stage, the gene dosage effect related to the
number of X chromosomes present during oogenesis is no longer present after blastulation, indicating that the increase in HGPRT
activity is determined by the embryonic genome (Epstein 1972).

The questions of immediate interest were whether both X chromosomes in female embryos function prior to the time of X inactivation, and, if so, when functional inactivation occurs. Therefore,
using the same reasoning as was applied to the study of X-chromosome function during oogenesis (Epstein 1969, 1972), numerous attempts were made to find a bimodal distribution of the activity of
HGPRT in single preimplantation mouse embryos. Such a finding would
be compatible with the conclusion that both female X chromosomes
function prior to inactivation. For various technical and methodo-
logical reasons, we were unable to demonstrate such a distribution,
although very recent work in several laboratories (Kratzer and
Gartler 1978; Chapman, West, and Adler 1978; Monk 1978) has now
shown that a bimodal distribution does exist. However, the validity of the gene-dosage approach for studying embryonic X-chromosome
expression was established when it was found that mouse teratocarcinoma cells known to have two X chromosomes have twice as much of
several X-linked enzymes as do teratocarcinoma cells with only one
X chromosome (Martin, Epstein, Travis, Tucker, Yatziv, Martin,

261

Clift, and Cohen 1978). Because of the probable equivalence of the teratocarcinoma cells to embryonic ectoderm (Martin, Smith, and Epstein 1978), these findings also suggested that it should be possible to find a similar gene-dosage effect in normal preimplantation embryos of known sex.

Since no unequivocal method for non-destructively sexing intact preimplantation mouse embryos is yet known, we decided to make use of a strategy based on the creation of identical twin embryos (Epstein, Smith, Travis, and Tucker 1978). This approach, which is shown schematically in Figure 1, permits one member of each pair to be used for sex determination by chromosome analysis, and the other for biochemical assay. By storing the half-embryos to be assayed while the karyotyping is being performed, it is possible to pool the half-embryos into groups of sufficient size (usually 5 to 7) to make the enzyme assays technically convenient and reliable.

The separated blastomeres develop a little more slowly into half-blastocysts (Fig. 2) than do whole control embryos cultured

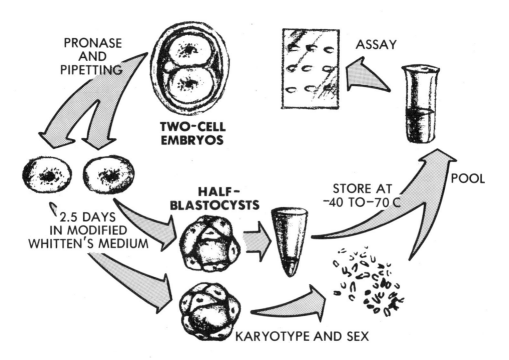

FIGURE 1. Preparation of half-blastocysts. General strategy for the production and analysis of half-blastocysts for experiments requiring knowledge of karyotype or sex. The technical details are described in Epstein *et al.* (1978).

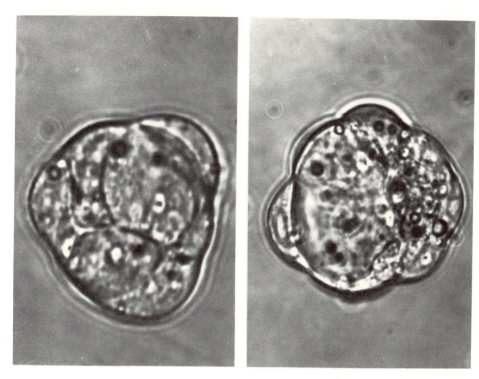

FIGURE 2.   Half-blastocysts.   Phase contrast.

in parallel, with blastulation occurring about 4 hours later. Both
members of a pair blastulate 71% of the time which, when combined
with a karyotyping success rate of 47%, gives an overall efficiency
of 33%. At the time of karyotyping, male and female embryos had an
identical number of cells, and the standard deviations of the cell
numbers were also the same (Table 1). The male to female sex ratio
was 0.89.

TABLE 1.   Number of cells in half blastocysts

Mixed male and female half-blastocysts	29.8 ± 2.7* cells
Known male half-blastocysts	30.0 ± 2.6 cells
Known female half-blastocysts	29.6 ± 2.7 cells

* Standard deviation

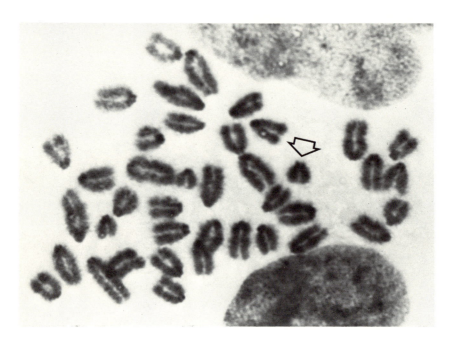

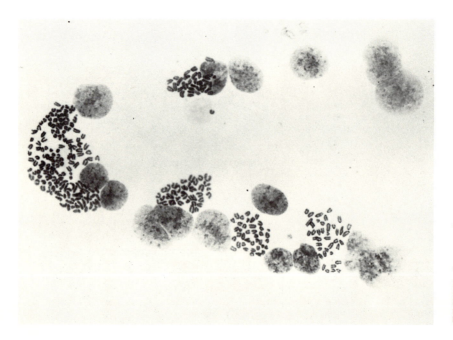

FIGURE 3. Left: Spread of whole male half-blastocyst, showing several metaphases. Right: Higher magnification of single metaphase, with Y chromosome indicated by arrow.

One half-blastocyst from each pair was frozen for assay within 2 hours of the time of blastulation, and the other karyotyped (Fig. 3) to determine the sex of the embryo. The embryos were then pooled and assayed for HGPRT or APRT by the method of Kratzer and Gartler (1978). While there was no difference between males and females in mean activities of the autosomally controlled APRT, the mean HGPRT activity of the female embryos was 2.2 times that of the males (Fig. 4). Of interest, although unexplained, is the fact that the spread of individual values was greater for the female embryos than for the male embryos for both the APRT and HGPRT determinations.

When later half-blastocysts, obtained 12—18 hours after blastulation, were assayed for HGPRT activity, no significant difference between male and female embryos was found. Again, the greater variability of the female activities was apparent (Fig. 4). Since this represented the same stage at which the cell number determinations were done, the sex difference in variability cannot be attributed to a greater variability in the number of cells in female embryos.

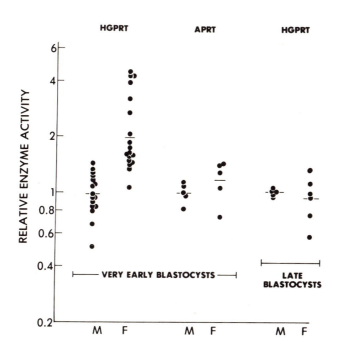

FIGURE 4. HGPRT and APRT activities in very early and in late blastocysts of known sex. The activities are plotted logarithmically to reduce the spread. The technical details are described in Epstein *et al.* (1978).

   We interpret our findings as indicating that both female X chromosomes function prior to the time of inactivation. Although the failure to find a dosage effect in late blastocysts could be interpreted to mean that inactivation has occurred, the fact that HGPRT activity may be falling during this period (Epstein 1970) makes such an inference hazardous, particularly since it is at variance with the teratocarcinoma results (Martin *et al.* 1978a). Therefore, experiments are now in progress to examine the activities of X-linked enzymes in sexed inner cell masses and embryos at later stages of development.

REFERENCES

Chapman, V. M., J. D. West and D. A. Adler. 1978. Bimodal distribution of α-galactosidase activity in mouse embryos. In Genetic Mosaics and Chimeras in Mammals, Liane B. Russell, Ed., Plenum Press, New York and London.

Epstein, C. J. 1969. Mammalian oocytes: X-chromosome activity. Science 163: 1078-1079.

Epstein, C. J. 1970. Phosphoribosyltransferase activity during early mammalian development. J. Biol. Chem. 245: 3289-3294.

Epstein, C. J. 1972. Expression of the mammalian X-chromosome before and after fertilization. Science 175: 1467-1468.

Epstein, C. J., S. Smith, B. Travis and G. Tucker. 1978. Both X-chromosomes function prior to X-chromosome inactivation in female mouse embryos. Nature, in press.

Kratzer, P. G. and S. M. Gartler. 1978. HGPRT expression in early mouse development. In Genetic Mosaics and Chimeras in Mammals, Liane B. Russell, Ed., Plenum Press, New York and London.

Martin, G. R., C. J. Epstein, B. Travis, G. Tucker, S. Yatziv, D. W. Martin, Jr., S. Clift and S. Cohen. 1978a. X-chromosome inactivation during differentiation of female teratocarcinoma stem cells *in vitro*. Nature 271: 329-333.

Martin, G. R., S. Smith and C. J. Epstein. 1978. Protein synthetic patterns in teratocarcinoma stem cells and mouse embryos at early stages of development. Develop. Biol., in press.

Monk, M. 1978. Biochemical studies on X-chromosome activity in preimplantation mouse embryos. In Genetic Mosaics and Chimeras in Mammals, Liane B. Russell, Ed., Plenum Press, New York and London.

This work was supported by grants from the National Institutes of Health (HD 03132) and the National Foundation – March of Dimes. C.J.E. is an Investigator of the Howard Hughes Medical Institute. Valuable technical assistance was provided by Ms. Estrella Lamela and Ms. Teodosia Zamora.

USE OF TERATOCARCINOMA STEM CELLS AS A MODEL SYSTEM FOR THE STUDY

OF X-CHROMOSOME INACTIVATION *IN VITRO*

Gail R. Martin[1], Charles J. Epstein[2], and David W. Martin, Jr.[3]

[1]Department of Anatomy and Cancer Research Institute, [2]Departments of Pediatrics and of Biochemistry and Biophysics, [3]Departments of Medicine and of Biochemistry and Biophysics, University of California, San Francisco, Calif. 94143

INTRODUCTION

One of the main obstacles to the study of the mechanism of X-chromosome differentiation or "X inactivation" is the difficulty of obtaining a population of embryonic cells in which both X chromosomes are functioning. The primary reason for this is that male embryos cannot be easily distinguished from female embryos, and therefore half of any random population of embryos will be males that contain only one X chromosome. Furthermore, since it is now apparent that X inactivation probably does not occur in all the cells of the embryo at the same time, there would be the additional difficulty of identifying and separating those cells in which both X chromosomes are active, even if a pure population of female embryos could be obtained. Since teratocarcinoma stem cells are closely similar to normal early embryonic cells and they are available in almost unlimited quantities, the goal of the research described here was to determine whether it might be possible to use clonal cultures of female teratocarcinoma stem cells, in place of embryonic cells, to study the phenomenon of X-chromosome inactivation. The results of this study have been described previously (Martin, Epstein, Travis, Tucker, Yatziv, Martin, Clift, and Cohen 1978).

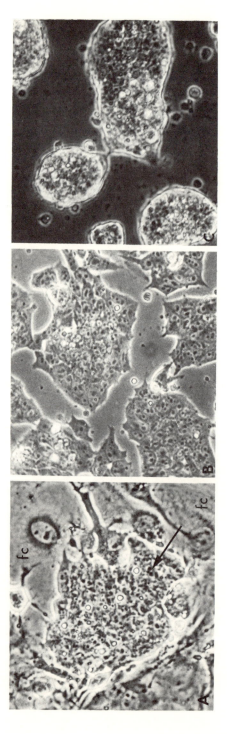

FIGURE 1

Similarities between teratocarcinoma cells and embryonic cells

    The analogy between mouse teratocarcinoma stem cells (embryo-
nal carcinoma cells) and the cells of the normal early embryo is
well documented (reviewed by Martin 1975, 1978; Graham 1977). The
fundamental similarity is that the tumor stem cells, like early
embryonic cells, are pluripotent. They are capable of proliferation in the undifferentiated state, and of differentiation to a
wide variety of cell types, both *in vivo* and *in vitro*.

    The full extent of their developmental capacity *in vivo* has
been dramatically demonstrated by experiments in which these tumor
stem cells were injected into a host mouse blastocyst and the ope-
rated embryo placed in the uterus of a foster mother. Many of the
animals born in these experiments have been shown to be chimeric
and to contain a variety of tissues derived from the injected embryonal carcinoma cells as well as from the host blastocysts (Brinster 1974, 1975; Mintz and Illmensee 1975; Illmensee and Mintz
1976; Papaioannou, McBurney, Gardner, and Evans 1975; Papaioannou,
Gardner, McBurney, Babinet, and Evans 1978; Dewey, Martin, Martin,
and Mintz 1977). Most striking were the results which showed that
embryonal carcinoma cells are able to form functional germ cells
in the chimeric animals (Mintz and Illmensee 1975; reviewed by
Illmensee 1978).

Behavior of teratocarcinoma stem cells in vitro

    The ability to behave like normal embryonic cells *in vitro* is
also retained by some established teratocarcinoma stem cell lines.
In particular, certain clonal embryonal carcinoma cell lines will

←———————————————————————

FIGURE 1.   Phase contrast photomicrographs of embryonal carcinoma
        cells (approx. 350 x). (Reduced 35% for purposes of reproduction)
        (A) Stem cell colony (arrow) on a fibroblastic feeder cell
        layer (fc).
        (B) Embryonal carcinoma cells shortly after passage to a cul-
        ture dish without feeder cells. Even when the cells are care-
        fully disassociated and are plated as a single-cell suspen-
        sion, they rapidly adhere to each other and form colonies
        which flatten on the tissue-culture surface. The boundaries
        between the individual cells are indistinct. Each cell is
        rounded or slightly bipolar, with a large, pale nucleus con-
        taining one or two distinct nucleoli.
        (C) Embryonal carcinoma cells approximately four days after
        passage to a culture dish without feeders. The cells have
        proliferated; and, as the colonies grow larger, they become
        rounder and less well attached to the tissue-culture sub-
        stratum.

differentiate in a manner that closely parallels the normal early postimplantation development of the mouse (Martin and Evans 1975*a, b*; Martin, Wiley, and Damjanov 1977). Such cell lines are maintained in the undifferentiated state by frequent subculture to a confluent fibroblastic feeder cell layer (Figs. 1, 2). This culture procedure probably acts in three nonspecific ways to inhibit differentiation. First, the feeder cells may provide factors that stimulate embryonal carcinoma cells to proliferate more rapidly (Martin and Evans 1975*b*). Such rapid growth may, in some way, be incompatible with a switch to differentiated functions. Second, it has been observed that when embryonal carcinoma cells are disaggregated and re-plated, they rapidly form aggregates that assume a more flattened geometry when cultured on a confluent feeder-cell layer. Since the process of forming a more rounded, three-dimensional structure apparently triggers differentiation (see below), the feeder effect of flattening the aggregates probably inhibits differentiation. Third, frequent subculture prevents the colonies of cells from becoming very large and rounding up, a process that would trigger their differentiation even in the presence of feeder cells (Evans and Martin 1975).

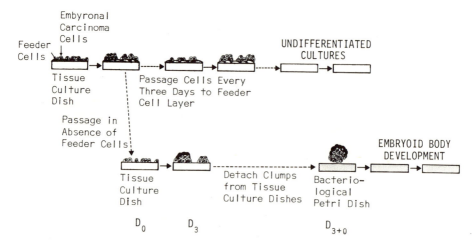

FIGURE 2. Diagram of culture regime for feeder-dependent embryonal carcinoma cells that form embryoid bodies *in vitro*. [From Martin *et al*. 1978*a*, reproduced by permission.]

To initiate differentiation, the cells are seeded in the absence of a feeder layer, and the clumps that form are not disaggregated. Instead, they are detached and cultured in suspension
(by plating in bacteriological petri dishes to which they do not
adhere). This allows the clumps to become very rounded (Fig. 2).
When this occurs, they begin the differentiative process known as
"embryoid body" formation (Pierce and Dixon 1959; Stevens 1959).
The first stage in the process, similar to that of the first stage
in the development of the mouse inner cell mass, is the differentiation of an outer layer of endoderm. When this culture regime
is followed, virtually every cell clump in the population synchronously forms such a two-layered "simple" embryoid body (Fig.
3).

Almost all of the pluripotent embryonal carcinoma cell lines
that we have isolated form simple embryoid bodies *in vitro*. While
some of these cell lines form embryoid bodies that remain as simple, two-layered structures when kept in suspension, other embryonal

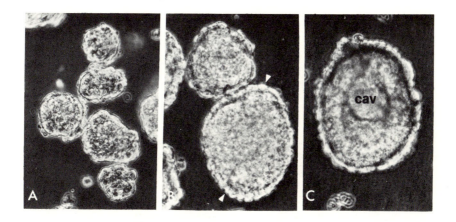

FIGURE 3. Embryoid body formation, as observed in the phase con-
    trast microscope (approx. 175 x).
    (A) Clumps of embryonal carcinoma cells formed in the ab-
    sence of feeder cells, at the time of detachment from the
    tissue culture substratum.
    (B) After 2 days in suspension, the embryonal carcinoma
    cell clumps have become simple embryoid bodies. Pointers
    indicate the outer layer of endoderm.
    (C) The simple embryoid bodies formed by some embryonal car-
    cinoma cell lines will continue to develop when cultured in
    suspension, forming cystic embryoid bodies with a central
    cavity (cav).
    [From Martin, Wiley, and Damjanov 1977; reproduced by per-
    mission.]

carcinoma cell lines form embryoid bodies that continue to differentiate when cultured in suspension. This more complex pattern of
differentiation, known as "cystic" embryoid body formation,
parallels the development of the inner cell mass and its derivatives during the early postimplantation phase of embryonic development (Figs. 3, 4).

Origin of mouse teratocarcinomas

In order to study the phenomenon of X-chromosome inactivation
in teratocarcinoma stem cells, cell lines obviously must be isolated from a female teratocarcinoma. Such tumors can be obtained
in two ways. First, they arise spontaneously in the ovary from
oocytes that have been parthenogenetically activated *in situ* (Stevens and Varnum 1974). Such ovarian oocytes have already completed
the first meiotic division (Eppig, Kozak, Eicher, and Stevens 1977)
and, following activation, they undergo a brief period of normal
embryonic development. Subsequently, their growth becomes disorganized and they form a tumor in the ovary. While most of the
tumors that form in this way are benign teratomas and consist of
only differentiated embryonic tissues, some are malignant teratocarcinomas which contain undifferentiated pluripotent stem cells
in addition to the differentiated cell types. This process of
spontaneous parthenogenesis, embryonic development, and subsequent
ovarian tumor formation occurs with high frequency in the LT strain
of mouse, and it has been found that approximately 50% of all adult
LT females have such ovarian tumors (Stevens and Varnum 1974).

It is also possible to induce female teratocarcinomas by
transplanting female embryos of any age up to 7.5 days of development to an extrauterine site such as the kidney or the testis of
an adult mouse. Like the spontaneous parthenogenetic embryos which
find themselves in an ectopic site (the ovary), the experimentally
transplanted embryos grow into disorganized tissue masses that are
either benign teratomas or malignant stem-cell-containing teratocarcinomas. Unlike the spontaneous ovarian tumors, the experimentally induced tumors are not parthenogenetic in origin (unless
experimentally activated parthenotes are grafted, as in the work
of Iles, McBurney, Bramwell, Deussen, and Graham 1975). In fact,
normal transplanted mouse embryos, derived from fertilized eggs
of either sex, will give rise to such tumors. Experimentally-
induced tumors have been obtained in this way from embryos of
several different inbred strains (Stevens 1968, 1970; Solter,
Skreb, and Damjanov 1970; Damjanov and Solter 1974).

Tumors can also form spontaneously in male mice. In contrast
to the spontaneous ovarian and embryo-derived tumors, testicular
tumors apparently do not arise as disorganized embryos. Instead

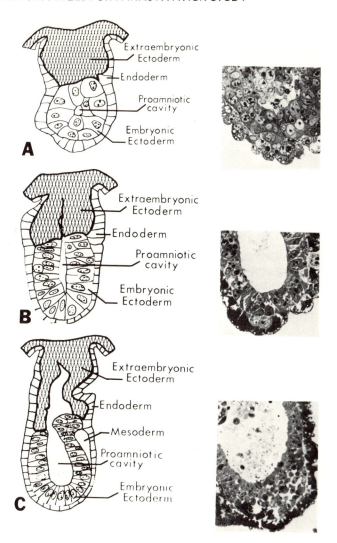

FIGURE 4. Similarity between cystic embryoid body development and normal early postimplantation development. A, B, and C are schematic representations of normal embryos at approximately 5, 6, and 7 days of development, respectively. To the right of each are sections of morphologically similar stages in the development of cystic embryoid bodies formed by embryonal carcinoma cells. (Magnification approx. 250 x for A and B; 200 x for C.)
[From Martin 1978; reproduced by permission.]

they are initiated when primordial germ cells begin abnormal proliferation during the development of the fetal testis (reviewed
by Stevens, 1975). However, aside from this difference in ontogeny,
no consistent biochemical, morphological, or behavioral differences
have as yet been detected between the stem cell of spontaneous
testicular tumors and the stem cells of either ovarian or embryo-
derived teratocarcinomas. Once stem-cell-containing tumors are
generated, either spontaneously or by experimental manipulation,
pluripotent embryonal carcinoma cell lines can be established from
them.

RATIONALE

The premise upon which we based our experiments is that, in
biochemical terms, X-chromosome differentiation is indeed an inactivation process, and that therefore both X chromosomes are genetically active in the embryo prior to X-chromosome differentiation.
There is now experimental evidence to support this hypothesis
(Epstein, Smith, Travis, and Tucker 1978; Chapman, West, and Adler
1978; Kratzer and Gartler 1978; Epstein, Travis, Tucker, and Smith
1978; Monk 1978).

If female teratocarcinoma stem cells are similar to the undifferentiated cells in the embryo at a time prior to X inactivation,
these cells should also contain two genetically active X chromosomes. If both X chromosomes are producing gene products in a
dosage-dependent manner, the level of any X-linked gene products
in the female teratocarcinoma stem cells with two X chromosomes
should be twice that in comparable male cells with one X chromosome. On the other hand, autosomal gene products should be present
in the same amount in the female and male cells, because both
should contain the same number of copies of these genes. To test
this, we isolated appropriate cell lines and measured the levels
of X-linked and autosomal gene products in these cells.

RESULTS

Description of cell lines isolated

Ideally we would like to study the X-chromosome activity in
female teratocarcinoma stem cells derived from tumors of both
spontaneous parthenogenetic and normal embryo origin. To this end
we isolated embryonal carcinoma cells from one spontaneous ovarian
(LT strain) and two embryo-derived tumors (AKR and 129 strains),
in the hope that one or both of the latter would be female. Also,
to obtain a male embryonal carcinoma cell line we isolated cells

from a spontaneous testicular tumor of the Large (LG) strain. In all cases, the isolation procedures described by Martin and Evans (1975*a, b*) were employed. The cells thus obtained were pluripotent clonal lines the growth of which in the undifferentiated state is feeder-dependent. All of these cell lines begin their differentiation with the formation of endoderm when they are cultured as described above (Fig. 2).

Cytogenetic analysis showed that, as expected, the ovarian LT tumor stem cells contained two X chromosomes. However, the other three cell lines each contained only one X chromosome; and none had a Y chromosome, even though the LG cell line was derived from a spontaneous testicular tumor and was thus definitely male in origin. It is possible that one or both of the embryo-derived embryonal carcinoma cell lines may have been female in origin and have lost an X chromosome either during growth in the tumor or following culture *in vitro*; however, it is equally possible that they were male and lost a Y chromosome. Figure 5 shows that each of the four cell lines examined has a diploid, or near-diploid, modal chromosome number, and that each has some chromosomal abnormalities. This is consistent with the observation that embryonal carcinoma cells are unusual among mouse cells in that they remain diploid, or near-diploid, even after long periods in culture. This observation led to the assumption that embryonal carcinoma cells generally remained euploid in culture; but more recently, when careful cytogenetic analysis was carried out, almost all established embryonal carcinoma cell lines were found to have small aneuploidies (reviewed by Graham, 1977).

In spite of its chromosomal abnormalities, the XX-LT cell line we isolated is appropriate for our purposes because simple autosomal aneuploidy does not interfere with X-chromosome differentiation (Gartler and Andina 1976). The three XO cell lines are also appropriate for comparison with the female cells, because they each contain only one X chromosome and for our purposes could thus be considered "males."

Evidence for two genetically active X chromosomes
in undifferentiated female teratocarcinoma stem cells

To test our hypothesis that both X chromosomes are genetically active in the female teratocarcinoma cells, we measured the levels of ten different enzymes in the XX-LT and XO cell lines. Of the enzymes tested, three are known to be X-linked in the mouse (Kozak, Nichols, and Ruddle 1975; Chapman and Shows 1976): glucose-6-phosphate dehydrogenase (G6PD, EC 1.1.1.49), α-galactosidase (α-gal, EC 3.2.1.22), and hypoxanthine-guanine phosphoribosyl transferase (HGPRT, EC 2.4.2.8). Of the other seven, five are known to be autosomal in the mouse (Kozak *et al.* 1975; Mouse News Letter 1977):

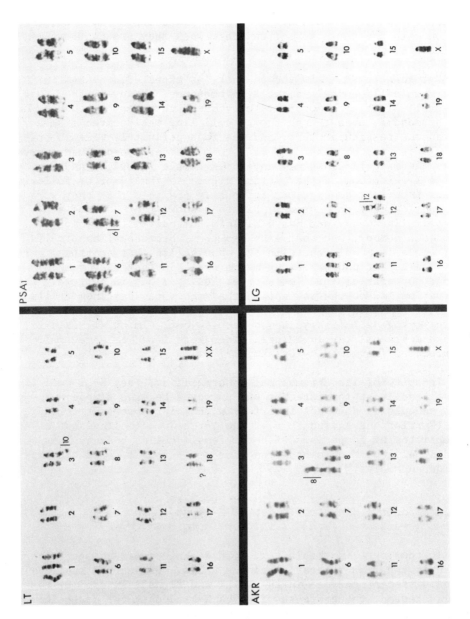

Figure 5

isocitrate dehydrogenase (Id-1; ICDH, EC 1.1.1.41), β-galactosi-
dase (β-gal, EC 3.2.1.23), β-glucuronidase (β-gluc, EC 3.2.1.31),
adenine phosphoribosyl transferase (APRT, EC 2.4.2.7), and 6-phos-
phogluconate dehydrogenase (6PGD, EC 1.1.1.44); the remaining two
are considered to be autosomal by analogy with man: adenosine
kinase (AK, EC 2.7.1.20) and β-N-acetyl-glucosaminidase (β-NAC-
gluc, EC 3.2.1.30).

The specific activities of these enzymes are shown in Table 1.
Although the actual specific activities varied as much as three-
fold, the ratio of specific activities in the XX-LT cells to those
in the XO cells was constant for each enzyme from one experiment
to the next (Fig. 6). For all seven autosomal enzymes tested in
the cell lines, the levels were the same in the XX-LT as in the XO
cells (APRT was not tested in the AKR and LG cells). In contrast,
the levels of all three X-linked enzymes were twice as high in the
XX-LT cells as in the XO cells.

It seems unlikely that these results are related to the aneuploid chromosome constitution of the different cell lines. The
same results were obtained when the XX-LT cells were compared with
XO teratocarcinoma stem cells from three unrelated mouse strains,
LG, AKR and 129, each of which had a different chromosomal abnormality (Fig. 5). Moreover, similar results were obtained with a
second LT cell line (clone 2, Table 1B), chromosomally different
from the first. This cell line, isolated from the same tumor as
the LT cells (clone 1) described above, has a modal chromosome
number of 40 (trisomic for chromosome 11 and monosomic for chromosome 6, with a few small autosomal rearrangements).

These results are consistent with the hypothesis that certain
genes on both X chromosomes are being expressed in the undifferentiated female teratocarcinoma stem cells. Presumably these are
the genes that are normally expressed early in mouse peri-implan-
tation development. We have still to determine whether this is
also true for other X-linked genes. For example, we have yet to
assay phosphoglycerate kinase (PKG 2.7.2.3), an X-linked enzyme
that is known to be induced during the early postimplantation
development of the mouse (Kozak and Quinn 1975). Still other
X-linked genes, such as that for ornithine carbamoyltransferase
(EC 2.1.3.3; DeMars, LeVan, Trend, and Russell 1976) are unlikely
to be transcribed from either X chromosome in the undifferentiated
teratocarcinoma cells, because they are specific to certain differentiated tissues.

FIGURE 5. Giemsa-banded karyotypes of teratocarcinoma stem cell
      lines. [From Martin et al. 1978a; reproduced by permission.]

TABLE 1. Specific activities* of enzymes in undifferentiated teratocarcinoma stem cells [From Martin et al. 1978]

$A^{\dagger}$		LT-XX (clone 1)	PSA1-XO	LG-XO	AKR-XO	Ratio§ $\frac{\text{LT(clone 1)}}{\text{PSA1}}$
X-linked Enzymes:						
G6PD	Expt. 1**	148.	73.	72.	75.	1.93 ± 0.04
	2**	52.	27.	32.	25.	
HGPRT	Expt. 1	4.6	2.3	2.4	3.8	2.16 ± 0.07
	2	3.1	1.7	1.6	2.2	
α-gal	Expt. 1	5.8	3.2	3.3	3.5	1.73 ± 0.06
	2	5.3	3.2	2.8	2.5	
Autosomal Enzymes:						
ICDH	Expt. 1	20.	21.	22.	20.	0.94 ± 0.08
	2	46.	44.	43.	40.	
β-gal	Expt. 1	2.5	2.7	2.0	3.2	0.95 ± 0.08
	2	2.8	3.5	2.8	2.5	
β-gluc	Expt. 1	2.7	2.9	1.9	1.9	0.86 ± 0.11
	2	1.9	3.0	2.8	2.3	
β-NAC-gluc	Expt. 1	75.	72.	73.	58.	0.99 ± 0.04
	2	68.	68.	66.	70.	

B‡		LT-XX (clone 1)	LT-XX (clone 2)	PSA1-XO	Ratio§ $\frac{\text{LT (clone 2)}}{\text{PSA1}}$
X-linked Enzymes:					
G6PD	Expt. 1	162.	145.	78.	1.88 ± 0.02
	2	192.	170.	92.	
HGPRT	Expt. 1	4.0	4.2	2.0	1.94 ± 0.15
	2	5.8	4.7	2.9	
Autosomal Enzymes:					
APRT	Expt. 1	4.8	3.9	4.6	0.77 ± 0.04
	2	3.5	3.2	4.5	
AK	Expt. 1	1.4	1.5	1.7	0.93 ± 0.11
	2	1.6	1.6	1.9	
6PGD	Expt. 1	95.	108.	107.	1.03 ± 0.04
	2	133.	140.	123.	

* Specific activities are expressed as nmoles product formed per min/mg protein.

† Enzymes assayed in all four of the cell lines shown in Fig. 5.

†† Comparison of specific activities of five enzymes in two independent clones derived from LT tumor 72484. The karyotype of clone 1 is shown in Figure 5. Clone 2 differs as described in the text.

§ The ratios given are based on the data from at least three independent experiments, including the two shown. They are reported with their standard errors.

** The data shown from two independent experiments in each case represent the extreme variation between experiments.

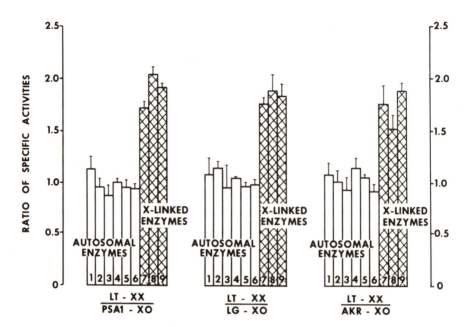

FIGURE 6. Mean ratios (with s.e.m.) of specific activities of
    enzymes in undifferentiated XX–LT cells compared with XO
    embryonal carcinoma cells.
    1, adenosine kinase; 2, β–galactosidase; 3, β–glucuronidase;
    4, β–N–Ac–glucosaminidase; 5, isocitrate dehydrogenase;
    6, 6–phosphogluconate dehydrogenase; 7, α–galactosidase;
    8, hypoxanthine–guanine phosphoribosyl transferase; 9, glu-
    cose–6–phosphate dehydrogenase.
    [From Martin *et al.* 1978*a*; reproduced by permission.]

*Evidence for X–chromosome inactivation during
differentiation of LT cells in vitro*

    If both X chromosomes are active in undifferentiated LT cells,
it can be inferred that these tumor stem cells are similar to
embryonic cells at a stage before X–chromosome inactivation.
Because the teratocarcinoma stem cells are very much like inner-
cell-mass cells or embryonic ectoderm (Martin, Smith, and Epstein
1978) during the early postimplantation period, when X inactivation
is probably occurring *in vivo,* it seemed likely that these cells
would undergo changes in X–chromosome activity if they differen-

tiated *in vitro*. To test this, we cultured both the XX–LT cells
and the XO–PSA1 (strain 129) cells in parallel. The PSA1 cell
line was chosen as a representative "male" because, of the three
XO cell lines described here, PSA1 cells and their derivatives
have been the most extensively characterized (Martin *et al.* 1977;
Dewey *et al.* 1977). Separate samples of the LT and PSA1 cells
were maintained in the undifferentiated state, or cultured in conditions conducive to differentiation (as described above, Fig. 2).
At 2–3 day intervals, all cells were assayed and the ratios of
specific activities of two X-linked and two autosomal enzymes were
determined in the XX compared with the XO cells.

The results of a typical experiment (Fig. 7) were those expected if X inactivation occurs during differentiation *in vitro*.
A striking change occurred in the ratio of XX to XO cells with respect to X-linked enzyme activity, beginning approximately 9 days
after plating the LT and PSA1 cells in the absence of feeders (i.e.,
the initiation of the differentiative process). The ratio of,
first, G6PD and then of HGPRT dropped from 2.0 to 1.0. In contrast, the ratios of activities of these X-linked enzymes remained
constant at 2.0 if the LT and PSA1 cells were maintained in the
undifferentiated state. Also, as expected, the ratios of activities
of autosomal enzymes remained 1.0, whether or not the cells differentiated. Similar results were obtained when the levels of G6PD
in the differentiating XX–LT cells were compared with those in the
other two XO cell lines (AKR and LG; HGPRT was not measured in these
experiments.

Figure 8 shows that the change in X-linked enzyme activity was
specific to the differentiative process. Samples of LT and PSA1
cells were allowed to differentiate, while the parent cultures were
maintained in the undifferentiated state. When G6PD activity in
the former had decreased, indicating X-chromosome inactivation,
second samples of the undifferentiated LT and PSA1 parent cultures
were subcultured in conditions conducive to differentiation. In
both cases, the decrease in activity began approximately 9 days
after the initiation of differentiation. No change in the karyotype of the LT cells occurred during differentiation.

                              DISCUSSION

The simplest hypothesis that is completely consistent with the
data described above is that both X chromosomes are active in undifferentiated stem cells derived from a spontaneous ovarian
teratocarcinoma, and that inactivation occurs when the cells are
allowed to differentiate *in vitro*. This interpretation of the
data assumes the validity of the premise that the amount of gene
product present in a cell is directly proportional to the number
of active genes.

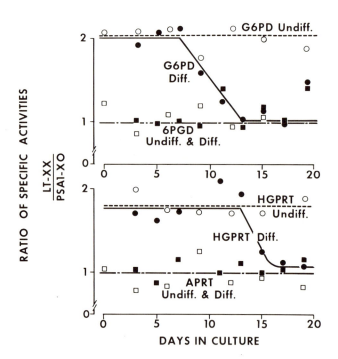

FIGURE 7.   Levels of X-linked gene products during differentiation
of teratocarcinoma stem cells *in vitro*.
Cultures of LT and PSA1 cells were maintained in the undifferentiated state, or were subcultured (at day 0) in the
absence of feeder cells to begin differentiation. At various
times during the subsequent three weeks, samples of XX-LT and
XO-PSA1 cells were collected and enzyme levels assayed. The
data shown are typical of the results obtained in two other
such experiments.
-o-, X-linked enzymes in undifferentiated cells
-●-, X-linked enzymes in differentiating cells
-□-, autosomal enzymes in undifferentiated cells
-■-, autosomal enzymes in differentiating cells
[From Martin *et al*. 1978*a*; reproduced by permission.]

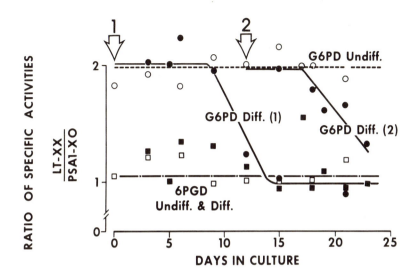

FIGURE 8.   Relationship between levels of X-linked gene products
   and the initiation of differentiation.
   Cultures of LT and PSA1 cells were maintained in the undifferentiated state. At day 0 (arrow 1), one sample of XX-LT cells
   and one of XO-PSA1 cells were subcultured in the absence of
   feeder cells to initiate differentiation. At day 12 (arrow
   2), a second sample of undifferentiated LT and of PSA1 cells
   was subcultured in the absence of feeder cells to begin differentiation. Portions of each cell population were collected
   at various times, and enzyme specific activities were determined.
   -o-, X-linked enzymes in undifferentiated cells
   -•-, X-linked enzymes in differentiating cells
   -□-, autosomal enzymes in undifferentiated cells
   -■-, autosomal enzymes in differentiating cells
   [From Martin *et al.* 1978*a*; reproduced by permission.]

Gene dosage as a measure of chromosome activity

     There is increasing evidence that, under appropriately con-
trolled conditions, quantification of enzyme activity can provide
a valid estimate of the number of functional genes or chromosomes.
Thus, when the loci under study have been mapped to specific
chromosomes by independent means, it has been possible to show

that the specific activity of each of several autosomal enzymes
is directly proportional to the number of autosomes present in the
cells which carry that locus (Marimo and Giannelli 1975; Magenis,
Koler, Lovrien, Bigley, DuVal, and Overton 1975; George and Francke
1976; Epstein, Tucker, Travis, and Gropp 1977; Feaster, Kwok, and
Epstein 1977; Eicher and Coleman 1977), or proportional to the
number of loci present (Bernstine, Russell, and Cain 1978). The
only important exception was found when blood cells from humans
with trisomy-21 were analyzed and found to have significantly increased levels of several enzymes, from which it was erroneously
concluded that the genes for these enzymes were on chromosome 21.
However, in that instance, the activities of appropriate control
enzymes, including one (G6PD) determined by an X-linked locus, were
also found to be altered (Baikie, Loder, DeGrouchy, and Pitt 1965),
thereby illustrating the difficulty of interpreting dosage effects
when the loci have not been mapped to specific chromosomes.

In terms of X-linked gene expression during development, the
precedent for the experiments described here is the assessment of
X-chromosome activity in developing oocytes by quantification of
gene dosage (Epstein 1969, 1972; Mangia, Abbo-Halbasch, and Epstein 1975). Those experiments were performed by taking advantage
of the existence of fertile female mice that are lacking an X-
chromosome (i.e. "XO" mice with only 39 chromosomes). Using two
of the three X-linked markers employed in the present study, G6PD
and HGPRT, it was demonstrated that oocytes from female mice with
two X chromosomes had twice the enzyme activity as did oocytes
from the XO females. This was true both during and at the completion of oogenesis. Similar studies carried out by Kozak, McLean,
and Eicher (1974) indicated that oocytes containing two X chromosomes had twice the level of PGK activity as did XO cells. In all
cases, the activities of the control autosomal enzymes were the
same in the two types of oocytes. The conclusion drawn from these
studies, that both X-chromosomes function during oogenesis, has
been confirmed by independent means in human oocytes (Gartler,
Liskay, Campbell, Sparkes, and Gant 1972; Migeon and Jelalian 1977).

Recently, several workers have been able to assay levels of
X-linked enzymes (HGPRT and α-gal) in individual preimplantation
embryos and have found evidence of a gene-dosage effect: a bimodal
distribution of activities was observed, with presumptive female
embryos having twice the activity of presumptive males (Chapman
et al. 1978; Monk 1978; Kratzer and Gartler 1978). In other
experiments using pools of half-blastocysts of known sex, the females had twice the activity of HGPRT as did the males (Epstein
et al. 1978a and b). Further studies on the level of PGK activity
in individual embryos developed from fertilized XX- and XO-derived
eggs indicated that, by 6 days of development, there is apparently
no dosage effect (Kozak and Quinn 1975). From this it was concluded that X inactivation had probably already occurred by this

stage of development. Taken together, these results suggest that measures of gene dosage of known X-linked markers represent an adequate means of monitoring X-chromosome activity in oocytes and developing embryos. Given the consistency of our results with all X-linked and control autosomal enzymes except isocitrate dehydrogenase (Id-1; see below), it seems likely that our experiments represent a valid approach to the study of X-chromosome function in teratocarcinoma stem cells.

Having thus presented the justification for using gene dosage as a measure of chromosome activity, it is necessary to point out an apparent exception that we have noted in our experiments. One of the autosomal control enzymes we measured was Id-1, governed by a locus on chromosome 1. Recent experiments have shown that trisomy for chromosome 1 results in a proportional increase in Id-1 activity in midgestation embryos (Epstein *et al.* 1977). However, the LT cell line (clone 1) described here is also trisomic for chromosome 1, but no similar dosage effect was noted. There are many possible reasons for the failure to find a dosage effect when one might be expected, and we do not believe this exception invalidates the interpretation we have placed on our other findings.

Alternative means of studying X-chromosome activity in teratocarcinoma stem cells

It would obviously be preferable to use a more direct measure of X-chromosome activity to prove that our interpretation of the data is correct and that female teratocarcinoma stem cells do contain two genetically active X chromosomes. Perhaps the best way to do this would be to make use of electrophoretic variants of X-linked markers. It is this approach which was originally used to demonstrate that only one X chromosome functions in female somatic cells such as fibroblasts (Davidson, Nitowsky, and Childs 1963). When the object is to demonstrate the simultaneous activity of both X chromosomes, the strategy is to make use of cells that are heterozygous for an electrophoretic variant of an X-linked enzyme that exists as a dimer or high multimer. If both X chromosomes are active within the same cell, the two electrophoretic variants of the gene products will be able to combine and form multimers with intermediate electrophoretic mobilities. This generally occurs only if both electrophoretic variants are synthesized within one cell, and does not occur if the two electrophoretic types are mixed *in vitro*.

Unfortunately, at present teratocarcinomas heterozygous for electrophoretic variants of X-linked markers are not yet available. It may, however, in the future be possible to obtain such tumors and to isolate stem cells from them. There is now one known

electrophoretic variant of an X-linked enzyme in the laboratory
species of mouse (*Mus musculus*). This is the variant of PGK
described by Nielsen and Chapman (1977). When this gene, found
in a wild stock of M. *musculus*, is backcrossed to inbred laboratory stocks, it should be possible experimentally to induce teratocarcinomas by grafting heterozygous embryos to extrauterine sites.
Clones of stem cells could then be isolated from such tumors, and
if these cells contain two active X chromosomes they will be synthesizing both electrophoretic variants of the enzyme. Since PGK
does not exist as a multimer, recloning experiments would have to
be carried out to demonstrate that undifferentiated subclones also
produce both electrophoretic forms of the enzyme. Presumably,
following differentiation, the individual cells would be producing
only one electrophoretic form of the enzyme.

X-chromosome activity in embryo-derived teratocarcinoma stem cells

The hypothetical experiments described above are based on the
assumption that the stem cells of embryo-derived teratocarcinomas
are similar to those of spontaneous parthenogenetic origin and
presumably contain two active X chromosomes. There are, however,
some data that suggest that this may not be the case.

McBurney and Adamson (1976) have also studied X-chromosome
activity in female teratocarcinoma stem cells. One of the cell
lines they examined (C86) apparently contains only one active X
chromosome, as judged both by cytogenetic criteria (presence of a
late-replicating chromosome) and by measures of gene dosage (the
levels of X-linked enzymes were the same in the female cells as in
male cells). Another cell line (C145a) apparently contains one
active and one partially active X chromosome, since there was no
late-replicating X chromosome in the C145a cells, and one of the
four X-linked enzymes measured (a-gal) showed a gene dosage
effect. One possible explanation for the difference between the
results reported by McBurney and Adamson and our results described
here involves the nature of the tumor cells *per se*. The tumors
from which they isolated stem cells were obtained by ectopic transfer of embryos of approximately 6.5 days gestation. Thus, the
tumors they generated may have arisen from embryonic cells in which
X inactivation had already occurred. In contrast, the LT cell
lines we used were derived from a spontaneous ovarian tumor.
Although the specific stage of normal development from which the
LT tumor cells were derived is not known, it may be intrinsically
different (for example preinactivation) from that of the embryo-
derived tumors.

It is also possible that the parthenogenetic origin of the LT
cells is of significance. The LT tumor cells almost certainly

arose from haploid ovarian eggs that had already undergone the
first meiotic division, and the near-diploid chromosomal complement of these cells is most likely a consequence of retention of
the second polar body, following parthenogenetic activation of the
egg (Eppig *et al.* 1977). Thus, in the LT cells both X chromosomes
are derived from cells that have undergone oogenesis, rather than
from one cell that has undergone oogenesis and one that has undergone spermatogenesis. In view of the fact that there is apparently some mechanism for chromosome "marking" which makes preferential paternal inactivation possible in some tissues of the mouse
(Takagi and Sasaki 1975; West, Frels, and Chapman 1977), this
atypical similarity between the two X chromosomes in the LT cells
may in some way account for their both being genetically active.
However, the fact that one of the two X chromosomes in these cells
can apparently undergo inactivation during embryo-like differentiation *in vitro* suggests that, even if both X chromosomes are
active as a consequence of an abnormal situation, their subsequent
behavior is normal.

An alternative possibility is that there are no intrinsic
differences between spontaneous parthenogenetic and embryo-derived
teratocarcinoma stem cells, and that the differences between our
results and those obtained by McBurney and Adamson are the consequences of some secondary event, perhaps related to culture of the
cells *in vitro*. Experiments are in progress to distinguish between
these two possibilities.

Potential uses of the LT teratocarcinoma stem cells

If our conclusion is correct, that the LT cells described here
contain two active X chromosomes and can undergo X-chromosome
inactivation *in vitro*, there are a number of ways in which these
cells can be used to study X-chromosome activity.

For example, these LT cells should provide a new means of preliminary mapping of X-linked markers. The levels of enzymes, or
even structural proteins suspected of being X-linked, could be
assayed in the XX-LT and XO-PSA1 cells. If evidence is found for
a two-fold difference between undifferentiated female and male
cells, this would suggest that the gene in question is X-linked,
and differentiation experiments of the type described above could
then be performed. We have, in fact, already used this technique
to obtain evidence for the X linkage in mouse of the gene for pyro-
phosphoribosylphosphate synthetase (PPrP S; EC 2.7.6.1; Martin,
Clift, and Martin, in preparation). It will of course be necessary
to confirm this by some independent means. It is significant that
Yen *et al.* (1978) have recently obtained evidence that this gene is
X-linked in man.

The LT cells described here could also be used to study the relationship between the biochemical and cytological aspects of X chromosome inactivation. The heterochromatic nature of the inactive X chromosome has always been considered a cytogenetic marker of the X-inactivation process. Although mice do not have the Barr body, which is a cytological manifestation of the heterochromatic inactive X chromosome in human females, it is well established that the inactive X chromosome of female mouse cells replicates late in the S phase of the cell cycle (reviewed by Lyon, 1972). However, the temporal relationship between late replication and genetic inactivity in biochemical terms has never been studied. The LT cells described here should provide an excellent model system for determining whether biochemical inactivation precedes or follows the onset of late replication. We have already determined that in the undifferentiated LT cells both X chromosomes replicate at the same time, and we are currently investigating whether the changes in enzyme activity found in the LT cells following their differentiation are accompanied by changes in the time of replication of one of the two X chromosomes in these cells.

In the long term, the LT cells will probably prove most useful in studies of the regulation of X-chromosome inactivation. At present, they provide the only source of the large quantities of cells that are needed for experiments to determine the molecular mechanisms involved in the inactivation of the X chromosome. In this context, it is of interest to note that our results show that, during the course of differentiation, the drop in activity of G6PD always preceded by four or five days the drop in activity of another X-linked enzyme, HGPRT. This could be interpreted as an indication that inactivation does not occur along the whole length of the X chromosome at one time, and that the G6PD locus is closer to an initiation site of X inactivation than is the HGPRT locus. (The exact location of these genes on the mouse X chromosome is not yet known.) Alternatively, it may be that the whole X chromosome undergoes inactivation at once, but that either the message for enzyme synthesis, or the enzyme itself, is considerably more stable in the case of HGPRT than in the case of G6PD. Experiments to distinguish between these possibilities should lead to a better understanding of the molecular mechanims of X-chromosome inactivation.

This work was supported by grants from the California Division of the American Cancer Society and the National Science Foundation (to G.R.M.) and the NIH (to C.J.E. and D.W.M.). C.J.E. and D.W.M. are Investigators of the Howard Hughes Medical Institute.

REFERENCES

Baikie, A. G., P. B. Loder, G. C. De Grouchy and D. B. Pitt. 1965. Phosphohexokinase activity of erythrocytes in mongolism: another possible marker for chromosome 21. Lancet 1, 412–414.

Bernstine, E. G., L. B. Russell and C. S. Cain. 1978. Effect of gene dosage on the expression of mitochondrial malic enzyme activity in the mouse. Nature 271: 748–750.

Brinster, R. L. 1974. The effect of cells transferred into the mouse blastocyst on subsequent development. J. Exp. Med. 140: 1049–1056.

Brinster, R. L. 1975. Can teratocarcinoma cells colonize the mouse embryo? In Roche Symposium on Teratomas and Differentiation, M. Sherman and D. Solter, Eds. Academic Press, New York, pp. 51–58.

Chapman, V. M. and T. B. Shows. 1976. Somatic cell genetic evidence for X-chromosome linkage of three enzymes in the mouse. Nature 259: 665–667.

Chapman, V. M., J. D. West and D. A. Adler. 1978. Bimodal distribution of α-galactosidase activities in mouse embryos. In Genetic Mosaics and Chimeras in Mammals, Liane B. Russell, Ed., Plenum Press, New York and London.

Damjanov, I. and D. Solter. 1974. Host-related factors determine the outgrowth of teratocarcinomas from mouse egg-cylinders. Z. Krebsforsch. 81: 63–69.

Davidson, R. G., H. M. Nitowsky and B. Childs. 1963. Demonstrations of two populations of cells in the human female heterozygous for glucose-6-phosphate dehydrogenase variants. Proc. Nat. Acad. Sci. USA 50: 481–485.

DeMars, R., S. L. LeVan, B. L. Trend and L. B. Russell. 1976. Abnormal ornithine carbamoyltransferase in mice having the sparse-fur mutation. Proc. Nat. Acad. Sci. USA 73: 1693–1697.

Dewey, M. J., D. W. Martin, Jr., G. R. Martin and B. Mintz. 1977. Mosaic mice with teratocarcinoma-derived mutant cells deficient in hypoxanthine phosphoribosyl transferase. Proc. Nat. Acad. Sci. USA 74: 5564–5568.

Eicher, E. M. and D. L. Coleman. 1977. Influence of gene duplication and X-inactivation on mouse mitochondrial malic enzyme activity and electrophoretic patterns. Genetics 85: 647–658.

Eppig, J. J., L. P. Kozak, E. M. Eicher, and L. C. Stevens. 1977. Ovarian teratomas in mice are derived from oocytes that have completed the first meiotic division. Nature 269: 517-518.

Epstein, C. J. 1969. Mammalian oocytes: X-chromosome activity. Science 163: 1078-1079.

Epstein, C. J. 1972. Expression of the mammalian X-chromosome before and after fertilization. Science 175: 1467-1468.

Epstein, C. J., G. Tucker, B. Travis and A. Gropp. 1977. Gene dosage for isocitrate dehydrogenase in mouse embryos trisomic for chromosome 1. Nature 247: 615-616.

Epstein, C. J., S. Smith, B. Travis and G. Tucker. 1978a. Both X-chromosomes function prior to X-chromosome inactivation in female mouse embryos. Nature, in press.

Epstein, C. J., B. Travis, G. Tucker and S. Smith. 1978b. The direct demonstration of an X-chromosome dosage effect prior to inactivation. In Genetic Mosaics and Chimeras in Mammals, Liane B. Russell, Ed., Plenum Press, New York and London.

Evans, M. J. and G. R. Martin. 1975. The differentiation of clonal teratocarcinoma cell cultures *in vitro*. In Roche Symposium on Teratomas and Differentiation, M. Sherman and D. Solter, Eds., Academic Press, New York, pp. 237-250.

Feaster, W. W., L. Kwok and C. J. Epstein. 1977. Dosage effects for superoxide dismutase-1 in nucleated cells aneuploid for chromosome 21. Amer. J. Hum. Genet. 24: 563-570.

Gartler, S. M. and R. J. Andina. 1976. Mammalian X-chromosome inactivation. Adv. in Hum. Genet. 7: 99-140.

Gartler, S. M., R. M. Liskay, B. K. Campbell, R. Sparkes and N. Gant. 1972. Evidence for two functional X-chromosomes in human oocytes. Cell Differ. 1: 215-218.

George, D. L. and U. Francke. 1976. Gene dosage effect: regional mapping of human nucleoside phosphorylase on chromosome 14. Science 194: 851-852.

Graham, C. F. 1977. Teratocarcinoma cells and normal mouse embryogenesis. In Concepts in Mammalian Embryogenesis, M. Sherman, Ed., MIT Press, Cambridge, Mass., pp. 315-394.

Iles, S. A., M. W. McBurney, S. R. Bramwell, Z. A. Deussen and C. F. Graham. 1975. Development of parthenogenetic and fertilized mouse embryos in the uterus and in extrauterine sites. J. Embryol. exp. Morph. 34: 387-405.

Illmensee, Karl. 1978. Reversion of malignancy and normalized differentiation of teratocarcinoma cells in chimeric mice. In, Genetic Mosaics and Chimeras in Mammals, Liane B. Russell, Ed. Plenum Press, New York and London.

Illmensee, K. and B. Mintz. 1976. Totipotency and normal differentiation of single teratocarcinoma cells cloned by injection into blastocysts. Proc. Nat. Acad. Sci. USA 73: 549-553.

Kozak, L. P. and P. J. Quinn. 1975. Evidence for dosage compensation of an X-linked gene in the 6-day embryo of the mouse. Devel. Biol. 45: 65-73.

Kozak, L. P., G. K. McLean and E. M. Eicher. 1974. X-linkage of phosphoglycerate kinase in the mouse. Biochem. Genet. 11: 41-47.

Kozak, C., E. Nichols and F. H. Ruddle. 1975. Gene linkage analysis in the mouse by somatic cell hybridization: assignment of adenine phosphoribosyltransferase to chromosome 8 and α-galactosidase to the X chromosome. Somatic Cell Genet. 1: 371-382.

Kratzer, P. G. and S. M. Gartler. 1978. HGPRT expression in early mouse development. In, Genetic Mosaics and Chimeras in Mammals, Liane B. Russell, Ed., Plenum Press, New York and London.

Lyon, M. F. 1972. X-chromosome inactivation and developmental patterns in mammals. Biol. Rev. 47: 1-35.

Magenis, R. E., R. D. Koler, E. Lovrien, R. H. Bigley, M. C. DuVal and K. M. Overton. 1975. Gene dosage: evidence for assignment of erythrocyte acid phosphatase locus to chromosome 2. Proc. Nat. Acad. Sci. USA 72: 4526-4530.

Mangia, F., G. Abbo-Halbasch and C. J. Epstein. 1975. X-chromosome expression during oogenesis in the mouse. Devel. Biol. 45: 366-368.

Marimo, B. and F. Giannelli. 1975. Gene dosage effect in human trisomy 16. Nature 256: 204-206.

Martin, G. R. 1975. Teratocarcinomas as a model system for the study of embryogenesis and neoplasia: Review. Cell 5: 229-243.

Martin, G. R. 1978. Advantages and limitation of teratocarcinoma stem cells as models of development. In, Development in Mammals, Vol. 3, M. Johnson, Ed. Elsevier/North-Holland Biomedical Press, in press.

Martin, G. R., C. J. Epstein, B. Travis, G. Tucker, S. Yatziv, D. W. Martin, Jr., S. Clift, and S. Cohen. 1978a. X-chromosome inactivation during differentiation of female teratocarcinoma stem cells *in vitro*. Nature 271: 329-333.

Martin, G. R. and M. J. Evans. 1975a. The differentiation of clonal lines of teratocarcinoma cells: formation of embryoid bodies *in vitro*. Proc. Nat. Acad. Sci. USA 72: 1441-1445.

Martin, G. R. and M. J. Evans. 1975b. The formation of embryoid bodies *in vitro* by homogeneous embryonal carcinoma cell cultures derived from isolated single cells. In, Roche Symposium on Teratomas and Differentiation, M. Sherman and D. Solter, Eds. Academic Press, New York, pp. 169-187.

Martin, G. R., S. Smith, and C. J. Epstein. 1978b. Protein synthetic patterns in teratocarcinoma stem cells and mouse embryos at early stages of development. Devel. Biol., in press.

Martin, G. R., L. M. Wiley and I. Damjanov. 1977. The development of cystic embryoid bodies *in vitro* from clonal teratocarcinoma stem cells. Devel. Biol. 61: 230-244.

McBurney, M. W. and E. D. Adamson. 1976. Studies on the activity of the X chromosomes in female teratocarcinoma cells in culture. Cell 9: 57-70.

Migeon, B. R. and K. Jelalian. 1977. Evidence for two active X chromosomes in germ cells of female before meiotic entry. Nature 269: 242-243.

Mintz, B. and K. Illmensee. 1975. Normal genetically mosaic mice produced from malignant teratocarcinoma cells. Proc. Nat. Acad. Sci. USA 72: 3585-3589.

Monk, Marilyn. 1978. Biochemical studies on X-chromosome activity in preimplantation mouse embryos. In Genetic Mosaics and Chimeras in Mammals, Liane B. Russell, Ed., Plenum Press, New York and London.

Mouse News Letter 56: 4-28, 1977.

Nielson, J. T. and V. M. Chapman. 1977. Electrophoretic variation for X-chromosome-linked phosphoglycerate kinase (PGK-1) in the mouse. Genetics 87: 319-325.

Papaioannou, V. E., M. W. McBurney, R. L. Gardner and M. J. Evans. 1975. Fate of teratocarcinoma cells injected into early mouse embryos. Nature 258: 70-73.

Papaioannou, V. E., R. L. Gardner, M. W. McBurney, C. Babinet and
M. J. Evans. 1978. Participation of cultured teratocarcinoma
cells in mouse embryogenesis. J. Embryol. Exp. Morph., in press.

Pierce, G. B. and F. J. Dixon. 1959. Testicular teratomas. I.
Demonstration of teratogenesis by metamorphosis of multipotential
cells. Cancer 12: 573-583.

Solter, D., N. Skreb and I. Damjanov. 1970. Extrauterine growth
of mouse egg cylinders results in malignant teratoma. Nature 227:
503-504.

Stevens, L. C. 1959. Embryology of testicular teratomas in strain
129 mice. J. Nat. Cancer Inst. 23: 1249-1295.

Stevens, L. C. 1968. The development of teratomas from intratesticular grafts of tubal mouse eggs. J. Embryol. Exp. Morph.
20: 329-341.

Stevens, L. C. 1970. The development of transplantable teratocarcinomas from intratesticular grafts of pre- and postimplantation
mouse embryos. Develop. Biol. 21: 364-382.

Stevens, L. C. 1975. Comparative development of normal and parthenogenetic mouse embryos, early testicular and ovarian teratomas, and embryoid bodies. In Roche Symposium on Teratomas and
Differentiation, M. Sherman and D. Solter, Eds., Academic Press,
New York, pp. 17-32.

Stevens, L. C. and D. S. Varnum. 1974. The development of teratomas from parthenogenetically activated ovarian mouse eggs.
Devel. Biol. 37: 369-380.

Takagi, N. and M. Sasaki. 1975. Preferential inactivation of the
paternally derived X chromosome in the extraembryonic membranes
of the mouse. Nature 256: 640-642.

West, J. D., W. I. Frels and V. M. Chapman. 1977. Preferential
expression of the maternally derived X-chromosome in the mouse yolk
sac. Cell 12: 873-882.

Yen, R. C. K., W. B. Adams, C. Lazar and M. A. Becker. 1978. Evidence for X-linkage of human phosphoribosylpyrophosphate synthetase.
Proc. Nat. Acad. Sci. USA 75: 482-485.

THE STABILITY OF X-CHROMOSOME INACTIVATION: STUDIES WITH MOUSE-HUMAN CELL HYBRIDS AND MOUSE TERATOCARCINOMAS

Brenda Kahan

Department of Zoology, University of Wisconsin,
Madison, Wisconsin 53706

The control scheme for the expression of X chromosomes in female mammals can be considered to consist of two parts (Lyon 1972, 1974). The first of these involves the initiation of inactivation of one X chromosome (Kratzer and Gartler 1978; Monk 1978; Chapman, West, and Adler 1978). This initial choice may be either random, as it is in eutherian embryonic somatic tissues, or preferential, as occurs in extraembryonic components of some species (Takagi 1978; West, Papaioannou, Frels, and Chapman 1978) and in somatic tissues of marsupial mammals (Cooper, Johnston, Murtagh, Sharman, VandeBerg, and Poole 1975). This report will focus on the second part of the problem of X-chromosome differentiation: how genetic repression of the inactive X is maintained and propagated. It will consider specifically some of the insights into the regulatory mechanisms involved in the maintenance of repression that may be gained from experiments designed to derepress genes on the inactive X.

Although few specific chemical or physical differences are known to exist between active and inactive X chromosomes, there are two general features of the inactive X we must ultimately be able to account for. One of these is that inactivation is an exceedingly stable state: re-expression of inactive X alleles in somatic cells has never been observed previously, though specific attempts to derepress X chromosomes have been made using cultured cells (Comings 1966; Von Kap-Herr and Mukherjee 1977), including those with methods sensitive enough to have detected derepression in diploid human cells had it occurred at frequencies even as low as 10^{-6} (Migeon 1972; Sato, Slesinki, and Littlefield 1972; Felix 1971). The somatic X remains inactive irrespective of the state of differentiation or tumorigenicity of the cell (Romeo and Migeon 1975).

Regardless of the apparent permanence in somatic cells of X
inactivation, it is probable that inactivation is totally reversible — at least in the germ line (see review by Gartler and Andina 1976). There is cytological evidence to suggest that female
primordial germ cells of the mouse initially contain an inactive
X, but that reactivation of this X occurs around the time the
migrating germ cells reach the ovary (Ohno 1964). There is genetic evidence that two active X's exist in human oocytes (Gartler,
Liskay, Campbell, Sparkes, and Gant 1972), and that both X's are
active even in premeiotic stages (Migeon and Jelalian 1977) at a
time when the germ cells are still vigorously dividing mitotically.
(Kangaroo germ cells however do not have two active X's, at least
in early oocytes [Johnston, Robinson, and Sharman 1976]).

Thus an attack on the problem of maintaining X-chromosome
inactivation may feasibly be broached from two different angles:
that of the permanence of somatic X inactivation; and the reversibility, or reactivation, of inactive X's in the mammalian ovary.

LOCALIZED DEREPRESSION OF THE HUMAN INACTIVE X CHROMOSOME

IN MOUSE-HUMAN CELL HYBRIDS

Dr. Robert DeMars and I considered we might be able to derepress genes on the human inactive X in somatic hybrid cells made
between mouse cells and human female cells (Kahan and DeMars 1975)
because of two events that occur frequently in these hybrid cells,
but are potentially lethal, or very rare, in the organism or in
cultured diploid cells. One is the preferential (and sometimes
very extensive) loss of human chromosomes; though it should be
emphasized that, after an initial, cataclysmic loss, there can be
an extended period of relative stability in which some hybrids
retain large numbers of human chromosomes over long periods of
time (Ruddle 1972; DeMars and Kahan, unpublished observations).
The other phenomenon common to interspecific hybrids is the frequent fragmentation, or breakage and rearrangement, that can occur
in the remaining human chromosomes. Indeed, evidence from experiments in which cells from different cell-cycle stages were fused
suggests that late-replicating segments may even be preferentially
fragmented (Johnson and Rao 1970).

Our reasoning was the following: if repression is maintained
by *trans*-acting signals that originate from either the autosomes,
the active X, or even distant portions of the inactive X, then the
loss of these chromosomes may lead to X derepression. Alternatively, if repression is propagated *cis* on the chromosome from one
or more inactivation sites, then derepression may occur only in
cells with fragmented X chromosomes.

The simple outline of our experiment then, was to fuse mouse male L cells with human female fibroblasts and ask: can we detect the expression of alleles which we know to be present only on the human inactive X; and, if so, is this expression correlated with specific patterns of chromosome segregation and breakage? There were, however, special refinements on this basic scheme that were crucial to the success of our experiment.

BASIS OF HYBRID SELECTION SCHEME:

PROPERTIES OF THE PARENTAL CELLS

First, we did not merely screen the hybrids for inactive X expression; rather, we applied a very strong selective pressure capable of detecting even very rare derepression events, on the order of 10^{-6}. The principle in brief is as follows. Cell growth in medium where *de novo* purine synthesis is blocked is dependent upon the utilization of an exogenous purine; if hypoxanthine is the purine supplied, the X-linked enzyme hypoxanthine phosphoribosyl transferase (HPRT) can be specifically required for survival (likewise if adenine is given, the analogous adenine phosphoribosyl transferase [APRT] becomes essential). We chose as our mouse parental cells a clone of 1D L cells with a nonreverting HPRT deficiency (Kahan, Held, and DeMars 1974): we then created human female cells that were also phenotypically highly deficient in HPRT by X-irradiating fibroblasts with 250 roentgens to increase their mutation rate (Albertini and DeMars 1973) and selecting for cells resistant to azaguanine (AG) or thioguanine (TG), toxic analogues of HPRT substrates (DeMars and Held 1972). We

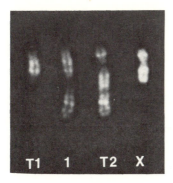

FIGURE 1.   X-chromosome translocation of the human female cells. The translocated X, T2, includes most of the long arm of chromosome no. 1. Quinacrine-band patterns show no apparent X-chromosome segment on T1, the remainder of chromosome no. 1.

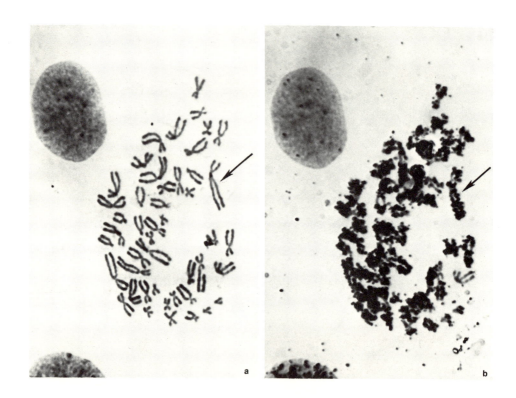

Figure 2

FIGURE 2.   Autoradiograph of human female cell.
    (a) Orcein stained chromosomes before application of emulsion.
The translocated X chromosome, T2, is indicated by an arrow.
(b) Same cell after development of silver grains. The T2
chromosome is labeled along with the autosomes. The single
unlabeled chromosome in the otherwise heavily labeled cell
(characteristic early-S replication pattern) is the normal X.

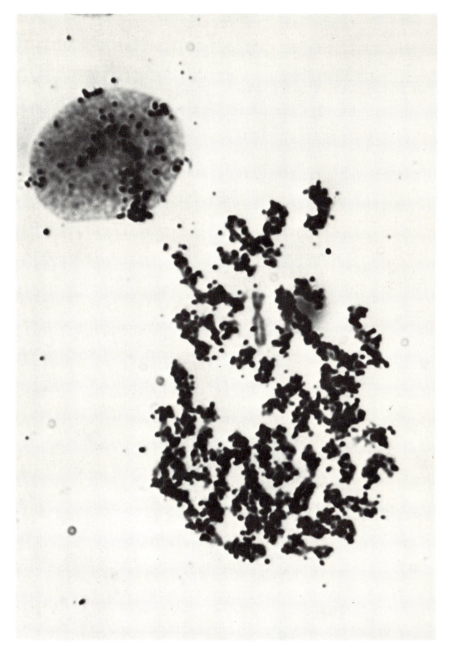

FIGURE 3.   Autoradiography of a second human female cell showing
     clearly the normal X morphology of the late-replicating
     chromosome.

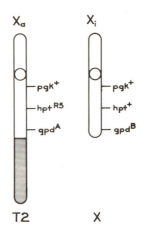

FIGURE 4. Interpretation of the two human X chromosomes. The
translocated X, T2, is the active X (X_a) and carries the
alleles for human PGK and G6PD-A. The hpt^{R5} allele on T2
denotes the particular HPRT deficiency of this clone designated R5. The inactive X (X_i) is morphologically normal
and carries the normal, unexpressed alleles for PGK, HPRT,
and G6PD-B enzymes.
[From Kahan and DeMars 1975.]

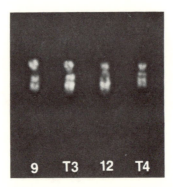

FIGURE 5. The 9-12 translocation of the human female cells.
Quinacrine-band patterns indicate a reciprocal exchange
between the distal portions of the long arms of chromosomes
nos. 9 and 12. T3 has the short arm, centromere, and proximal long-arm region of no. 9; while T4 has the short arm,
centromere, and proximal long-arm segment of no. 12.

could therefore fuse mouse and human cells, both phenotypically
HPRT deficient, and select for hybrids in a medium, HAS (hypoxanthine plus azaserine), in which neither parental cell type could
grow. Hybrid cells, also, would not grow in HAS, unless hybridization resulted in X-chromosome derepression. If this occurred,
hybrid cells that could now express the normal HPRT allele on the
human inactive X would survive.

Fortuitously, among the clones of TG-resistant human cells
was one in which an X-autosome translocation had occurred (Fig. 1).
This created yet another, morphological, marker for distinguishing
the two human X chromosomes in hybrid cells. The morphologically
normal X in this clone is the inactive X. The translocated X
clearly replicates in synchrony with the rest of the autosomes
(Fig. 2) while the morphologically normal X is clearly the asynchronously replicating X (Figs. 2 and 3) and is the inactive X.

The X chromosomes of the human parent are interpreted as
follows (Fig. 4): The translocated X is the active X and expresses
human PGK and G6PD-A. It has the altered HPRT allele of this
particular clone, R5. The morphologically normal X is the inactive
X. Since other clones from this G6PD heterozygote expressed
G6PD-B, HPRT, and PGK, we presume these alleles are present on the
inactive X. Thus there are at least three differences between the
two X's, and it should be easy to distinguish two different classes
of hybrids having either one or the other human X chromosomes.

There was another chromosome translocation pair in the human
clone, between a no. 9 and a no. 12 chromosome (Fig. 5). This was,
however, probably not significant in our experiment except that the
translocation chromosome T4, present in some of our hybrids, is a
marker indicating that the hybrids were in fact made with cells of
this particular human clone.

A second very important feature of our experiment was that we
did not require the immediate functioning of HPRT. Instead, we
initially isolated hybrids on the basis of adenine utilization,
which requires APRT activity (Fig. 6). The mouse cells were doubly
deficient — in APRT and HPRT activity; hybrids that retained human
chromosome no. 16, containing the human APRT gene (Tischfield and
Ruddle 1974; Kahan *et al.* 1974), grew up on a "lawn" of human fibroblasts. These were isolated, expanded to approximately 3-9 x 10^6
cells, and a portion was then reselected in hypoxanthine. This
first "permissive" step for hybrid formation was essential: if
we immediately selected with hypoxanthine, no hybrids formed.
Evidently, this time is required to reach a population size in
which a very rare event may occur.

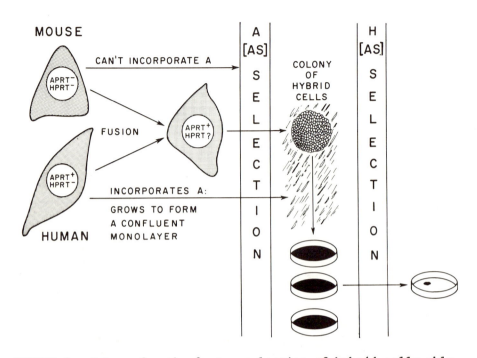

FIGURE 6. Scheme for the 2-step selection of hybrid cells able
to utilize hypoxanthine. The first step selects for hybrids
able to utilize adenine via the human APRT enzyme. A portion
of the cells of each hybrid is then subjected to hypoxanthine
selection; from some of the adenine-selected hybrids, a rare
cell with HPRT activity will give rise to a colony in HAS
medium.

PROPERTIES OF THE HYBRID CELLS

Approximately 10% of hybrids isolated in adenine gave rise to
colonies in hypoxanthine at frequencies of $1-2 \times 10^{-6}$. The six
HAS colonies (hereafter referred to as DX hybrids) represent six
independent events that restored the ability to utilize hypoxanthine.

The first point we established was that each of the six hybrids had HPRT activity that was distinctly human. Anti-human
HPRT antibody does not crossreact with mouse HPRT but precipitates
hybrid enzyme as effectively as human enzyme (Kahan and DeMars
1975).

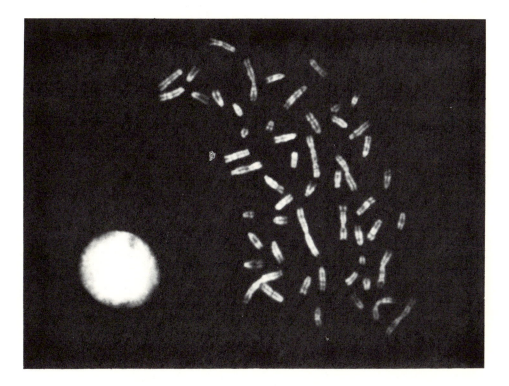

FIGURE 7. Quinacrine fluorescent metaphase of the mouse parental
     line, D7. The mode of 52 chromosomes includes 8 large meta-
     centrics, each easily distinguishable from the two human X's.

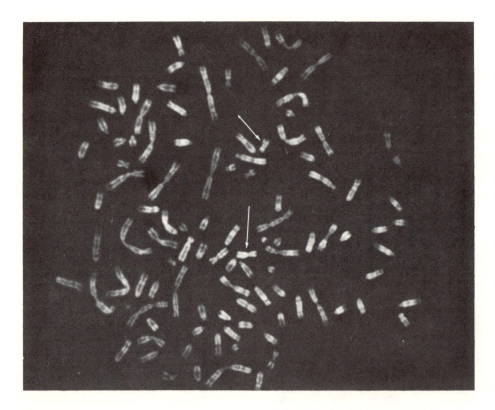

FIGURE 8. Quinacrine-fluorescent metaphase of hypoxanthine-
    selected hybrid DX10-2. Many human chromosomes are present,
    but only one X chromosome, namely, the morphologically
    normal one indicated by the lower arrow. The human marker
    chromosome T4 is identified by the upper arrow.

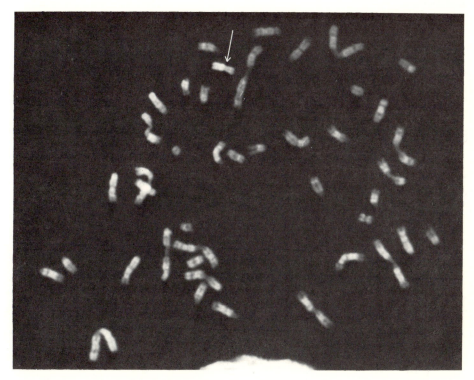

FIGURE 9. Quinacrine-fluorescent metaphase of hypoxanthine-selected hybrid DX36-2. Few, if any, human chromosomes — other than the normal X chromosome indicated by the arrow — are present in cells of this hybrid.

The second important observation was that each clone isolated in hypoxanthine did contain a human X chromosome. The mouse karyotype includes eight metacentrics, each clearly distinguishable from either of the two human X chromosomes (Fig. 7). The karyotype of the six DX hybrids ranged from one extreme in which nearly 60% of the human chromosome pairs were represented, including only one X chromosome (Fig. 8), to the other in which few, if any, human chromosomes, except an X chromosome, were present (Fig. 9). In each of the six DX hybrids, only one of the two human X's was present; and in each case it was the morphologically normal X chromosome, known to be the inactive X of the human fibroblasts.

The important question is: is the human HPRT gene that is active in these cells located on the normal X chromosome, also present in nearly all DX cells? The chromosome source of HPRT can be determined by selecting cells able to grow in TG and correlating the loss of HPRT activity with loss of a specific human chromosome. Fluctuation tests, performed with control hybrids containing an active X chromosome, indicate that during the second, slow, phase of chromosome elimination the human X is lost with a probability of about 10^{-3} per cell generation in nonselective medium (Kahan, unpublished results). In TG survivors of DX hybrids, which arose at incidences of $4-8 \times 10^{-3}$, the concordant loss of HPRT activity and the normal X chromosome occurs. In four DX10-2-1 subclones isolated in hypoxanthine and five in TG, the normal X is the only chromosome specifically present in nearly all cells of the former, and absent in all cells of the latter (Table 1). In an even more stringent criterion of association, two clones (discussed again below) had an average of 3.8 and 1.7, respectively, normal human X's per cell, yet all their TG-selected cells contained no human X chromosomes (Kahan and DeMars, in preparation). The complete agreement between the presence of HPRT activity and the X chromosome, and their simultaneous loss, is good evidence for locating the active HPRT allele on the morphologically normal X chromosome, and suggests that this allele has been derepressed on the formerly inactive X.

It was a common observation, especially in subclones isolated from the six DX hybrids, that more than one morphologically normal X chromosome was present in a single cell (Kahan and DeMars, in preparation). In Fig. 10, a hybrid metaphase containing one complement of mouse chromosomes includes six identical, normal human X's. This is reminiscent of an observation made by Green, Wang, Kehinde, and Meuth (1971) that human chromosomes retained by specific selection in mouse-human hybrid cells sometimes exist in multiple copies. These investigators found that such chromosomes can be preferentially increased by nondisjunction by growing the cells in low substrate concentration for the enzyme under active selection. Specifically, they found up to eight copies of chromosome

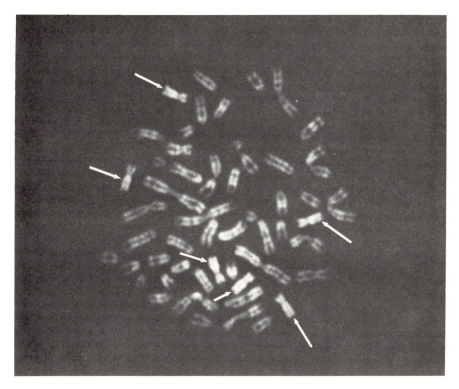

FIGURE 10.   Fluorescent metaphase of hypoxanthine-selected hybrid,
    DX12, clone 1-6.   The six morphologically normal X chromosomes
    are marked by arrows.

TABLE 1. Human chromosomes present in hypoxanthine- or TG-selected clones of hybrid subclone DX10-2-1*

Human chromosome	HAS-1	HAS-2	HAS-3	HAS-4	TG-1	TG-2	TG-3	TG-4	TG-5
1									
2									
3									58
4	38	83	72						
5									
6									
7	57	83	72	82	50		84	71	67
8	10	92	64	71	50		84	57	
9									
10				76					
11									
12		75	9	94	86		76	71	
13	76	92	64	94	86	25	100	93	92
14	38	83	27	94	79		69	86	75
15									
16	10	75	91	94	71		92	79	50
17									
18									

19									
20	5	83	64	76	86		100	57	100
21	95	75	100	88	79	83	84	93	100
22		83	100	100					
X	95	83	100	100					
T1									
T2									
T3									
T4	10	75	75	82	28		62	64	67
No. of X chromosomes/cell mode (range)	1 (0–3)	1 (0–1)	2 (1–2)	1 (1)	0 (0)	0 (0)	0 (0)	0 (0)	0 (0)
No. of human chromosomes/cell mode (range)	5 (2–10)	11 (9–12)	8 (6–10)	10 (8–13)	8 (3–12)	2 (0–4)	8 (6–10)	8 (5–10)	6 (4–9)
Total No. of chromosomes/cell mode (range)	— (77–94)	88 (74–92)	— (81–89)	91 (79–95)	93 (65–93)	— (65–110)	— (69–88)	— (82–97)	81 (79–86)
Total No. of metaphases	21	12	11	17	14	12	13	14	12

* Percentage of cells in which a specific chromosome can be identified.

no. 17, specifying thymidine kinase (TK), in clones isolated in
low thymidine concentrations in HAT (hypoxanthine, aminopterin, and
thymidine) medium. One possible explanation for our observation of
multiple X chromosomes is that the DX hybrids may have had low HPRT
activity initially, possibly resulting from only partial derepression of the HPRT gene; however, their HPRT enzyme levels are not
different from those of control hybrids retaining an active human
X. Although HPRT activities of both types of hybrids range from
27—75% that of HPRT positive mouse L cells, similar X duplication
has not been seen in the control hybrids. Alternatively, inactive
X chromosome material may be inherently more susceptible to nondisjunction events in interspecific hybrids.

A further important consideration is the qualitative extent of
X-chromosome derepression. Are other alleles (e.g., PGK and
G6PD-B) on the inactive X expressed? An important control, an
adenine-selected hybrid (57-3-1) that retained the active X chromosome (T2) in about 50% of the cells (Fig. 11), but not the inactive
X, did express both G6PD-A (Fig. 12) and human PGK (Fig. 13).
Other control hybrids with an active X chromosome also invariably
expressed G6PD and PGK. To our surprise, not one of the DX hybrids
expressed either human G6PD or PGK (Figs. 12 and 13), even though
the X chromosome is apparently intact and present in nearly every
cell. Either enzyme would have been easily detectable at a level
of 10% of the total activity.

We believe the simplest interpretation of these results is
that the HPRT gene on the inactive X has been derepressed; in each
of six cases, the derepression is local and does not extend into
the flanking regions containing the G6PD or PGK genes. We infer
from this that there may be at least three separately repressible
units on the human inactive X, containing PGK, HPRT, and G6PD,
respectively. Alternatively, the localized derepression in somatic
cells may be unable to spread into adjacent regions, just as
derepression from active, autosomal regions translocated to the X
chromosome is not propagated into the inactive X segment (Russell
1963). Instead, repression from the inactive X portion extends for
some distance into the autosomal DNA.

HUMAN CHROMOSOMES PRESENT IN HYBRIDS HAVING A

LOCALLY DEREPRESSED X CHROMOSOME

Can we ascribe the X-chromosome derepression results obtained
in mouse-human cell hybrids to a particular pattern of human
chromosomes present, or absent, in the DX hybrids? Several points
emerge from the tabulated results.

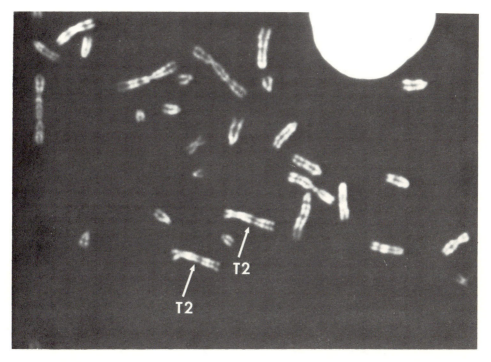

FIGURE 11.   Portion of a fluorescent metaphase of adenine-selected
     hybrid 57-3-1. The translocated, active X chromosomes are
     identified by arrows.

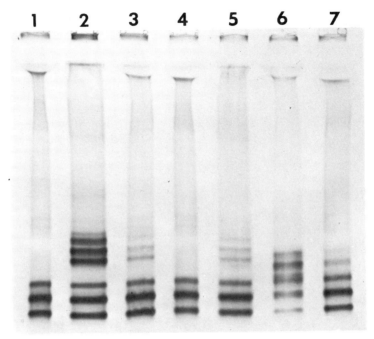

FIGURE 12. Electrophoresis of G6PD from mouse, human, and hybrid
clones in an acrylamide slab gel. (1) Mouse D7; (2) 1:1
mixture of mouse D7:human 356, expressing human G6PD-B;
(3) 9:1 mixture of mouse D7:human 356; (4) hybrid DX10-4;
(5) 9:1 mixture of hybrid DX10-4:human 356; (6) hybrid 713.6:
mouse-human cell hybrid with an active human X expressing
G6PD-A; (7) hybrid 57-3-1: mouse-human cell hybrid containing the active X chromosome, T2, of human R5 cells, expressing G6PD-A.

(1) All hybrids have *only* the normal X chromosome, present in
nearly every cell (Table 2), except hybrid DX36-2, which could be
separated into clones with a normal X in most cells (Table 2, last
column), or clones without a recognizable X in any cell (unpublished results). Presumably, breakage of the normal X occurred in
some cells of hybrid DX36-2. However, breakage of the X is not
required for HPRT derepression.

(2) There is variability in the autosomes present. However,
no autosome is consistently present in most cells of all hybrids.
Therefore, no particular chromosome is required to maintain the
repression of the PGK and G6PD alleles: they remain repressed in
the absence of a particular autosome or the active X (Table 2).

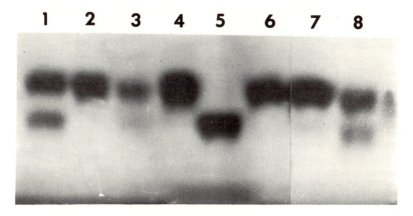

FIGURE 13. Cellogel electrophoresis of PGK from mouse, human, and
  hybrid clones. (1) 1:1 mixture of mouse D7:human 356; (2)
  hybrid DX36-2; (3) hybrid 57-3-1: mouse-human cell hybrid
  containing the active X chromosome, T2, of human R5 cells,
  expressing human PGK; (4) mouse D7; (5) human 356; (6) hybrid
  DX10-2; (7) 9:1 mixture of hybrid DX10-2:human 356; (8) hybrid D78.9: mouse-human cell hybrid with an active human X,
  expressing human PGK.

(3) Similarly, the loss of the active X or of a particular
autosome is not sufficient to result in the expression of the inactive X, since the spectrum of human chromosomes present before and
after X-chromosome derepression is essentially the same, in both
distribution and frequency (Table 3).

(4) The chromosome patterns of four DX hybrids — DX10-2 and
DX10-4 (Table 2), DX10-1 (not shown), and DX10-3 (not shown) —
are essentially identical and probably reflect a common origin,
since the corresponding adenine-selected hybrids were isolated
from the same petri dish. Nonetheless, each of the four hypoxanthine-selected hybrids represents an independent derepression
event.

(5) The active X, T2, is absent in all cells examined both
before and after HPRT derepression (Tables 2 and 3). Furthermore,
T2 is not present in adenine-selected hybrids, even in the rare
cell in which derepression occurs, as shown by subcloning experiments (Kahan and DeMars, unpublished results). Two considerations

TABLE 2. Human chromosomes present in hypoxanthine−selected hybrids*

Human chromosome	DX10-2	DX10-4	DX12	DX36-2	DX36-2 subclone 7
1					
2					
3			9		
4	97	100		13	35
5					
6					
7	97	97	91	9	
8	89	100			
9					
10	92	97	17		
11	100	100			
12	92	97			
13	100	100			
14	100	97	59		
15					
16	100	100	2	13	
17					
18	86	97			
19					
20	97	97			
21	89	97			
22				13	30
X	94	100	93	59	95
T1					
T2					
T3					
T4	94	97			
No. of X chromosomes/cell mode (range)	1 (0-2)	1 (1)	1 (0-5)	1 (0-2)	1 (0-3)
Total No. of chromosomes/cell mode (range)	16 (13-17)	16 (13-17)	4 (1-8)	1 (0-4)	2 (0-4)
Total No. of chromosomes/cell mode (range)	108 (95-111)	108 (101-109)	52 (37-57)	— (39-55)	— (40-58)
Total No. of metaphases	35	35	92	32	20

* Percentage of cells in which a specific chromosome can be identified.

TABLE 3. Comparison of human chromosomes present in hybrid cells before and after X-chromosome derepression*

Human chromosome	Adenine-selected hybrid 10-4	Hypoxanthine-selected hybrid DX10-4	Adenine-selected hybrid 36-2	Hypoxanthine-selected hybrid DX36-2
1				
2				
3				
4	100	94	20	13
5				
6				
7	97	93	18	9
8	100	94		
9				
10	97	99	10	
11	100	93		
12	97	83		
13	100	100		
14	97	97		
15				
16	100	100	18	13
17				
18	97	94	5	
19				
20	97	93		
21	97	94		
22			28	13
X	97	97	60	59
T1				
T2				
T3				
T4	97	91		
No. of X chromosomes/cell mode (range)	1 (1-2)	1 (1)	1 (0-3)	1 (0-2)
Total No. of chromosomes/cell mode (range)	110 (90-114)	108 (101-109)	52 (41-59)	— (39-55)
Total No. of metaphases	69	35	40	32

* Percentage of cells in which a specific chromosome can be identified.

are evoked. One, it is extremely unlikely that the active X
chromosome is the source of the human HPRT enzyme in DX hybrids.
Two, are we, however, overlooking a repressive effect that the
active X chromosome might have on the inactive X when the two are
present in the same cell? We can more directly demonstrate an
apparent lack of interaction between the active X and the partially
derepressed, inactive X by reintroducing the human active X into
the DX hybrids in the following way: DX10-4 hybrids were fused
with their human parental R5 cells. New "secondary" hybrids could
be obtained in HAT medium, as DX10-4 is TK deficient and R5 is
HPRT deficient (Kahan and DeMars, in preparation). Of ten newly
isolated hybrids, three expressed HPRT and G6PD-A and contained
both the active X (T2) and the presumptive inactive, but partially
derepressed, X chromosome in the same cell (Fig. 14). Thus, the
presence of the human active X in these hybrids does not result in
the repression, or inactivation, of the HPRT allele expressed by
the otherwise inactive human X chromosome.

We can find no evidence in these experiments to support the
idea of *trans*-acting human repression of the inactive X chromosome,
emanating either from the autosomes or the active X. Alternatively,
the proposal of *trans*-acting repressors emanating from the mouse
genome also seems unlikely. DX10-4 hybrid cells may also be fused
with other HPRT deficient mouse cells or hybrid cells, made between
mouse D7 cells and human male cells. Viable "secondary" hybrids
selected in HAT result in frequencies comparable to that of adenine-
selected D7 and human R5 hybrid cells (Kahan and DeMars, in preparation), indicating that the human HPRT allele remains active
even in the presence of the added mouse chromosomes.

BEHAVIOR OF AN LT OVARIAN TERATOCARCINOMA IN THE MOUSE

Ovarian teratomas in the mouse are common in the LT strain
(Stevens and Varnum 1974). *In vitro* clones were derived from an
LT teratocarcinoma no. 74115 kindly supplied by Dr. Leroy Stevens
by methods described previously (Kahan and Ephrussi 1970). When
cells of one LT embryonal clone (clone 8) were injected intraperitoneally (IP) into female LT mice, an extraordinary pattern of
growth was observed. In most of the females, large, rapidly growing tumors were found that were located exclusively in the ovaries
and were bilateral in many of the animals (Fig. 15). Although
extraovarian tumors do form in a few animals, these are usually
small and few in number and are limited exclusively to females;
males inoculated IP with the same number of cells have no tumors
(Table 4).

The ovarian tumors consist largely of undifferentiated teratocarcinoma embryonal cells, with areas of normal ovary scattered
among the tumor cells. The ovarian tumors appear to be derived

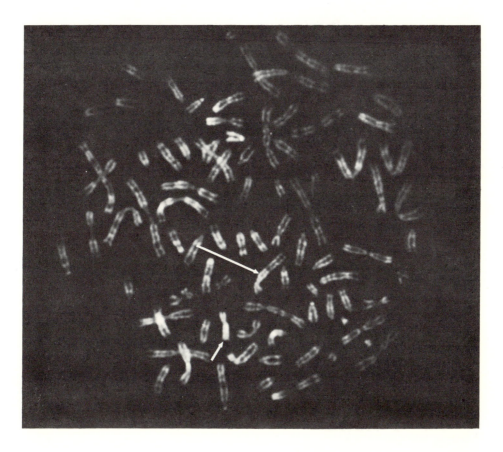

FIGURE 14. Fluorescent metaphase of a cell hybrid between hypoxanthine-selected hybrid DX10-4 cells and the human female cells
(clone R5) that were the human parental cells of hybrid DX10-4.
Two human chromosomes are present in cells of this hybrid R-3,
subclone 1: the active X, T2, marked by the long arrow; and
a morphologically normal X chromosome, indicated by the short
arrow, presumed to be the inactive, but partially derepressed
X chromosome.

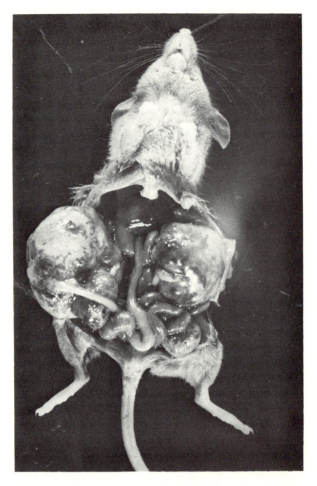

FIGURE 15.   Female LT mouse with large bilateral ovarian tumors
      following intraperitoneal injection of LT clone 8 cells.

only from the injected cells, as both have the same karyotype of
39 chromosomes, including one metacentric. The growth is encap-
sulated within the bursa, and is probably initiated by tumor cells
arriving in the ovary via the bloodstream.

How general this pattern of tumor growth is among various
teratocarcinoma tumors is not yet known. Although some teratocarcinoma No. 6050 sublines show ovarian growth as well as massive
IP growth, other 6050 sublines selected by Dr. Robert Auerbach for
spleen growth (Auerbach 1977) do not produce ovarian tumors. A
malignant endodermal line derived from the same LT tumor, and clone

TABLE 4. Tumor incidence in LT mice inoculated intraperitoneally with 2-4 x 10^6 cells of clone 8, an LT embryonal cell clone.

Females with ovarian tumors	18/29 = 62%
Females with bilateral ovarian tumors	8/18 = 44%
Females with exclusively ovarian tumors	13/18 = 72%
Females with 1-3 other IP tumors	3/18 = 17%
Females with generally disseminated IP tumor growth	2/18 = 11%
Males with IP tumors	0/10 = 0%

ID fibrosarcoma cells also produce some ovarian tumors, though again, not exclusively. Still other tumor lines show no ovarian growth (Kahan, unpublished results). What is remarkable about the LT embryonal line is the *specificity* with which these cells arrive at and grow only in the ovary, perhaps reflecting the specificity shown by normal germ cells, from which the tumor is derived, in their migration to the embryonic ovary. The basis for such specificity is unknown, though preferential cell adhesions are implicated in other model systems of tumor metastasis (Nicholson, Winkelhake, and Nussey 1976) and similar findings have been obtained with these LT and other teratocarcinoma cells (Kahan, manuscript in preparation). Nevertheless, this observation suggests a new approach for assessing the influence of the ovarian environment on X-chromosome expression in teratocarcinoma cells, as well as in other cell types, and possibly even at various stages of ovarian developmental growth.

X-CHROMOSOME BEHAVIOR IN *IN VITRO* TERATOCARCINOMA EMBRYONAL CELLS

To characterize the state of X-chromosome differentiation in embryonal carcinoma cells, an investigation of teratocarcinomas derived from different sources has been initiated. Though the results represent only a few experiments, X-chromosome mutation frequencies indicate that some female teratocarcinoma cells have a single active X chromosome (Table 5). McBurney and Adamson (1976) have found that XX embryonal cells derived from six- and seven-day female embryos (Iles 1977) have only a single active X, as determined by gene-dosage, cytogenetic, and mutational studies. However, Martin, Epstein, Travis, Tucker, Yatziv, Martin, Clift, and Cohen (1978) and Martin, Epstein, and Martin (1978) have found

TABLE 5. Incidence of TG-resistant colonies in embryonal cell lines derived from teratocarcinomas of various sources

Cells	Type	No. of experiments	No. of TG colonies	Cloning efficiency (CE)	Incidence (corrected for CE)
6050	XY male, from a 6-day strain-129 embryo*	2	2, 3	20%	2×10^{-6} 1×10^{-6}
T6-11	XY male, from a 7-day strain-T6 embryo[+]	1	11	13%	1.5×10^{-6}
T6-4	XX female, from a 7-day strain-T6 embryo[+]	1	3	12%	2.3×10^{-6}
Clone 8	XX female, from an LT ovarian tumor	1	5	10%	5×10^{-6}

* Stevens 1970

[+] Kahan, unpublished

by gene dosage analysis that XX embryonal lines derived from an
ovarian teratocarcinoma appear to have two active X's. They suggest that this difference may reflect the state of X-chromosome
determination present in the normal cell(s) at the time of tumor
initiation, inactivation having already occurred in six- and seven-
day embryonic cells, but not in cells derived from oocytes that
have completed their first meiotic division (Eppig, Kozak, Eicher,
and Stevens 1977); or, alternatively, that culture conditions (e.g.
growth on plastic) may initiate X inactivation. It should also
be noted that parthenogenetically activated oocytes in the LT ovary
may proceed for quite some time in an apparently normal fashion —
some showing normal tissue relationships of the equivalent day-seven
embryo before disorganization sets in and results in a teratoma
(Stevens and Varnum 1974). X inactivation is known to occur in
normal diploid parthenogenetic mouse embryos of 7.5—8.5 equivalent
days of gestation (Kaufman, Guc-Cubrilo, and Lyon 1978). It may be,
then, that ovarian-derived teratocarcinomas can have either one or
two active X chromosomes, if the tumors originate at different
developmental points.

    Karyotype analyses of the female lines in Table 5 confirm
the presence of two X's in the TG-derived cells (Fig. 16). In
agreement with McBurney and Adamson (1976), XX embryonal cells
from a seven-day embryo-derived tumor show a mutation frequency
suggesting single-allele expression. In contrast to Martin *et al*.
(1978*a*, *b*), LT ovary-derived clone 8 also has a frequency of TG-
resistant cells suggesting X inactivation. As previously mentioned,
it may be possible to obtain both types of ovarian tumors — having

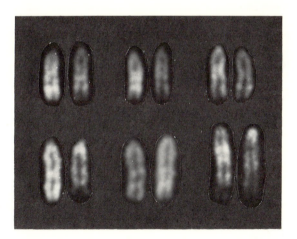

FIGURE 16. The two X chromosomes present in TG-resistant embryonal
            cells. The pair from three metaphases of cells derived from
            LT clone 8 (top row) and T6-4 clone 2 (bottom row) is shown.

either one or two active X's. McBurney and Adamson (1976) have
suggested, however, that there may be a third and very intriguing
explanation for X differences among different teratocarcinoma
clones. In their six-day embryo-derived tumor (day of plug = day
0), not all criteria of X inactivation were met: a late-replicating X could not be found, and enzyme levels of α-galactosidase
were double those found in other XX or XO lines. It may be that
total X genetic inactivation and the accompanying parameters (late
replication, early prophase condensation, interphase Barr body
formation) do not occur simultaneously; and, indeed, studies on
the normal embryo also suggest developmental asynchrony (Issa,
Blank, and Atherton 1969; Takagi 1974; see also review by Gartler
and Andina 1976). If teratocarcinoma stem cells are arrested at
different developmental stages of this process, different tumors
may express different parts of the whole phenomenon that do not
necessarily have to exist simultaneously. It is perhaps too early
to generalize about X-chromosome behavior in different embryonal
clones, as each may represent a different stage of the X-inactivation process.

Experiments have been undertaken to determine whether X-
chromosome reactivation in teratocarcinoma stem cells can occur.
TG-resistant subclones of clone 8 were injected into female mice
and the resulting ovarian tumors were cloned in various selective
media to determine the frequency of hypoxanthine-utilizing derivatives. Clones able to survive in HAT have been obtained, though
no *in vitro*-maintained cells able to utilize hypoxanthine have
been found in 2×10^8 cells. Work to further characterize these
cells is in progress. Karyotype results indicate they are derived
from the injected cells, but the basis for their ability to survive
in HAT is unknown at present. Teratocarcinoma stem cells and normal female germ cells have important properties in common — most
significantly, their apparent totipotentiality (Illmensee and Mintz
1976; and Illmensee 1978), and also cell surface antigens (Gooding
and Edidin 1974; Gooding, Hsu, and Edidin 1976). It would be a
pleasing analogy to find that, just as their normal counterparts
appear to do when they migrate into the embryonic ovary, so female
teratocarcinoma stem cells "recycled" through the ovary also reac-
tivate an X chromosome.

In conclusion, there is now a variety of systems to investigate the initiation of X-inactivation (Martin *et al.* 1978), the
maintenance of the inactivated state, and perhaps even the reactivation step thought to occur in the ovary. Together with new
molecular cloning techniques, these should increase our understanding of this important developmental problem of chromosome and
gene structure and function.

I would like to express my appreciation to Dr. Robert Auerbach and Dr. Robert DeMars for their support and stimulation. I am grateful to Mrs. Mary Nousek for superb culture assistance. Ms. Beth Trend assisted in the HPRT and PGK analyses. This work was supported by grants from the National Institutes of Health to B.K. (CA18994) and to Robert DeMars (GM-06983 and GM-15422).

REFERENCES

Albertini, R. J. and R. DeMars. 1973. Somatic cell mutation: detection and quantification of X-ray-induced mutation in cultured, diploid human fibroblasts. Mutation Res. 18: 199-244.

Auerbach, R. 1977. Toward a developmental theory of immunity: selective differentiation of teratoma cells. In Cell and Tissue Interaction, J. W. Lash and M. M. Burger, Eds. Raven Press, New York, pp. 47-55.

Chapman, V. M., J. D. West, and D. A. Adler. 1978. Bimodal distribution of α-galactosidase activities in mouse embryos. In Genetic Mosaics and Chimeras in Mammals, Liane B. Russell, Ed. Plenum Press, New York and London.

Comings, D. E. 1966. The inactive X chromosome. Lancet ii: 1137-1138.

Cooper, D. W., P. G. Johnston, C. E. Murtagh, G. B. Sharman, J. L. VandeBerg, and W. E. Poole. 1975. Sex-linked isozymes and sex chromosome evolution and inactivation in kangaroos. In Isozymes, III — Developmental Biology, L. Markert, Ed. Academic Press, New York, pp. 559-573.

DeMars, R. and K. Held. 1972. The spontaneous azaquanine-resistant mutants· of diploid human fibroblasts. Humangenetik 16: 87-110.

Eppig, J. J., L. P. Kozak, E. M. Eicher and L. C. Stevens. 1977. Ovarian teratomas in mice are derived from oocytes that have completed the first meiotic division. Nature 269: 517-518.

Felix, J. S. 1971. Genetic studies on cultured cells bearing the Lesh-Nyhan mutation (hypoxanthine-guanine phosphoribosyl-transferase deficiency) with attempts to derepress the inactive X chromosome in heterozygous female cells. Ph.D. Thesis, University of Wisconsin, Madison.

Gartler, S. M. and R. J. Andina. 1976. Mammalian X-chromosome inactivation. Adv. Hum. Genet. 7: 99-140.

Gartler, S. M., R. M. Liskay, B. K. Campbell, R. Sparkes and N. Gant. 1972. Evidence for two functional X chromosomes in human oocytes. Cell Diff. 1: 215-218.

Gooding, L. R. and M. Edidin. 1974. Cell surface antigens of a mouse testicular teratoma. J. Exp. Med. 140: 61-78.

Gooding, L. R., Y. Hsu and M. Edidin. 1976. Expression of teratoma-associated antigens on murine ova and early embryos. Dev. Biol. 49: 479-486.

Green, H., R. Wang, O. Kehinde and M. Meuth. 1971. Multiple human TK chromosomes in human-mouse somatic cell hybrids. Nature New Biol. 234: 138-140.

Iles, S. A. 1977. Mouse teratomas and embryoid bodies: their induction and differentiation. J. Embryol. Exp. Mprph. 38: 63-75.

Illmensee, Karl. 1978. Reversion of malignancy and normalized differentiation of teratocarcinoma cells in chimeric mice. In, Genetic Mosaics and Chimeras in Mammals, Liane B. Russell, Ed. Plenum Press, New York and London.

Illmensee, K. and B. Mintz. 1976. Totipotency and normal differentiation of single teratocarcinoma cells by injection into blastocysts. Proc. Nat. Acad. Sci. USA 73: 549-553.

Issa, M., C. E. Blank and G. W. Atherton. 1969. The temporal appearance of sex chromatin and of the late-replicating X chromosome in blastocysts of the domestic rabbit. Cytogenetics 8: 219-237.

Johnson, R. T. and P. N. Rao. 1970. Mammalian cell fusion: induction of premature chromosome condensation in interphase nuclei. Nature 226: 717-722.

Johnston, P. G., E. S. Robinson and G. B. Sharman. 1976. X chromosome activity in oocytes of kangaroo pouch young. Nature 264: 359-360.

Kahan, B. and R. DeMars. 1975. Localized derepression on the human inactive X chromosome in mouse-human cell hybrids. Proc. Nat. Acad. Sci. USA 72: 1510-1514.

Kahan, B. and B. Ephrussi. 1970. Developmental potentialities of clonal *in vitro* cultures of mouse testicular teratoma. J. Natl. Cancer Inst. 44: 1015-1036.

Kahan, B., K. R. Held and R. DeMars. 1974. Genes for human adenine phosphoribosyltransferase on chromosome No. 16. Genetics
78: 1143-1156.

Kaufman, M. H., M. Guc-Cubrilo and M. F. Lyon. 1978. X-chromosome
inactivation in diploid parthenogenetic mouse embryos. Nature 271:
547-549.

Kratzer, P. G. and S. M. Gartler. 1978. HGPRT expression in early
mouse development. In Genetic Mosaics and Chimeras in Mammals,
Liane B. Russell, Ed. Plenum Press, New York and London.

Lyon, M. F. 1972. X-chromosome inactivation and developmental
patterns in mammals. Biol. Rev. 47: 1-35.

Lyon, M. F. 1974. Mechanisms and evolutionary origins of variable
X-chromosome activity in mammals. Proc. Roy. Soc. Lond. B. 187:
243-268.

Martin, G. R., C. J. Epstein and D. W. Martin, Jr. 1978a. Use of
teratocarcinoma stem cells as a model system for the study of X-
chromosome inactivation in vitro. In Genetic Mosaics and Chimeras
in Mammals, Liane B. Russell, Ed. Plenum Press, New York and London.

Martin, G. R., C. J. Epstein, B. Travis, G. Tucker, S. Yatziv,
D. W. Martin, S. Clift and S. Cohen. 1978b. X-chromosome inactivation during differentiation of female teratocarcinoma stem cells
in vitro. Nature 271: 329-333.

McBurney, M. W. and E. D. Adamson. 1976. Studies on the activity
of the X chromosomes in female teratocarcinoma cells in culture.
Cell 9: 57-70.

Migeon, B. R. 1972. Stability of X-chromosomal inactivation in
human somatic cells. Nature 239: 87-89.

Migeon, B. R. and B. R. Jelalian. 1977. Evidence for two active
X chromosomes in germ cells of female before meiotic entry. Nature
269: 242-243.

Monk, Marilyn. 1978. Biochemical studies on X-chromosome activity
in preimplantation mouse embryos. In Genetic Mosaics and Chimeras
in Mammals, Liane B. Russell, Ed. Plenum Press, New York and London.

Nicholson, G. L., J. L. Winkelhake and A. C. Nussey. 1976. An
approach to studying the cellular properties associated with metastasis: Some in vitro properties of tumor variants selected in

vivo for enhanced metastasis. In Fundamental Aspects of Metastasis, L. Weiss, Ed. North-Holland Publ. Co., Amsterdam. pp. 291-303.

Ohno, S. 1964. Life history of female germ cells in mammals. Proc. 2nd Int. Conf. Congenital Malformations Natl. Found. 36-40.

Romeo, G. R. and B. R. Migeon. 1975. Stability of X chromosomal inactivation in human somatic cells transformed by SV-40. Humangenetik 29: 165-170.

Ruddle, F. H. 1972. Linkage analysis using somatic cell hybrids. Adv. Human Genetics 3: 173-235.

Russell, L. B. 1963. Mammalian X chromosome action: inactivation limited in spread and in region of origin. Science 140: 976-978.

Sato, K., R. R. Slesinski and J. W. Littlefield. 1972. Chemical mutagenesis at the phosphoribosyltransferase locus in cultured human lymphoblasts. Proc. Nat. Acad. Sci. USA 69: 1244-1248.

Stevens, L. C. 1970. The development of transplantable teratocarcinomas from intratesticular grafts of pre- and postimplantation mouse embryos. Dev. Biol. 21: 364-382.

Stevens, L. C. and D. S. Varnum. 1974. The development of teratomas from parthenogenetically activated ovarian mouse eggs. Dev. Biol. 37: 369-380.

Takagi, N. 1974. Differentiation of X chromosomes in early female mouse embryos. Exp. Cell Res. 86: 127-135.

Takagi, N. 1978. Preferential inactivation of the paternally derived X chromosome in mice. In Genetic Mosaics and Chimeras in Mammals, Liane B. Russell, Ed. Plenum Press, New York and London.

Tischfield, J. A. and F. H. Ruddle. 1974. Assignment of the gene for adenine phosphoribosyltransferase to human chromosome 16 by mouse-human somatic cell hybridization. Proc. Nat. Acad. Sci. USA 71: 45-49.

Von Kap-Herr, C. and B. B. Mukherjee. 1977. Stability of inactive X-chromosome in mouse embryoid body-mule cell and transformed mouse cell-mule cell heterokaryons. Exp. Cell Res. 104: 369-376.

West, J. D., V. E. Papaioannou, W. I. Frels and V. M. Chapman. 1978. Preferential expression of the maternally derived X chromosome in extraembryonic tissues of the mouse. In Genetic Mosaics and Chimeras in Mammals, Liane B. Russell, Ed. Plenum Press, New York and London.

STUDIES OF HUMAN-MOUSE CELL HYBRIDS WITH RESPECT TO X-CHROMOSOME

INACTIVATION

Barbara R. Migeon, Joyce A. Sprenkle, and Tai T. Do

Department of Pediatrics, Johns Hopkins University
School of Medicine, Baltimore, Maryland 21205

As a means of obtaining insights into the mechanisms for maintaining X-chromosome inactivation, we have carried out a series of
experiments in an attempt to reverse the process. To identify cells
in which the silent X has been derepressed, we have developed a
model based on the one described by Comings (1966) using human
fibroblasts heterozygous for the common A electrophoretic variant
of glucose-6-phosphate dehydrogenase ($G6PD_A$). In our model, however, the cells are also heterozygous for the Lesch-Nyhan mutation
specifying deficiency of hypoxanthine guanine phosphoribosyl transferase ($HGPRT^-$), so that we can select for *rare* cells in which
reactivation has occurred (Migeon 1972). Clonal populations of
skin fibroblasts from females heterozygous for both $G6PD_A$ and
$HGPRT^-$, but expressing only the alleles on the active X, are subjected to a variety of treatments, and the phenotype with regard
to both loci is ascertained following treatment. The resultant
phenotype is interpreted according to Table 1. The G6PD heteropolymer, because it is never found in mixtures of the two cells under
conditions used for these studies, is a sensitive indicator of two
functional X chromosomes within the same cell, while the presence
of variants at two X-linked loci helps distinguish reactivation
from other events such as reversion, somatic crossing over, or contamination with cells of other phenotype.

With this model, we have examined the effect of a variety of
treatments. Clones have been subcultured under the usual culture
conditions for as many as 14 transfers without observable change in
G6PD phenotype. Exposure to cold shock (4°C) for various periods
of time resulted eventually in cell death, with no alteration in
X-linked phenotype. Sustained exposure to pharmacological doses of

329

TABLE 1. Model for X-inactivation studies

Clonal genotype[†]	Phenotype	Interpretation
	$G6PD_A$ $HGPRT^-$	No effect.
	$G6PD_{AB}$ $(\equiv)$* $HGPRT^+$	Activation of Xi.
$Xa = G6PD_A$ $HGPRT^-$ $\}$ $R_X \dashrightarrow$	$G6PD_A$ $HGPRT^+$	Mutation or somatic exchange.
$Xi = g6pd_B$ $hgprt^+$	$G6PD_B$ $HGPRT^-$	Mutation or somatic exchange.
	$G6PD_B$ $HGPRT^+$	Activation of Xi, plus functional loss of Xa. OR, contamination[§] with $G6PD_B$ $HGPRT^+$ cells.
	$G6PD_{AB}(=)$[‡] $HGPRT^+$	Activation of Xi, plus functional loss of Xa. OR, contamination[§] with $G6PD_B$ $HGPRT^+$ cells.

[†] Xa = active X; Xi = inactive X.

* AB heteropolymer.

[‡] No heteropolymer.

[§] Other polymorphic markers needed to distinguish between alternatives, i.e., HLA.

a variety of hormones (tri-iodo thyronine, cortisol, testosterone, and estradiol), and to dimethyl sulfoxide and bromodeoxyuridine also were ineffective (unpublished observations). Strong selective pressure favoring alleles on the inactive X was ineffective in inducing reactivation even when cell survival depended on expression of alleles on the inactive X* (Migeon 1972). Transformation of these clones by Simian Virus 40 (SV40) did not affect the X-linked enzyme phenotype (Romeo and Migeon 1974).

Stimulated by observations of Harris, Watkins, Ford, and Schoefl (1966) that relatively differentiated nuclei, in which the synthesis of DNA, RNA, or both has been suppressed, can be induced to resume synthesis of nucelic acids by fusion with less differentiated cells of another species, we explored the possibility that fusion with mouse cells might influence the activity of genes on the inactive X. Our initial studies of mouse-human hybrids provided evidence for the stability of X-chromosome inactivation in human cells (Migeon 1972; Table 2, mating #1, this paper). In that mating, the human parent was heterozygous only at the G6PD locus, both X chromosomes having normal HGPRT alleles, so that there was no selective pressure for reactivation of the inactive X. Therefore, we have undertaken other experiments designed to test the effect of interspecific hybridization, utilizing medium that favors the proliferation of cells with a derepressed X.

Table 2 summarizes the experiments that have been carried out: With the exception of mating #1, the human parent cell, in each case, has been a clone heterozygous at both G6PD and HGPRT loci. The mutation at the HGPRT locus has been studied extensively and no revertants have been found among more than 10^8 cells tested. The mouse parental cells were L-cell variants having selectable markers. In one set of experiments (Table 2, mating #2), the human fibroblast clone expressing $G6PD_A$ and the HGPRT mutant allele (with $G6PD_B$ and the HGPRT wild-type allele on the inactive X chromosome) was hybridized to mouse A9 cells lasking HGPRT, and the hybrids were selected in HAT. Since both parent cells were HGPRT deficient, neither could proliferate in HAT, and the growth of hybrids required activation of the HGPRT+ allele on the inactive X chromosome. From this mating, we isolated three HAT-resistant colonies which proved to be mouse cell revertants; no human-mouse hybrids were obtained.

Another mating (Table 2, mating #3) was designed to select for neither human X but for the human chromosome E-17 instead. This was done in hopes of obtaining hybrids that lose the active human

---

* In HAT medium, which blocks *de novo* purine synthesis, activation of the normal HGPRT allele (on the inactive X) is essential for survival of these heterozygous cells (see Model, Table 1).

TABLE 2. Results of hybridization between human skin fibroblast clones and mouse L cells.

Mating	Parent cells		Selection favors retention of:	Results
	Mouse	Human*		
1	Ag: $G6PD_M$ $HGPRT^-$	$Xa = G6PD_A$ $HGPRT^+$ $Xi = g6pd_B$ $hgprt^+$	Either human X	4 hybrid clones: 4, $G6PD_{M+A}^+$ 0, $G6PD_B$
2	Ag: $G6PD_M$ $HGPRT^-$	$Xa = G6PD_A$ $HGPRT^-$ $Xi = g6pd_B$ $hgprt^+$	Human inactive X	0 hybrid clones
3	Cl-1D: $G6PD_M$ $HGPRT^+$ TK^-	$Xa = G6PD_A$ $HGPRT^-$ $Xi = g6pd_B$ $hgprt^+$	Human E-17	14 hybrid clones: 8, $G6PD_M$ only 6, $G6PD_{M+A}^+$ 0, $G6PD_B$ 0, Human HGPRT
4	Ag: $G6PD_M$ $HGPRT^-$	$Xa = G6PD_B$ $HGPRT^+$ $Xi = g6pd_A$ $hgprt^-$	1) Human active X	28 hybrid clones: 28, $G6PD_{M+B}^+$
			2) Human inactive X	25 hybrid clones: 25, $G6PD_M$ 0, $G6PD_A$

* Xa = active X; Xi = inactive X.

+ Including interspecies heteropolymers.

X while retaining the inactive one. Eight of the resulting 14 hybrids were identified as hybrid on the basis of expressing human
lactate dehydrogenase (LDH), but had neither human G6PD nor human
HGPRT, having lost the active X. The remaining 6 hybrid clones
had human G6PD and the interspecies heteropolymer but, in each case,
the G6PD isozyme was the one specified by the active X of the human
parent cell (G6PD$_A$). In no hybrid was there evidence for derepression of the inactive X. The failure to observe re-expression of
the inactive chromosome cannot be attributed to precocious application of selection for the HGPRT allele. In this mating, human
HGPRT was not essential, even in HAT medium, because the mouse
parent cell has normal HGPRT activity, so that gratuitous growth
of the hybrid cells could take place; in fact, the hybrid clones
that retained a human X kept the one expressing the HGPRT$^-$ allele
(the active X). Derepression did not occur, even though the conditions were favorable.

The last set of hybridizations, which explored the possibility
that loss of the human active X in hybrids might turn on the inactive X chromosome, was stimulated by the suggestions of Kahan and
DeMars (1975) that localized derepression of this type occurs once
the active X chromosome is lost. In mating #4, the human parental
clone expressed the G6PD$_B$ and HGPRT wild-type alleles, whereas
G6PD$_A$ and the mutant HGPRT allele were on the inactive X. Cells
were hybridized with A9 lacking HGPRT, and hybrids were selected
in HAT + ouabain (HOT). This time, selection favored the active X
chromosome; 28 hybrids were obtained, and all expressed the human
G6PD allele as well as the interspecies heteropolymers (Table 2,
mating #4; Figure 1a). One week following isolation, each hybrid
clone was taken out of selective medium and permitted one week's
growth under nonselective conditions. 10^6 cells from each clone
were then plated into medium containing 6-thioguanine in order to
select for the hybrid cells that had lost the active X chromosome.*
Results of these experiments are presented in further detail in
Table 3. All 28 hybrid clones gave rise to populations of cells
able to proliferate in 6-thioguanine; when analyzed for G6PD phenotype, cells from each of these clones had lost the human active X
chromosome, as indicated by the loss of G6PD$_B$, the interspecific
heteropolymer (Fig. 1b), and human phosphoglycerate kinase (PGK).
Yet, no clones expressed the G6PD$_A$ allele or the expected interspecies heteropolymers between G6PD$_A$ and mouse G6PD$_M$. Therefore,
in none of the 28 hybrid clones did loss of the active X chromosome
result in the expression of the alleles on the inactive X.

_____

* The purine analog, 6-thioguanine, is toxic to cells with HGPRT
  activity.

TABLE 3. Summary of results of mating #4.*

No. of clones analyzed	Selective medium	Enzymes present					
		G6PD		PGK		LDH	
		mouse	human	mouse	human	mouse	human
28	HOT	28	28	28	28	NT	NT
28	6TG	28	0	28	0	28	24

* See Table 2.

We conclude from these studies of man-mouse hybrids that two X chromosomes may be expressed in a single cell — evident from the presence of interspecies heteropolymers for G6PD. This is true also for intraspecific human hybrids which express heteropolymers made up of reassociation of $G6PD_A$ and $G6PD_B$ subunits (Migeon, Norum, and Corsaro 1974; Corsaro and Migeon 1978). However, neither interspecies fusion nor loss of the active X chromosome induces reactivation of the genetically inert X.

Since cell fusion of this kind often activates genes that have been turned off in differentiated cells (Harris *et al.* 1966; Peterson and Weiss 1972), the means of inactivating these genes probably differ from that involved in the repression of genes on the silent X.

Our studies also suggest that the inactive X chromosome is not retained in hybrids, presumably because it is not derepressed and hence contributes little selective advantage to a hybrid cell. It is likely that the loss of sex chromatin observed in heteroploid tumors (Tavares 1966), or following SV_{40} transformation (Romeo and Migeon 1975), is also attributable to loss of the inactive X.

MATERIALS AND METHODS

Media. The nonselective medium was MEM supplemented with nonessential amino acids and 15% fetal calf serum. Selective media were nonselective medium enriched with amethopterin, hypoxanthine thymidine, and glycine (HAT) or with 6 x 10^{-5} M 6-thioguanine (6TG), or with HAT supplemented with 10^{-6} M ouabain (HOT) (Corsaro and Migeon 1978).

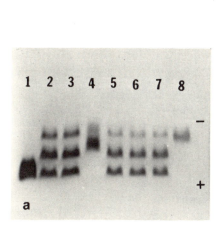
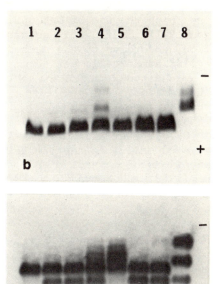

FIGURE 1. Cellulose acetate electrophoresis of hybrids derived
from mating #4 (see Table 2).
(a) G6PD of hybrids selected in HOT.
Parents: Slot 1 (A9); slot 8 (G6PD$_B$ HGPRT$^+$: g6pd$_A$ hgprt$^-$)
Hybrids: Slots 2–3, 5–7
G6PD$_{AB}$ control: Slot 4
(b) G6PD (top) and LDH (bottom) of hybrids re-selected in
6-thioguanine
Parents: Slot 1 (A9); slot 8 (g6PD$_B$ HGPRT$^+$; g6pd$_A$ hgprt$^-$)
Hybrids: Slots 2–7 (one hybrid colony, slot 4, still has
nonviable remnants of the original population of hybrids —
which disappeared on subsequent subcultures).
Note that hybrids, having lost the active X chromosome, still
expressed human LDH, but did not derepress the inactive X.

Cells. Parental cell lines were LMTK$^-$ Cl-1D, deficient in
thymidine kinase; and A9, deficient in HGPRT. Fibroblast strains
#81 and #76 were derived from skin biopsies of females heterozygous
for the G6PD$_{AB}$ alleles, as well as for a nonreverting mutation
resulting in HGPRT deficiency. The human parental clones were obtained by plating 10 cells into 60 mm petri dishes containing HOT
or 6TG, establishing clonal cultures by isolating well-separated
colonies with stainless steel cylinders.

Cell hybridization. Hybrids for the first three matings were obtained with the use of β-propriolactone inactivated sendai virus (Migeon 1972). Mating #4 was carried out using PEG 6000, 50% solution, according to the method of Davidson and Gerald (1976). 10^6 A9:10^5 human cells per 60 mm petri dish were cocultivated. Cells were exposed to PEG 24 hours later and dishes were refilled with HOT medium.

Enzyme studies. The species origin of G6PD, LDH (Corsaro and Migeon 1978), PGK, and HGPRT was identified by means of electrophoresis on cellulose acetate gels. Assays for HGPRT and PGK were modifications of methods of Der Kaloustian, Byrne, Young, and Childs (1969) and Meera Khan (1971), respectively.

This work was supported by NIH grant HD 05465.

REFERENCES

Comings, D. E. 1966. The inactive X chromosome. The Lancet ii: 1137-1138.

Corsaro, C. M. and B. R. Migeon. 1978. Gene expression in euploid human hybrid cells: Ouabain-resistance is codominant. Somat. Cell Genet., in press.

Davidson, R. G., H. M. Nitowsky, and B. Childs. 1963. Demonstrations of two populations of cells in the human female heterozygous for glucose-6-phosphate dehydrogenase variants. Proc. Natl. Acad. Sci. USA 50: 481-485.

Davidson, R. and P. Gerald. 1976. Improved techniques for the induction of mammalian cell hybridization by polyethylene glycol. Som. Cell Genet. 2: 165-176.

Der Kaloustian, V. M., R. Byrne, W. J. Young, and B. Childs. 1969. An electrophoretic method for detecting hypoxanthine-guanine phosphoribosyl transferase variants. Biochem. Genet. 3: 299.

Harris, H., J. F. Watkins, C. E. Ford, and G. I. Schoefl. 1966. Artificial heterokaryons of animal cells from different species. J. Cell Sci. 1: 1-30.

Kahan, B. and R. DeMars. 1975. Localized derepression on the human inactive X chromosome in mouse-human cell hybrids. Proc. Natl. Acad. Sci. USA 72: 1510-1514.

Meera Khan, P. 1971. Enzyme electrophoresis on cellulose acetate gel: Zymogram patterns in man-mouse and man-uinen hamster somatic cell hybrids. Arch. of Biochem. and Biophys. 145: 470-483.

Migeon, B. R. 1972. Stability of X chromosome inactivation in human somatic cells. Nature 239: 87-89.

Migeon, B. R. and J. F. Kennedy. 1975. Evidence for the inactivation of X chromosome early in the development of the human female. Amer. J. of Hum. Genet. 27: 233-239.

Migeon, B. R., R. A. Norum, and C. M. Corsaro. 1974. Isolation and analysis of somatic hybrids from two human diploid cells. Proc. Natl. Acad. Sci. USA 71: 937-941.

Peterson, J. and M. Weiss. 1972. Expression of differentiated functions in hepatoma cell hybrids: Induction of mouse albumin production in rat hepatoma-mouse fibroblast hybrids. Proc. Nat. Acad. Sci. 69: 571-575.

Romeo, G. and B. R. Migeon. 1975. Stability of X chromosomal inactivation in human somatic cells transformed by SV-40. Humangenetik 29: 165-170.

Tavares, A. S. 1966. Sex chromatin in tumors. In, The Sex Chromatin, K. L. Moore, Ed. Saunders, Philadelphia, pp. 405-433.

X-Chromosome Nonrandomness:
Imprinting, Selection

PREFERENTIAL INACTIVATION OF THE PATERNALLY DERIVED X CHROMOSOME IN MICE

Nobuo Takagi

Chromosome Research Unit, Faculty of Science, Hokkaido
University, Sapporo, Japan

Random X-chromosome inactivation makes the female of placental
mammals a natural mosaic for clones of cells having either the
maternally derived X (X^m) or paternally derived one (X^p) genetically
inactivated (Lyon 1961). In marsupials, on the other hand, preferential inactivation of the paternally inherited X chromosome
seems to be a rule in most tissues (Sharman 1971; Cooper, Johnston,
Murtagh, Sharman, VandeBerg, and Poole 1975). There are, however,
instances in which inactivation is obviously not random in placental mammals (Lyon 1974). Nonrandomness was assessed from studies
made on differentiated cells remote from early embryonic cells in
which inactivation occurred. Thus it is not clear whether nonrandom inactivation, or a secondary event(s) after random inactivation,
was responsible for the ultimate nonrandom expression.

A cytological study in early female mouse embryos heterozygous
for the unbalanced form of Cattanach's translocation, T(X;7)1Ct
(Cattanach 1961), carried out at our laboratory (Takagi and Sasaki
1975), revealed that the asynchronously replicating X chromosome
was predominantly paternal in 6½-day postcoital (p.c.) embryos.
Bisection of 7½-day p.c. embryos demonstrated that the excess of
the allocyclic X^p was more pronounced in the extraembryonic half
than in the embryonic half. In a limited number of conceptuses at
8½ days of gestation, we showed that the over-representation of the
allocyclic X^p was restricted to the chorion and the yolk sac.
Later, Wake, Takagi, and Sasaki (1976) confirmed the predominance
of cells with the allocyclic X^p in the rat yolk sac; and West,
Frels, Chapman, and Papaioannou (1977) showed preferential expression of the maternal X-linked allele for phosphoglycerate kinase
(PGK-1) in the mouse yolk sac. Since both cell types were nearly

equally represented in the embryo proper, this phenomenon is evidently not due to a gene analogous to the O^{hv} mutation (Drews,
Blecher, Owen, and Ohno 1974; Ohno, Geller, and Kan 1974) or to the
Xce^a allele of the controlling element (Cattanach and Williams 1972;
Cattanach 1975), which makes the inactivation process nonrandom.
This finding seems closely relevant to various aspects of early embryonic development as well as to X-chromosome inactivation itself.
This chapter will give a brief account of further studies on the
subject.

IDENTIFICATION OF THE GENETICALLY INACTIVATED X CHROMOSOME

Identification of the inactivated X chromosome in our studies
is based primarily on replication late in the S phase. Rattazzi
and Cohen (1971) have proved by single-cell cloning of female mule
cells *in vitro* that the late-replicating X is indeed the genetically inactive one. The reverse may not always be true. The
late-replicating X chromosomes in embryonic and adult mouse cells
are identifiable by quinacrine (QM) fluorescence and by the acetic
saline Giemsa (ASG) technique (Takagi and Oshimura 1973). They
appear heterochromatic along their entire lengths, fluorescing
brightly after QM staining, and staining intensely after the ASG
procedure. A single heterochromatic X is detected by these techniques even when it is not easily identified by ^{3}H-thymidine
(^{3}H-TdR) autoradiography.

Incorporation of 5-bromodeoxyuridine (BUdR), followed by acridine orange fluorescence (Dutrillaux, Laurent, Couturier, and
Lejeune 1973), is adequate for demonstrating the inactive X
chromosome. After continuous treatment with BUdR, the asynchronously replicating X is easily distinguished as the one with weak
red (Fig. 1a) or bright green (Fig. 1b) fluorescence (Takagi and
Sasaki 1975), depending on the relative amount of incorporated
BUdR. For the sake of brevity, the terms "inactive" or "inactivated" will be used interchangeably with such terms as allocyclic,
late replicating, or asynchronously replicating. Similarly, the
term "active" will correspond to isocyclic or synchronously replicating.

X-INACTIVATION MOSAICISM IN VARIOUS REGIONS OF 8½-DAY EMBRYOS

Mosaic composition was examined in 60 embryos at 8½ days p.c.
from chromosomally normal females mated with males carrying Cattanach's translocation. This is the earliest stage at which some
definite embryonic portions can be isolated with relative ease; and,
at the same time, this is the last stage at which individual cells
of intact embryos can incorporate BUdR or ^{3}H-TdR *in vitro* and yield

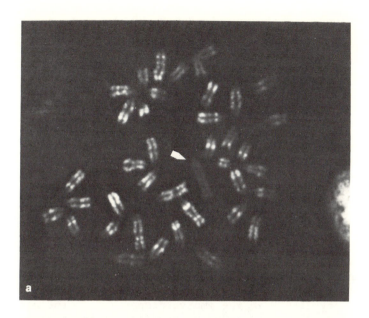

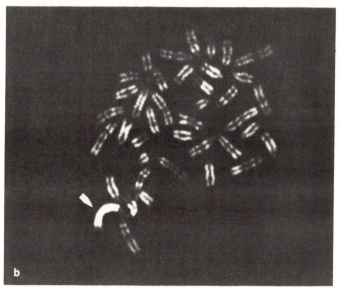

FIGURE 1. Two kinds of asynchronously-replicating X chromosomes
from 8½-day mouse embryos. Cells were allowed to incorporate
BUdR for 8 hours *in vitro* and then stained with acridine
orange. (a) The late-replicating X incorporated BUdR much
more than did the other chromosomes, and fluoresced weakly.
(b) The early-replicating allocyclic X incorporated much less
BUdR and fluoresced brightly.

a large number of metaphase cells without resort to tissue culture.
Usually, conceptuses were separated into the embryo proper, yolk
sac, allantois, and chorion immediately before slide preparation
(Wroblewska and Dyban 1969). When possible, the chorion was further divided into dorsal and ventral halves. The former three
regions were separated relatively free of contamination, but the
chorion could contain a small amount of the ectoplacental cone and
yolk sac.

Routinely, mosaic composition was determined on the basis of
50 metaphase cells; but when two kinds of cells appeared irregular-
ly, another 50 cells were scored. In case abnormality was suspected, we examined as many cells as possible. The allantois and the
chorion yielded fewer metaphases than the embryo proper and the
yolk sac. Data were omitted unless at least 20 cells were counted
in a sample.

The mosaic composition in each embryonic region, expressed as
the percentage of cells with the X^P allocyclic, is shown in Table
1. Cells with an allocyclic X^m were slightly in excess of those
with an allocyclic X^P in the embryo proper and in the allantois,
in contrast to our preliminary report (Takagi and Sasaki 1975).
The X^P-allocyclic cells outnumbered X^m allocyclics in the two extraembryonic regions, but the mosaic composition in the yolk sac was
considerably lower in this series than in that reported previously.
A t-test showed no significant difference in mosaic composition
between the embryo proper and the allantois. Differences are highly
significant between other regions. Correlation is statistically
significant between the embryo proper and the allantois ($p < 0.05$),
and between the embryo proper and the yolk sac ($p < 0.01$, Fig. 2);
whereas it is not significant between the allantois and yolk sac.

TABLE 1. Mosaic composition due to X-chromosome inactivation in
four embryonic regions from $8\frac{1}{2}$-day conceptuses produced by the
cross $X^n X^n$ x $X^t Y$*

Region	% of cells with allocyclic X^P
Yolk sac (n=60)	74.41 ± 1.64
Embryo proper (n=60)	47.74 ± 1.61
Allantois (n=14)	46.19 ± 5.02
Chorion (n=36)	98.43 ± 0.41

* X^n = normal X chromosome; X^t = X chromosome carrying a large
autosomal insertion (Cattanach's translocation)

Table 2 shows the mean mosaic composition in 63 heterozygous 8½-day embryos from the cross between heterozygous females and chromosomally normal males. These figures are essentially in accord with those obtained in the above 60 conceptuses. However, the mosaic composition in the yolk sac was more variable in this cross (Fig. 3) than in the other; and the correlation was not significant between the embryo proper and the yolk sac.

OVER-REPRESENTATION OF X^P-INACTIVE CELLS IN THE EXTRAEMBRYONIC

ECTODERM AND YOLK-SAC ENDODERM

The polar trophectoderm gives rise to the extraembryonic ectoderm (Gardner and Johnson 1975), the main constituent of the chorion. We may safely conclude that the extraembryonic ectoderm consists nearly exclusively of cells with the inactive X^P. The yolk sac comprises the extraembryonic mesoderm and endoderm derived from the primitive endoderm (Gardner and Papaioannou 1975). The allantois is composed solely of mesoderm (Snell and Stevens 1966) of the lineage common to the yolk-sac mesoderm (Fig. 4). The mosaic composition in the yolk-sac mesoderm may be similar, though not identical, to that in the allantois of the same conceptus. If this is the case, it should be the yolk-sac endoderm that accounts for the overrepresentation of X^P-inactive cells in the yolk sac as a whole. West *et al.* (1977) used an X-linked electrophoretic variant for PGK-1, recently reported by Nielsen and Chapman (1977), to estimate the relative proportions of the expression of X^m and X^P in the mouse yolk sac. They have shown that the paternally derived *Pgk-1* allele, and hence probably the whole X chromosome, is not expressed in the yolk-sac endoderm.

This obviously predicts correlation between the mosaic composition in the yolk sac and in the allantois. The failure to get a significant correlation coefficient between the two may be due to small sample size (14 pairs) and to the fact that the mosaic composition of the allantois had to be worked out on the basis of a relatively small number of metaphase cells. It is of special interest that the predominance of X^P-inactive cells was found in descendants of the trophectoderm and the primitive endoderm, the earliest two tissues that have differentiated from the totipotent cells forming the entire embryo.

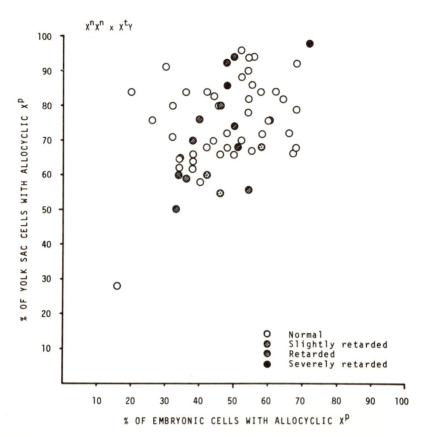

FIGURE 2. A scatter diagram showing mosaic composition in the embryo proper and the yolk sac in 60 female 8½-day embryos obtained from the cross X^nX^n x X^tY. Correlation is significant between the two regions. The regression line here is $Y = 0.43X + 53.66$.

TABLE 2. Mosaic composition in the embryo proper and the yolk sac from 8½-day conceptuses produced by the cross X^tX^n x X^nY

Region	% of cells with allocyclic X^P
Embryo proper (n=63)	48.32 ± 1.83
Yolk sac (n=63)	78.83 ± 2.32

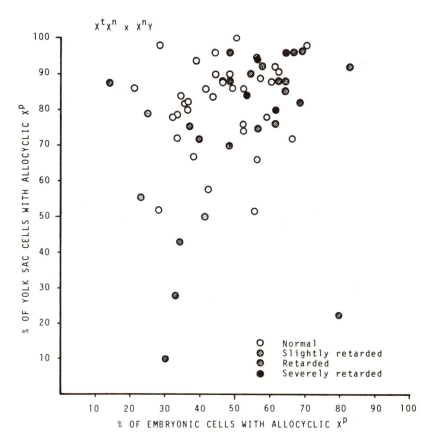

FIGURE 3. A scatter diagram showing mosaic composition in the embryo proper and the yolk sac in 63 female 8½-day embryos obtained from the cross X^tX^n x X^nY. Retarded embryos are more frequent in this cross than in the cross X^nX^n x X^tY, and correlation is not significant between the embryo proper and the yolk sac.

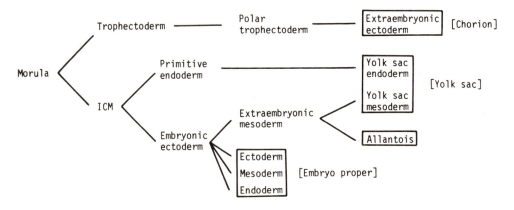

FIGURE 4. Cell lineages in embryonic regions cytogenetically
examined in the present study. This is based on the diagram
by Gardner and Papaioannou (1975).

EARLY-REPLICATING ALLOCYCLIC X CHROMOSOME IN THE CHORION

In the vast majority of cells, the allocyclic X in the chorion
is different from that in other regions. It is the brightest
element in the complement after continuous treatment of cells with
BUdR for as long as 8 hours. The proportion of cells with the
bright X chromosome varied in different conceptuses. Table 3 summarizes the results from 43 conceptuses. ^{3}H-TdR autoradiography
demonstrated that replication finished in this chromosome much earlier than in the rest of the complement. Silver grains, if any,
after continuous labeling with the radioactive TdR for 6 hours,
were restricted to the centromeric portion or, more frequently,
to the distal region of the fd X chromosome (an X chromosome with
a long autosomal insertion). A similar brightly fluorescent X
chromosome was also found in trophoblastic cells grown from 3½-day
blastocysts transplanted into the testis. In our earlier report
(Takagi 1974), we assumed, on the basis of autoradiographic data,
that the allocyclic X chromosome replicating early in the S phase
changes into a late replicator with fetal development. Although
we have evidence for such change in a proportion of cells (N. Wake
and N. Takagi, unpublished observation), it is more likely that the
early-replicating X is characteristic for trophectoderm derivatives.

TABLE 3. Mosaic composition and frequency of the early-replicating X chromosome in the chorion

Sample	% of cells with allocyclic X^P	% of early-replicating X
Dorsal half (n=12)	99.20 ± 0.39	56.87 ± 6.82
Ventral half (n=12)	97.15 ± 1.34	71.93 ± 7.97
Combined (n=12)	98.56 ± 0.50	70.78 ± 4.73
Whole (n=24)	98.44 ± 0.55	81.48 ± 4.04

It is unknown whether this early-replicating X has any functional significance in trophectoderm derivatives. In this context, it was of special interest to find a retarded conceptus (Fig. 6d) in which 94% of chorionic cells had a late-replicating X chromosome, rather than an early-replicating one. It may be worth-while to explore the control mechanism of replication and the possible modification of genetic activity in early- and late-replicating X chromosomes.

PREFERENTIAL INACTIVATION OF X^P IN THE TROPHECTODERM

There are at least 4 possible ways to bring about the unbalanced mosaicism in the yolk sac and chorion: (1) preferential inactivation of X^P; or (2) random inactivation, followed by either (a) selective growth of cells in which X^m is active, or (b) preferential sampling of X^m-active cells as foundation cells, or (c) reactivation of the inactive X^m with simultaneous inactivation of the active X^P.

The elegant study of Gardner and Lyon (1971) on coat color of mice developed from blastocysts injected with a single inner-cell-mass (ICM) cell from 3½-day blastocysts established that inactivation has not occurred at 3½ days. Their further study, injecting single 4½-day ICM cells, yielded evidence indicating the two X chromosomes have not yet differentiated at 4½ days. Our own study (Takagi 1974) has demonstrated that each X chromosome from XX morulae shows a QM fluorescent pattern identical to that of the X chromosome from a male cell. A heterochromatic, brightly fluorescent X chromosome is found in metaphase cells from blastocysts consisting of more than 40 cells. Concomitant appearance of a heteropycnotic element, most probably an X, in prophase nuclei, strongly supports the view that the modified QM fluorescence reflects inactivation. Our study suggested, but, owing to its technical limitation, could not prove, that genetic inactivation had occurred at this stage. Recently, support for this view has come from measurements of the activity of hypoxanthine-guanine-phosphoribosyl transferase (HGPRT) in single preimplantation embryos. It has been demonstrated that both X chromosomes are active in preimplantation embryos, at least at the morula stage (Monk 1978), but that inactivation has occurred in most cells of the blastocyst on day 4 of gestation (Monk and Kathuria 1977). The number of cells in the ICM is small in comparison with that in the trophectoderm at this stage (Barlow, Owen, and Graham 1972). The chronological discrepancy between the time of inactivation assessed genetically, using injection chimeras, and that assessed cytologically or biochemically may be reconciled if one assumes that inactivation occurs earlier in the trophectoderm than in the ICM.

If inactivation in the trophectoderm in fact precedes that in the ICM, it would be possible to assess whether the initial decision process is random in the former without microdissection of the blastocysts. On this assumption, we tried to examine parental origin of the heterochromatic X chromosome in preparations made from intact $3\frac{1}{2}$ to 4-day blastocysts heterozygous for Cattanach's translocation (Takagi, Wake, and Sasaki 1978). Of 205 chromosomally ascertained heterozygous blastocysts, 89 possessed at least one metaphase with a brightly fluorescent X chromosome (Fig. 5). The cell number ranged from 32 to 96 in these embryos. Parental origin of the heterochromatic X chromosome is summarized in Table 4. The number of informative cells was not large, yet it is evident that the paternally derived X was heterochromatic in most cases. The heterochromatic X chromosome at this stage is not late replicating (Takagi 1974), resembling the early-replicating X chromosome in the chorion. Cytogenetic similarities between the blastocysts and the chorion tempt us to suggest that the over-representation of the X^P-inactive cells in the chorion reflects preferential inactivation in the trophectoderm, though the final conclusion must await observations on the separated trophectoderm and ICM.

PREFERENTIAL INACTIVATION OF X^P IN THE PRIMITIVE ENDODERM

At $4\frac{1}{2}$ days, differentiation of the primitive endoderm on the blastocoelic surface of the ICM may be deduced from morphological appearance as well as from the specific patterns of chimerism when this tissue is injected into host blastocysts (Gardner and Papaioannou 1975). There is also evidence to suggest that determination of progenitor cells of the primitive endoderm has occurred at $3\frac{1}{2}$ days (Gardner and Papaioannou 1975). Since X inactivation has not occurred at this stage (Lyon 1974), it is likely that inactivation takes place independently in the primitive endoderm and in the

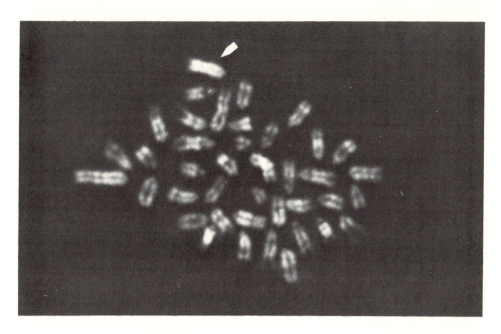

FIGURE 5. A QM-stained metaphase spread from a 3½-day blastocyst. The paternally derived X^n is heterochromatic and fluorescing brightly. [Reproduced, by permission, from Cytogenet. Cell Genet. <u>20</u>: 240-248. (Karger, Basel 1978)]

TABLE 4. Parental influence on heterochromatization of the X chromosome in $X^n X^t$ blastocysts. [From Cytogenet. Cell Genet. <u>20</u>: 240-248 (Karger, Basel 1978)]

Cross	Heterochromatic	
	X^t	X^n
$X^t X^n \times X^n Y$	4	26
$X^n X^n \times X^t Y$	86	11

non-endoderm of the ICM. Thus, cellular differentiation precedes
or coincides with X-chromosome inactivation in the primitive endoderm as in the trophectoderm. In the absence of evidence to the
contrary, this seems to indicate that nonrandom sampling of foundation cells after random inactivation does not account for over-
representation of X^p-inactive cells in the yolk-sac endoderm.

The possible role of reversal of inactivation has been examined
by double labeling of 6½ to 7½-day embryos with ^{3}H-TdR in the first
cell cycle *in vitro*, followed by BUdR in the next (Takagi 1976).
The asynchronously-replicating X chromosome identified by autoradiography always corresponded to the chromosome identified by fluorescence microscopy in the same cell, providing no evidence for
the reversal of inactivation at the critical period of yolk-sac
formation.

West *et al*. (1977) have examined the relative proportions of
PGK-1 isozymes in the yolk sac of heterozygous progeny of *Pgk-1^a/*
Pgk-1^b females mated with either *Pgk-1^a*/Y or *Pgk-1^b*/Y males. In
each cross, the maternally inherited allele was preferentially
expressed in the yolk sac (i.e., *Pgk-1^b* in the cross *Pgk-1^a/Pgk-1^b*
x *Pgk-1^a*/Y, and *Pgk-1^a* in the cross *Pgk-1^a/Pgk-1^b* x *Pgk-1^b*/Y), even
though the progeny from the two crosses had developed in similar
heterozygous uteri. This appears to rule out cell selection, based
on differences in genetic makeup of two X chromosomes, as a cause
of preferential expression of the maternally derived *Pgk-1* allele.

There is still a possibility that the maternal environment, as
such, exerts selection pressure against X^p-active cells. We examined this possibility indirectly by exposing embryos to male
environment. The 3½-day blastocysts were individually grafted
under the testis capsule of adult male mice, and explants recovered 7—8 days later were subjected to cytogenetic examination. At
least 20 metaphases could be scored in 15 female explants. The
inactive X was predominantly paternal in 14 embryos, whereas it
was predominantly maternal in the largest embryo we have ever
recovered from the testis. The X^m-inactive cells in this large
embryo predominated in both the embryonic and extraembryonic
regions. Although full evaluation of this case has to await further data, we may tentatively conclude that the mosaicism is not
affected in the male environment and possibly not in the female
either.

Several conceptuses examined at 8½ days have low mosaic compositions in the yolk sac as well as in the embryo proper (Figs 2—3,
Table 5). Assuming mosaic composition is similar in the embryo
proper and in the yolk-sac mesoderm, and about a half of the yolk-
sac cells are endodermal in origin, we have to postulate inactivation of X^m in a considerable proportion of endodermal cells in

TABLE 5. Mosaic composition in 5 exceptional conceptuses

| Embryo | Parents | Growth | % of cells with allocyclic X^P in | | |
			Yolk sac	Embryo	Chorion
71–11	$X^t X^n - X^n Y$	retarded	10.1	29.9	—
112–8	$X^t X^n \ X^n Y$	retarded	28.0	32.9	—
121–6	$X^t X^n \ X^n Y$	retarded	22.3	79.2	—
143–7	$X^t X^n \ X^n Y$	retarded	42.9	34.0	—
177–1	$X^n X^n \ X^t Y$	normal	28.6	16.0	90.0

such conceptuses. This suggests that the X^m-inactive cell itself
is not lethal or severely disadvantageous in the yolk-sac endoderm.
It is likely that the mosaic composition of the yolk-sac endoderm
at $8\frac{1}{2}$ days reflects, to a certain extent, the initial condition at
the time of inactivation. One may conclude, therefore, that inactivation is generally nonrandom in the primitive endoderm, but that
nonrandomness may be relaxed under certain conditions.

DEVELOPMENTAL IMPLICATION OF PREFERENTIAL INACTIVATION OF X^P

The eutherian type of random X inactivation is considered to
have evolved from the marsupial type of paternal-X inactivation
(Cooper 1971). It is possible to assume that the preferential inactivation of X^P in extraembryonic membranes of mice represents a
character inherited from the paternal-X-inactivation system. Alternatively, it may be an innovation following the establishment of
random inactivation in eutherians. The latter predicts certain
advantages of the X^m-active cells in embryonic development. But,
in the total absence of knowledge about the functional significance
of paternal-X inactivation in marsupials, the former cannot help to
favor either functional significance or neutrality of X^m-active
cells in mouse extraembryonic regions.

One possible way of assessing the significance of the preferential inactivation of X^P would be to examine the development of
exceptional embryos whose yolk sac or chorion is not predominated
by X^P-inactive cells. So far we have found five embryos with low
mosaic composition* in the yolk sac (Table 5). Four of them showed

---

* Low and high mosaic composition refer to the frequencies of
  cells with X^P allocyclic

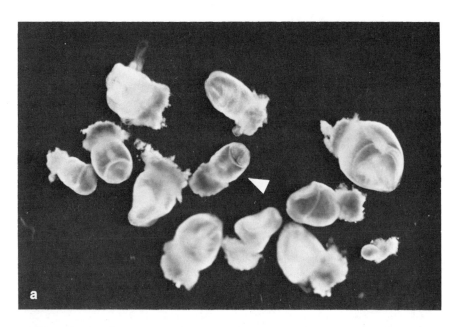

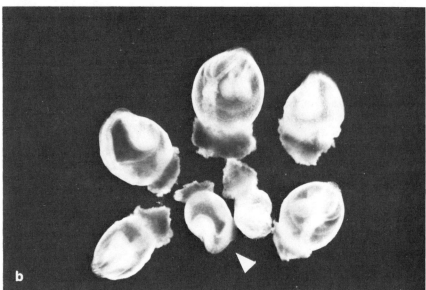

FIGURE 6. Cytogenetically exceptional embryos with their littermates before incubation with BUdR. Arrows indicate embryos
listed in Table 5, as follows: (a) embryo #121-6; (b) embryo
#143-7; (c) embryo #177-1; (d) embryo #158-2, in which 94%
of chorionic cells had a late-replicating X chromosome.

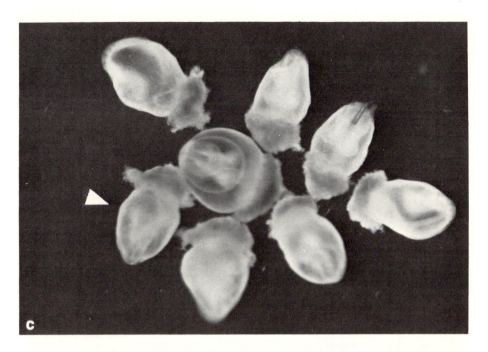

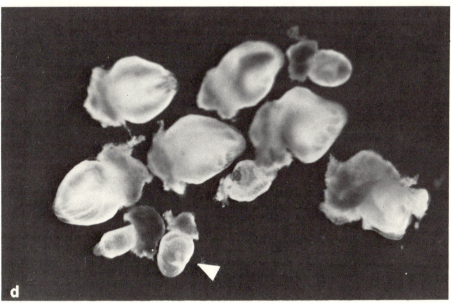

FIGURE 6 (CONTINUED)

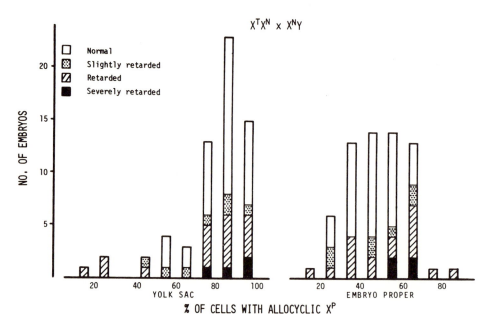

FIGURE 7.   Distribution of mosaic compositions in the yolk sac and
the embryo proper in 8½-day embryos from the cross $X^t X^n$ x $X^n Y$.
Low mosaic compositions in the yolk sac, but not in the embryo
proper, are apparently related to growth retardation.

growth retardation in comparison with their littermates (Fig. 6a—b),
but the remaining one was more or less normal in development (Fig.
6c). Mosaic composition was also low in the embryo proper in four
of them. That this is not a contributing factor to developmental
delay is apparent from several normally developed conceptuses with
low mosaic composition in the embryo proper, but with high mosaic
composition in the yolk sac (Figs. 2—3). A structural rearrangement of the X chromosome could evoke both nonrandom inactivation
and developmental delay, but scrutiny of karyotypes in each case
failed to show any evidence for a new rearrangement. The chorion
was not examined in 4 of the cases; but, in the remaining one, 90%
of chorionic cells were X^p-inactive.

Developmentally retarded embryos at 8½ days are not rare, especially in the cross $X^t X^n$ x $X^n Y$ (Fig. 7). However, the high incidence of growth regardation in conceptuses having a yolk sac of
low mosaic composition is statistically significant. One interpretation of this finding is that the predominance of X^p-active cells
in the yolk sac is responsible for growth retardation. Conversely,
the abnormal development may account for the predominance of X^m-

inactive cells in the yolk sac. Viable X^{P}O mice and androgenetic
mice experimentally produced by Hoppe and Illmensee (1977) may not
be consistent with the former view. In either case, further studies
in such abnormal embryos would be fruitful for a better understanding of the mechanism and the role of X-chromosome inactivation
in mammals.

CONCLUSION

     Several points of interest emerge from our cytogenetic studies
on pre- and postimplantation mouse embryos, and from the findings
of other laboratories.

     1. Over-representation of X^P-inactive cells in the chorion
and the yolk sac is due to the extraembryonic ectoderm and the
yolk-sac endoderm, respectively. However, this should be verified
by further studies.

     2. Differentiation of the trophectoderm and the primitive
endoderm precedes, or coincides with, X-chromosome inactivation in
each tissue. It is not known whether X inactivation occurs earlier
in the primitive endoderm than in the non-endoderm of the ICM.

     3. Preferential inactivation of X^P accounts for the over-
representation of X^P-inactive cells in the trophectoderm and primitive endoderm.

     4. Over-representation of X^m-inactive cells in the yolk sac
may somehow be related to abnormal embryonic development. It is
not known whether the former is the cause or result of the latter.

     5. The vast majority of the allocyclic X^P's in the chorion
(and possibly in other trophectoderm derivatives) is early replicating, rather than late replicating, and finishes replication much
earlier than any other chromosome in the complement. It would be
of interest to explore the control mechanism governing replication
time and the genetic difference between early- and late-replicating
allocyclic X chromosomes.

     The author wishes to thank Professor Motomichi Sasaki for
valuable advice and for a critical reading of the manuscript; and
Dr. Norio Wake for discussion and assistance. Our experimental
work was supported by grants from the Ministry of Education,
Science, and Culture, and the Ministry of Health and Welfare of
Japan.

REFERENCES

Barlow, P. W., D. Owen and C. F. Graham. 1972. DNA synthesis in the preimplantation mouse embryo. J. Embryol. exp. Morph. 27: 431-445.

Cattanach, B. M. 1961. A chemically-induced variegated-type position effect in the mouse. Z. VererbLehre 92: 165-182.

Cattanach, B. M. 1975. Control of chromosome inactivation. Ann. Rev. Genet. 9: 1-18.

Cattanach, B. M. and C. E. Williams. 1972. Evidence of nonrandom X chromosome activity in the mouse. Genet. Res. 19: 229-240.

Cooper, D. W. 1971. Directed genetic change model for X chromosome inactivation in eutherian mammals. Nature, Lond. 230: 292-294.

Cooper, D. W., P. G. Johnston, C. E. Murtagh, G. B. Sharman, J. L. VandeBerg and W. E. Poole. 1975. In Isozymes. Vol. III. Developmental Biology, C. L. Markert, Ed., pp. 559-573. San Francisco: Academic Press.

Drews, U., S. R. Blecher, D. A. Owen and S. Ohno. 1974. Genetically directed preferential X-activation seen in mice. Cell 1: 3-8.

Dutrillaux, B., C. Laurent, J. Couturier and J. Lejeune. 1973. Coloration des chromosomes humains par l'acridine orange apres traitement par le 5 bromodeoxyuridine. C. R. Acad. Sc. Paris 276: 3179-3181.

Gardner, R. L. and M. H. Johnson. 1975. Investigation of cellular interaction and development in the early mammalian embryo using interspecific chimaeras between the rat and mouse. In Cell Patterning (Ciba Found. Symp. 29), pp. 183-200. Amsterdam: Associated Scientific Publishers.

Gardner, R. L. and M. F. Lyon. 1971. X chromosome inactivation studied by injection of a single cell into the mouse blastocyst. Nature, Lond. 231: 385-386.

Gardner, R. L. and V. E. Papaioannou. 1975. Differentiation in the trophectoderm and inner cell mass. In The Early Development of Mammals, pp. 107-132. London: Cambridge University Press.

Hoppe, P. C. and K. Illmensee. 1977. Microsurgically produced homozygous-diploid uniparental mice. Proc. Natl. Acad. Sci. USA 74: 5657-5661.

Lyon, M. F. 1961. Gene action in the X-chromosome of the mouse (*Mus musculus* L.). Nature, Lond. 190: 372-373.

Lyon, M. F. 1974. Mechanisms and evolutionary origins of variable X-chromosome activity in mammals. Proc. roy. Soc. B. 187: 243-268.

Monk, M. 1978. Biochemical studies on X-chromosome activity in preimplantation mouse embryos. In Symposium on Genetic Mosaics and Chimeras in Mammals, Liane B. Russell, Ed. Plenum Press, New York and London.

Monk, M. and Kathuria, H. 1977. Dosage compensation for an X-linked gene in preimplantation mouse embryos. Nature, Lond. 270: 599-601.

Nielsen, J. T. and V. M. Chapman. 1977. Electrophoretic variation for sex-linked phosphoglycerate kinase (PGK-1) in the mouse. Genetics 87: 319-325.

Ohno, S., L. N. Geller and J. Kan. 1974. The analysis of Lyon's hypothesis through preferential X-activation. Cell 1: 175-184.

Rattazzi, M. C. and M. M. Cohen. 1971. Further proof of genetic inactivation of the X-chromosome in the female mule. Nature, Lond. 237: 393-395.

Sharman, G. B. 1971. Late DNA replication in the paternally derived X chromosome of female kangaroos. Nature, Lond. 230: 231-232.

Snell, G. D. and L. C. Stevens. 1966. Early embryology. In Biology of the Laboratory Mouse, 2nd edition, E. L. Green, Ed. New York: McGraw-Hill.

Takagi, N. 1974. Differentiation of X chromosomes in early female mouse embryos. Exptl. Cell Res. 86: 127-135.

Takagi, N. 1976. Stability of X chromosome differentiation in mouse embryos: reversal may not be responsible for the extreme X-inactivation mosaicism in extraembryonic membranes. Hum. Genet. 34: 207-211.

Takagi, N. and M. Oshimura. 1973. Fluorescence and Giemsa banding studies of the allocyclic X chromosome in embryonic and adult mouse cells. Exptl. Cell Res. 78: 127-135.

Takagi, N. and Sasaki, M. 1975. Preferential inactivation of the paternally derived X chromosome in the extraembryonic membranes of the mouse. Nature, Lond. 256: 640-642.

Takagi, N., N. Wake and M. Sasaki. 1978. Cytologic evidence for preferential inactivation of the paternally derived X chromosome in XX mouse blastocysts. Cytogenet. Cell Genet. 20: 240-248.

Wake, N., N. Takagi and M. Sasaki. 1976. Nonrandom inactivation of X chromosome in the rat yolk sac. Nature, Lond. 262: 580-581.

West, J. D., W. I. Frels, V. M. Chapman and V. E. Papaioannou. 1977. Preferential expression of the maternally derived X chromosome in the mouse yolk sac. Cell 12: 873-882.

Wroblewska, J. and A. P. Dyban. 1969. Chromosome preparation from embryos during early organogenesis: Dissociation after fixation, followed by air drying. Stain Technol. 44: 147-150.

PREFERENTIAL EXPRESSION OF THE MATERNALLY DERIVED X CHROMOSOME IN EXTRAEMBRYONIC TISSUES OF THE MOUSE

John D. West[1], Virginia E. Papaioannou[1], William I. Frels[2] and Verne M. Chapman[2]

[1]Department of Zoology, University of Oxford, South Parks Road, Oxford, OX1 3PS, England. [2]Department of Molecular Biology, Roswell Park Memorial Institute, 666 Elm Street, Buffalo, NY 14263, USA.

INTRODUCTION

Nonrandom X-chromosome expression in XX female mammals has been reported in several different situations. For example, when one X chromosome carries a deletion, only the normal X chromosome is expressed (Grumbach, Morishima, and Taylor 1963), but when one X chromosome is involved in a certain reciprocal X-autosome translocation* — Searle's translocation in mice (reviewed by Eicher 1970) — only the abnormal X chromosome is expressed. Similar exclusive expression of one X chromosome has been reported in the blood of certain human X-inactivation mosaics (Nance 1964; Gandini, Gartler, Angioni, Argiolas, and Dell'Acqua 1968), and this observation is most consistently made when the absent blood-cell population would express a deleterious X-linked gene, such as an HPRT deficiency (Nyhan, Bakay, Connor, Marks, and Keel 1970). Less extreme cases of nonrandom X-chromosome expression have been reported in some tissues of humans (Nance 1964; Ropers, Wienker, Grimm, Schroetter, and Bender 1977) and mules (Hook and Brustman 1971), and for various stocks of mice apparently heterozygous for an X-linked controlling-element locus (Cattanach and Isaacson 1965; Grahn, Lea, and Hulesch 1970; Krzanowska and Wabik 1971; Falconer and Isaacson 1972; Ohno, Christian, Attardi, and Kan 1973).

---

* See Russell and Cacheiro, this volume for analyses of randomness in other X-autosome translocations.

These examples of nonrandom X-chromosome expression appear to be a result of genetic heterozygosity which results in either non-random X-chromosome inactivation or a selective advantage to one of the two cell populations in the mosaic and are discussed elsewhere in this volume (Russell and Cacheiro 1978; Migeon 1978). In other cases, the parental origin of the X chromosomes, rather than the X-linked genotype, influences X-chromosome expression. This has been reported for various macropod marsupials (VandeBerg, Cooper, and Sharman 1973; Cooper, Johnston, Murtagh, and VandeBerg 1975) and for certain extraembryonic membranes of the mouse and rat (Takagi and Sasaki 1975; Wake, Takagi, and Sasaki 1976). In both of these situations, the maternally derived X chromosome (X^m) is preferentially expressed.

In this article we shall consider the expression of X chromosomes in the developing mouse embryo and its extraembryonic membranes.

CYTOGENETIC EXPERIMENTS

The first evidence for preferential expression of X^m in certain extraembryonic membranes was reported by Takagi and Sasaki (1975) for the mouse; and, a year later, a similar observation was made for the rat by Wake, Takagi, and Sasaki (1976). These authors identified X^m and X^p cytologically in mitotic preparations from conceptuses that were heterozygous for Cattanach's insertion in the mouse and heterozygous for a telocentric-subtelocentric dimorphism in the rat. The inactive X chromosome was assumed to be the asynchronously replicating (allocyclic) homologue, which was distinguished from its isocyclic partner using a specific staining technique. The results from these cytogenetic experiments are summarised in Table 1.

For both mouse and rat, X^p was asynchronously replicating (and presumably inactive) in about 50% of the mitotic spreads from the embryo and in about 90% of those from the yolk sac. The percentage for the mouse chorion was even higher than for the yolk sac, but the situation in the allantois was closer to that in the embryo. The nonrandom staining of the X chromosomes in the yolk sac and chorion was shown to be an effect of the parental origins of the chromosomes, rather than of the X-linked genotypes, by making reciprocal crosses where the marker chromosomes were introduced from the mother and father, respectively. These experiments provided cytogenetic evidence for preferential activity of X^m in the mouse chorion and in the yolk sacs of both mouse and rat.

TABLE 1. Parental influence on X-inactivation mosaic composition of 8½-day mouse embryos and 10½-day rat embryos
(Data from Takagi and Sasaki 1975; and Wake, Takagi, and Sasaki 1976)

Area examined	Mating type*	% with allocyclic X^P	
		Mouse	Rat
Embryo	I	—	55
	II	—	57
Anterior half of embryo	I	52	—
	II	52	—
Posterior half of embryo	I	55	—
	II	57	—
Allantois	I	77	—
	II	66	—
Yolk sac	I	90	95
	II	89	91
Chorion	I	97	—
	II	98	—

* The chromosome markers introduced from the male parent in mating-type I were introduced from the female parent in mating-type II.

GENETIC EXPERIMENTS

In our experiments we have used an electrophoretic variant of the X-linked enzyme phosphoglycerate kinase (PGK-1), discovered by Nielsen and Chapman (1977), to investigate the expression of X^m and X^P in the mouse embryo and yolk sac. These genetic experiments support and extend the cytogenetic evidence for preferential expression of X^m in the mouse yolk sac.

Fetuses and yolk sacs were dissected on the fourteenth day of gestation, coded, and analysed blind for the expression of PGK-1A and PGK-1B isozymes as described previously (West, Frels, Chapman, and Papaioannou 1977). Heterozygous fetuses were distinguished from homozygous and hemizygous fetuses by virtue of their two-banded PGK-1 phenotype. In all the experiments described below, we considered only the heterozygous female progeny (as defined by the PGK-1 isozyme pattern from fetal homogenates), unless stated otherwise. The proportions of the two PGK-1 isozyme bands were classified according to a five-point scale shown in Table 2 (footnote). Although this quantitation is subjective, the classification of three series of coded artificial mixtures of PGK-1A and PGK-1B male kidney homogenates suggests that the error is small. These mixtures indicate that the PGK-1A and PGK-1B isozymes stain with similar intensity on our gels, and that a minor isozyme band representing 5—10% of the homogenate mixture can be detected (West *et al.* 1977).

The first four crosses shown in Table 2 were designed to confirm the cytogenetic results of Takagi and Sasaki (1975). In these reciprocal crosses, the *Pgk-1^a* allele was introduced from a non-inbred background and the *Pgk-1^b* allele was introduced from either C3H/HeHa or DBA/2Ha inbred mice. In all four crosses, the mean PGK score for the fetus is close to 3, indicating balanced mosaicism. The yolk sacs, however, have a more unbalanced isozyme distribution. The reciprocal crosses show that the direction of this imbalance is not consistently toward the preferential expression of either the *Pgk-1^a* allele or the *Pgk-1^b* allele, but shows a preferential expression of the maternally derived allele.

Contamination of the yolk sac with maternal tissue (or maternal enzyme) would contribute to the unbalanced expression of PGK-1 in the yolk sacs of heterozygous progeny. This was ruled out as an explanation for our results, however, by experiments involving heterozygous mothers and embryo transfers. We also tested for the extent of maternal contamination by monitoring the expression of the autosomal, ubiquitous enzyme glucose phosphate isomerase (GPI-1). The details of these controls are discussed elwewhere (West *et al.* 1977). Thus, the results from the first four crosses shown in Table 2 support the results of the cytogenetic experiments reported by Takagi and Sasaki (1975); the expression of an X-linked gene and the asynchronous replication of one X chromosome both strongly suggest that the maternally derived X chromosome is preferentially expressed in the mouse yolk sac.

Influence of the maternal environment

Preferential expression of X^m could be a result of either (1) an intrinsic difference between X^m and X^p produced by a differential marking process dependent on the parental origins of the two X chromosomes, or (2) a selection pressure exerted by the maternal environment and dependent on the X-linked gene expression in the mother.

TABLE 2. Mean PGK scores for fetuses and yolk sacs from six crosses

Cross*		No. of conceptuses	Mean PGK score† (± S.E.)	
Female	Male		Fetuses	Yolk sacs
Experiment 1				
b/b(C3H)	a/Y	54	3.39 ± 0.07	1.96 ± 0.04
b/b(DBA)	a/Y	52	3.15 ± 0.06	1.94 ± 0.03
a/a	b/Y(C3H)	34	3.50 ± 0.09	4.56 ± 0.10
a/a	b/Y(DBA)	36	3.11 ± 0.08	4.25 ± 0.08
Experiment 2				
a/b	a/Y	25	3.24 ± 0.10	2.00 ± 0.00
a/b	b/Y(C3H)	34	3.53 ± 0.09	4.32 ± 0.09

* a/a = $Pgk\text{-}1^a/Pgk\text{-}1^a$; b/b = $Pgk\text{-}1^b/Pgk\text{-}1^b$; a/b = $Pgk\text{-}1^a/Pgk\text{-}1^b$; a/Y = $Pgk\text{-}1^a$/Y; b/Y = $Pgk\text{-}1^b$/Y; C3H = C3H/HeHa; DBA = DBA/2Ha.

† The proportions of PGK-1A and PGK-1B isozyme bands were scored on a five-point scale: 1, only PGK-1B detected; 2, PGK-1B > PGK-1A; 3, PGK-1B $\simeq$ PGK-1A; 4, PGK-1A > PGK-1B; 5, only PGK-1A detected.

We have tested the second possibility, that X-linked genes expressed in the maternal reproductive tract exert a selection pressure on the developing yolk sac, in two ways. The first test was to cross heterozygous females to either $Pgk-1^a$/Y or $Pgk-1^b$/Y hemizygous males. In each cross, half the female progeny were heterozygous and all the conceptuses developed in heterozygous mothers but the parental origins of the two $Pgk-1$ alleles differed between the crosses. In the $Pgk-1^a/Pgk-1^b$ x $Pgk-1^a$/Y cross, the heterozygous progeny receive the $Pgk-1^b$ allele from their mother; whereas in the heterozygous progeny from the $Pgk-1^a/Pgk-1^b$ x $Pgk-1^b$/Y cross, the $Pgk-1^a$ allele is of maternal origin. The results from these crosses are shown in Table 2. The PGK score for the yolk sacs again indicates unbalanced mosaicism. The two crosses with heterozygous females differ in the direction of the imbalance and show a preferential expression of the maternally derived allele, even though the progeny from the two crosses develop in similar heterozygous reproductive tracts, which were mosaic for $Pgk-1$ and probably for many other X-linked genes.

The second test was to transfer embryos surgically from matings between C3H/HeHa ($Pgk-1^b/Pgk-1^b$) females and $Pgk-1^a$/Y males and from the reciprocal crosses between $Pgk-1^a/Pgk-1^a$ females and C3H/HeHa ($Pgk-1^b$/Y) males to uteri of a third strain of mice [random-bred HA(ICR) strain] that were homozygous for $Pgk-1^b$. Female embryos from these matings were heterozygous (PGK-1AB phenotype) and implanted into PGK-1B uteri. Unbalanced mosaicism in the yolk sacs is again implied by the PGK scores shown in Table 3. The reciprocal crosses differ in the direction of the imbalance and indicate preferential expression of the maternally derived allele in the yolk sac. In the more informative cross, heterozygous embryos received a $Pgk-1^a$ allele from their $Pgk-1^a/Pgk-1^a$ mother but implanted into a PGK-1B uterus. In this case preferential expression of the maternal ($Pgk-1^a$) allele occurred in the yolk sac.

TABLE 3. Mean PGK scores for fetuses and yolk sacs after blastocysts from reciprocal crosses were transferred into the uteri of HA(ICR) strain females ($Pgk-1^b/Pgk-1^b$)

Cross*		HA(ICR) recipient female	No. of conceptuses	Mean PGK score (± S.E.)	
Female	Male			Fetuses	Yolk sacs
b/b(C3H)	a/Y	b/b	16	3.69 ± 0.12	2.00 ± 0.00
a/a	b/Y(C3H)	b/b	13	3.46 ± 0.14	4.15 ± 0.10

* a/a = $Pgk-1^a/Pgk-1^a$; b/b = $Pgk-1^b/Pgk-1^b$; a/Y = $Pgk-1^a$/Y;

  b/Y = $Pgk-1^b$/Y; C3H = C3H/HeHa.

Both these experiments show that the maternally derived *Pgk-1* allele is preferentially expressed in the yolk sac irrespective of the X-linked gene expression in the uterus. The crosses using heterozygous females also rule out the possibility of an influence of the maternal environment on earlier preimplantation-stage embryos. We therefore conclude that the parental origin of the *Pgk-1* allele determines the direction of the unbalanced expression in the yolk sac, and that X^m is intrinsically different from X^p.

Nature of the unbalanced mosaicism

The visceral yolk sac comprises two layers of cells, an outer layer of endoderm and an inner layer of mesoderm. We separated these two layers and analysed them independently to determine whether both layers showed the preferential expression of the maternally derived *Pgk-1* allele.

For this analysis we used conceptuses resulting from crosses between C3H/HeHa females (*Pgk-1^b/Pgk-1^b*) and *Pgk-1^a*/Y hemizygous males. We selected female conceptuses on the basis of sex chromatin staining of the amnion (Vickers 1967) and separated the yolk-sac endoderm from the yolk-sac mesoderm after limited digestion in trypsin and pancreatin (Levak-Švajger, Švajger, and Škreb 1969). To ensure adequate activity for electrophoretic analysis, yolk-sac fractions were pooled from three females. The sex of each of the three conceptuses was confirmed by a double banded PGK-1AB isozyme pattern for each fetus. The results of the analysis of eight groups of three heterozygous female conceptuses is shown in Table 4. Each row represents the five fractions analysed from a group of three conceptuses and comprises three individual fetuses (labeled A, B, and C), pooled yolk-sac mesoderm, and pooled yolk-sac endoderm.

The PGK scores for the mesoderm samples indicate that both *Pgk-1* alleles are expressed. In seven of the eight endoderm samples, however, we detected only the maternally derived isozyme (PGK-1B). We detected a minor PGK-1A component in one sample; but, when this sample was re-coded and analysed four more times, no PGK-1A band was seen. We do not know whether the original scoring was a result of some technical error, or whether this sample contained a very small PGK-1A component. The PGK scores for the yolk-sac mesoderm samples still indicate a perferential expression of the maternally derived *Pgk-1* allele compared to the fetuses. The possibility of contamination with yolk-sac endoderm, however, has still to be eliminated.

The results shown in Table 4 strongly suggest that the unbalanced mosaicism in the yolk sac is due to an extreme imbalance

TABLE 4. PGK scores for fetuses, yolk-sac mesoderm, and yolk-sac endoderm from $Pgk-1^b/Pgk-1^b$(C3H/HeHa) x $Pgk-1^a$/Y conceptuses

Fetuses			Yolk sacs (A, B and C pooled)	
A	B	C	Mesoderm	Endoderm
3	3	3	2	1
4	3	3	2	1
3	4	3	2	1
3	3	4	2	1
3	4	4	3	1
3	3	4	3	1
3	4	3	3	1
3	3	3	2	2

in the yolk-sac endoderm. It seems probable that the paternally derived *Pgk-1* allele (and probably the whole of X^P) is not expressed in the yolk-sac endoderm.

Specificity of the exclusive expression of the maternally derived Pgk-1 *allele*

The agreement between the results from the cytogenetic and genetic studies implies that the nonrandom expression of the *Pgk-1* locus in the mouse yolk sac is not specific to this locus but reflects the expression of other X-linked genes. *Mus musculus* x *Mus caroli* hybrids provide a useful system for testing this inference, since these hybrids are heterozygous for the X-linked genes responsible for glucose-6-phosphate dehydrogenase (G6PD) and hypoxanthine guanine phosphoribosyl transferase (HPRT), as well as for PGK (Chapman and Shows 1976). The expression of PGK in the yolk sacs and fetuses of hybrid conceptuses has been examined (West, Frels, and Chapman 1978). The results, shown in Table 5, indicate preferential expression of the maternally derived (*M. musculus*) *Pgk-1* allele, although for technical reasons reciprocal crosses have not been made. Preliminary experiments indicate that the *M. musculus* form of G6PD is also probably preferentially expressed in the yolk sacs of these hybrids (West, Frels, and Chapamn, unpublished), but this has yet to be confirmed.

TABLE 5. Preferential expression of the maternally derived X chromosome in the yolk sacs of female *Mus musculus* x *Mus caroli* hybrids
[From West, Frels, and Chapman 1978]

Developmental age (days)	Number of female hybrid conceptuses	Mean PGK score*	
		Fetuses	Yolk sacs
12½—13½	5	2.60 ± 0.24	4.00 ± 0
13½—14½	2	3.00 ± 0	4.00 ± 0
14½—15½	11	2.64 ± 0.15	4.00 ± 0.13
15½—16½	4	2.00 ± 0	4.25 ± 0.25
Total	22	2.54 ± 0.11	4.05 ± 0.08

* *Mus musculus* (M) and *Mus caroli* (C) bands of phosphoglycerate kinase were scored on the following five-point scale: 1, only C detected; 2, C > M; 3, C ≃ M; 4, M > C; 5, only M detected.

The tissue distribution of the preferential expression of X^m has not yet been fully established. Similarly, it is unknown whether this phenomenon is restricted to rats and mice or more widespread. The available cytogenetic and genetic data relevant to the tissue distribution in mice is presented in Tables 1 and 4, and summarised in Table 6. In Table 6, the tissues are listed according to their origin from one of the three layers of the 4½-day blastocyst (Gardner and Papaioannou 1975). Although the data are incomplete, the results are compatible with the idea that derivatives of the primitive ectoderm are mosaic and comprise both cells that express X^m and cells that express X^p, whereas derivatives of the other two cell lineages express only X^m. Experiments are now in progress to fill in the gaps in Table 6. Preliminary results indicate that X^p is not expressed in trophoblast (Frels and Chapman, unpublished) or chorionic ectoderm (Frels, Chapman, and Rossant, unpublished).

TABLE 6. Expression of X^m and X^p in mouse cell lineages*

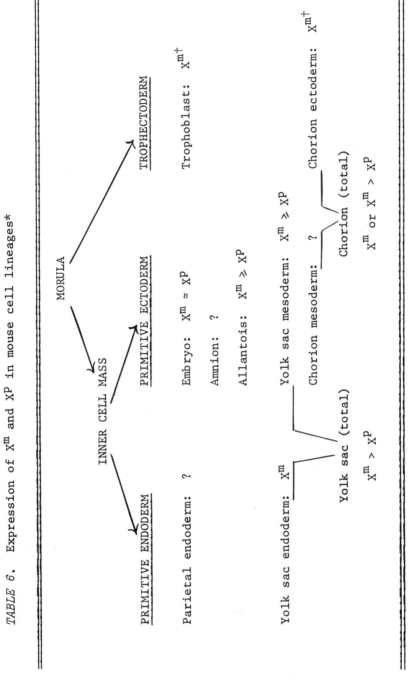

* Cell lineages based on Gardner and Papaioannou 1975.

† Unpublished results of Frels and Chapman (trophoblast) and Frels, Chapman, and Rossant (chorion ectoderm).

SOME INTERPRETATIONS AND SPECULATIONS

Although adult female eutherian mammals are functional mosaics (Lyon 1961) with two populations of cells, expressing X^m and X^P respectively, X^P is either not expressed or expressed in very few cells in the marsupials so far studied (VandeBerg, Cooper, and Sharman 1973; Cooper *et al.* 1975). The results discussed above indicate that X-chromosome expression in some extraembryonic tissues of mice and rats is similar to that described for the body tissues of marsupials. It seems reasonable, therefore, to look for a common mechanism for these two groups of observations. Any explanation for the observed preferential expression of X^m in certain extraembryonic membranes of mice and rats needs to take into account both the evidence that this involves some intrinsic difference between X^m and X^P and that this difference is interpreted in a tissue-specific way.

Although the tissue distribution of the expression of X^P has not been completely analysed, the division of the tissues of the conceptus into the three primary cell lineages shown in Table 6 provides a useful framework for further experimentation. Representative tissues from each of the lineages have been studied, and for the purposes of this discussion we shall assume that only the derivatives of the primitive ectoderm express both X^m and X^P, and that the derivatives of the other two lineages shown in Table 6 express only X^m.

The evidence that X^m and X^P are "marked" as different is open to several interpretations. We have argued elsewhere (West *et al.* 1977) that the most likely interpretation is that both X^m and X^P are active in all the cells of the early preimplantation embryo, but, at the time of X-chromosome inactivation, X^P is preferentially inactivated in the cells ancestral to the yolk sac endoderm. We shall now assume that this preferential inactivation occurs in all the cells of the primitive endoderm and trophectoderm. Lyon (1977) has suggested that the tissue specificity of preferential X-chromosome inactivation could be explained if the effect of the differential "marking" of X^m and X^P is relatively short-lived, and if X-chromosome inactivation occurs later in the primitive ectoderm than in the other two lineages. Thus, it is proposed that the differential "marking" of X^m and X^P "wears off" after X-chromosome inactivation in the trophectoderm and the primitive endoderm but before X-chromosome inactivation in the primitive ectoderm. (The timing of X-chromosome inactivation in the trophectoderm and primitive endoderm could coincide with the differentiation of these tissues on the fourth and fifth day, respectively.) This scheme can accommodate the observations on marsupials by postulating that X-chromosome inactivation in their primitive ectoderm normally occurs before the loss of the differential "marking" of X^m and X^P.

This "marking" of X^m and X^p as different is analogous to the concept of "chromosome imprinting" (Chandra and Brown 1975).

There is at least some circumstantial evidence that suggests that X-chromosome inactivation may not occur simultaneously throughout the embryo. Park (1957) suggested that sex chromatin is absent in preimplantation human and macaque embryos and begins to form after implantation, at first in the trophoblast and later in the embryo proper. Aitken (1974) showed that there was a gradual increase in the frequency of sex-chromatin-positive cells in the trophectoderm during delayed implantation in the roe deer. Although Plotnick, Klinger, and Kosseff (1971) claimed that sex chromatin formation begins in all regions of the preimplantation rabbit embryo at the same time, it is not clear whether the authors distinguished between trophectoderm and inner cell mass cells. The experiments involving X-chromosome function, although limited, are at least compatible with the idea that X-chromosome inactivation may occur later in the primitive ectoderm than in the other cell lineages. The experiments of Gardner and Lyon (1971) indicate that both X chromosomes in the primitive ectoderm are potentially active until at least the fifth day, whereas the distribution of activities of X-linked enzymes among individual morulae and blastocysts is compatible with earlier X-chromosome inactivation in at least some cells of the blastocyst (Adler, West, and Chapman 1977; Monk and Kathuria 1977). This topic is discussed in more detail by Chapman, West, and Adler (1978); Epstein, Travis, Tucker, and Smith (1978); Kratzer and Gartler (1978); and Monk (1978).

Takagi, Wake, and Sasaki (1978) have also recently suggested that X-chromosome inactivation might occur earlier in the cells of the trophectoderm than in the inner cell mass of the mouse blastocyst. These authors found that some mitotic spreads from XX blastocysts had no heterochromatic (inactive) X chromosome whereas others had a single heterochromatic X, predominantly of paternal origin. These observations are consistent with the idea, discussed above, that the paternally derived X chromosome is preferentially inactivated in cells in which X-chromosome inactivation occurs relatively early. This work is discussed in more detail by Takagi (1978).

CONCLUSIONS

Our results strongly suggest that only the maternally derived X chromosome is expressed in the mouse yolk-sac endoderm. We have demonstrated that the mother's X-linked genes that are expressed in the maternal reproductive tract do not cause this effect by exerting a selection pressure against embryonic cells that express X^p. We therefore conclude that the parental origins of X^m

and X^P somehow "mark" them as different from one another. This difference is expressed in a tissue-specific way, such that in the yolk-sac endoderm (and probably in other derivatives of the primitive endoderm and trophectoderm) only X^m is expressed, whereas the fetus (and probably other derivatives of the primitive ectoderm) is a mosaic of two mixed cell populations that, respectively, express X^m and X^P. The suggestion that the expression of X^P in a tissue may depend on a relatively late time of X-chromosome inactivation in cells that are ancestral to that tissue deserves further investigation.

SUMMARY

Cytogenetic experiments reported by Takagi and Sasaki (1975) provided the first evidence for preferential activity of the maternally derived X chromosome (X^m) in the mouse yolk sac and chorion. This has been confirmed using an electrophoretic variant of phosphoglycerate kinase (PGK-1) to study the expression of the two X chromosomes in female mouse conceptuses, heterozygous for the X-linked *Pgk-1* gene. In *Pgk-1^a/Pgk-1^b* heterozygous fetuses, the two isozymes of PGK-1 are detectable in almost equal proportions as expected for a balanced mosaic phenotype; but in the yolk sacs, the maternally derived form of PGK-1 predominates, suggesting unbalanced mosaicism. The possibility of a selection pressure exerted by the maternal reproductive tract against cells that express the paternally derived X chromosome (X^P) has been excluded. Preferential expression of the maternally derived allele occurred even when the mother was heterozygous, or when embryos were surgically transferred into the uteri of females homozygous for the other *Pgk-1* allele. These experiments indicate that the parental origins of X^m and X^P "mark" them as different from one another, and that this differential marking results in preferential expression of X^m in the yolk sac. Further experiments revealed that, although both PGK-1 isozymes were present in the yolk-sac mesoderm, the isozyme produced by the paternally derived allele was absent (or present at very low activity levels) in the yolk-sac endoderm.

The paternally derived *Pgk-1* allele (and therefore probably the whole of X^P) may be inactive in other tissues derived from the primitive endoderm and trophectoderm, and the tissue distribution of this effect is now being explored. The differential "marking" of X^m and X^P and the tissue specificity of this effect is not yet understood. One possibility is that differences in timing of X-chromosome inactivation among different tissues in the early embryo determine whether X^P may be expressed.

We are grateful to the National Institutes of Health and the Medical Research Council for financial support for our own work. V. E. Papaioannou also thanks the Cancer Research Campaign and the International Union Against Cancer for support.

REFERENCES

Adler, D. A., J. D. West and V. M. Chapman. 1977. Expression of α-galactosidase in preimplantation mouse embryos. Nature 267: 838–839.

Aitken, R. J. 1974. Sex chromatin formation in the blastocyst of the roe deer (*Capreolus capreolus*) during delayed implantation. J. Reprod. Fert. 40: 235–239.

Cattanach, B. M. and J. H. Isaacson. 1965. Genetic control over the inactivation of autosomal genes attached to the X chromosome. Z. VererbLehre 96: 313–323.

Chandra, H. S. and S. W. Brown. 1975. Chromosome imprinting and the mammalian X chromosome. Nature 253: 165–168.

Chapman, V. M. and T. B. Shows. 1976. Somatic cell genetic evidence for the X chromosome linkage of three enzymes in the mouse. Nature 259: 665–667.

Chapman, V. M., J. D. West and D. A. Adler. 1978. Bimodal distribution of α-galactosidase activities in mouse embryos. In Genetic Mosaics and Chimeras in Mammals, Liane B. Russell, Ed., Plenum Press, New York and London.

Cooper, D. W., P. G. Johnston, C. E. Murtagh and J. L. VandeBerg. 1975. Sex chromosome evolution and activity in mammals, particularly kangaroos. In Eukaryote Chromosome. W. J. Peacock and R. D. Brock, Eds., pp. 381–393. Camberra: Australian National University Press.

Eicher, E. M. 1970. X autosome translocations in the mouse: total inactivation versus partial inactivation of the X chromosome. Adv. Genet. 15: 175–259.

Epstein, C. J., B. Travis, G. Tucker and S. Smith. 1978. The direct demonstration of an X-chromosome dosage effect prior to inactivation. In Genetic Mosaics and Chimeras in Mammals, Liane B. Russell, Ed., Plenum Press, New York and London.

Falconer, D. S. and J. H. Isaacson. 1972. Sex-linked variegation modified by selection in Brindled mice. Genet. Res. 20: 291–316.

Gandini, E., S. M. Gartler, G. Angioni, N. Argiolas and G. Dell' Acqua. 1968. Developmental implications of multiple tissue studies in glucose-6-phosphate dehydrogenase-deficient heterozygotes. Proc. Nat. Acad. Sci. USA 61: 945-948.

Gardner, R. L. and M. F. Lyon. 1971. X chromosome inactivation studied by injection of a single cell into the mouse blastocyst. Nature 231: 385-386.

Gardner, R. L. and V. E. Papaioannou. 1975. Differentiation in the trophectoderm and inner cell mass. In The Early Development of Mammals, M. Balls and A. E. Wild, Eds., pp. 107-132. London: Cambridge University Press.

Grahn, D., R. A. Lea and J. Hulesch. 1970. Location of an X-inactivation controller gene on the normal X chromosome of the mouse. Genetics 64: 525.

Grumbach, M. M., A. Morishima and J. H. Taylor. 1963. Human sex chromosome abnormalities in relation to DNA replication and heterochromatinization. Proc. Nat. Acad. Sci. USA 61: 945-948.

Hook, E. B. and L. D. Brustman. 1971. Evidence for selective differences between cells with an active horse X chromosome and cells with an active donkey X chromosome in the female mule. Nature 232: 349-350.

Kratzer, P. G. and S. M. Gartler. 1978. HGPRT expression in early mouse development. In Genetic Mosaics and Chimeras in Mammals, Liane B. Russell, Ed., Plenum Press, New York and London.

Krzanowska, H. and B. Wabik. 1971. Selection for expression of sex-linked gene Ms (Mosaic) in heterozygous mice. Genetica Polonica 12: 537-544.

Levak-Švajger, B., A. Švajger and N. Škreb. 1969. Separation of germ layers in presomite rat embryos. Experentia 25: 1311-1312

Lyon, M. F. 1961. Gene action in the X chromosome of the mouse (Mus musculus L). Nature 190: 372-373.

Lyon, M. F. 1977. Chairman's address. In Reproduction and Evolution. Proceedings of the 4th Symposium on Comparative Biology of Reproduction (Australian Academy of Science) pp. 95-98.

Migeon, B. R. 1978. Selection and cell communication as determinants of female phenotype. In Genetic Mosaics and Chimeras in Mammals, Liane B. Russell, Ed., Plenum Press, New York and London.

Monk, M. 1978. Biochemical studies on X-chromosome activity in preimplantation mouse embryos. In, Genetic Mosaics and Chimeras in Mammals, Liane B. Russell, Ed. Plenum Press, New York and London.

Monk, M. and H. Kathuria. 1977. Dosage compensation for an X-linked gene in preimplantation mouse embryos. Nature 270: 599-601.

Nance, W. E. 1964. Genetic tests with a sex-linked marker: glucose-6-phosphate dehydrogenase. Cold Spring Harbor Symposia on Quantitative Biology 29: 415-425.

Nielsen, J. T. and V. M. Chapman. 1977. Electrophoretic variation for sex-linked phosphoglycerate kinase (PGK-1) in the mouse. Genetics 87: 319-325.

Nyhan, W. L., B. Bakay, J. D. Connor, J. F. Marks and D. K. Keel. 1970. Hemizygous expression of glucose-6-phosphate dehydrogenase in erythrocytes of heterozygotes of the Lesch-Nyhan syndrome. Proc. Nat. Acad. Sci. USA 65: 214-218.

Ohno, S., L. Christian, B. J. Attardi and J. Kan. 1973. Modified expression of the *testicular feminization* (*Tfm*) gene of the mouse by a "controlling element" gene. Nature New Biol. 245: 92-93.

Park, W. W. 1957. The occurrence of sex chromatin in early human and macaque embryos. J. Anat. 91: 369-373.

Plotnick, F., H. P. Klinger and A. L. Kosseff. 1971. Sex chromatin formation in preimplantation rabbit embryos. Cytogenetics 10: 244-253.

Ropers, H-H., T. F. Wienker, T. Grimm, K. Schroetter and K. Bender. 1977. Evidence for preferential X chromosome inactivation in a family with Fabry disease. Am. J. Hum. Genet. 29: 361-370.

Russell, L. B. and N. L. A. Cacheiro. 1978. The use of mouse X-autosome translocations in the study of X-inactivation pathways and nonrandomness. In Genetic Mosaics and Chimeras in Mammals, Liane B. Russell, Ed., Plenum Press, New York and London.

Takagi, N. 1978. Preferential inactivation of the paternally derived X chromosome in mice. In, Genetic Mosaics and Chimeras in Mammals, Liane B. Russell, Ed. Plenum Press, New York and London.

Takagi, N. and M. Sasaki. 1975. Preferential inactivation of the paternally derived X chromosome in the extraembryonic membranes of the mouse. Nature 256: 640-641.

Takagi, N., N. Wake and M. Sasaki. 1978. Cytologic evidence for preferential inactivation of the paternally derived X-chromosome in XX mouse blastocysts. Cytogenet. Cell Genet. 20: 240-248.

VandeBerg, J. L., D. W. Cooper and G. B. Sharman. 1973. Phosphoglycerate kinase. A polymorphism in the wallaby *Macropus parryi*: activity of both X chromosomes in muscles. Nature 243; 47-48.

Vickers, A. D. 1967. Amniotic sex chromatin and foetal sexing in the mouse. J. Reprod. Fertil. 14: 503-505.

Wake, N., N. Takagi and M. Sasaki. 1976. Nonrandom inactivation of X chromosome in the rat yolk sac. Nature 262: 580-581.

West, J. D., W. I. Frels and V. M. Chapman. 1978. *Mus musculus* x *Mus caroli* hybrids: mouse mules. J. Hered., in press.

West, J. D., W. I. Frels, V. M. Chapman and V. E. Papaioannou. 1977. Preferential expression of the maternally derived X chromosome in the mouse yolk sac. Cell 12: 873-882.

IN SEARCH OF NONRANDOM X INACTIVATION: STUDIES OF THE PLACENTA

FROM NEWBORNS HETEROZYGOUS FOR GLUCOSE-6-PHOSPHATE DEHYDROGENASE

Barbara R. Migeon and Tai T. Do

Department of Pediatrics, Johns Hopkins University
School of Medicine, Baltimore, Maryland 21205

The version of the X-inactivation hypothesis presented by
Lyon (1961, 1972) proposed that inactivation was a random event
with respect to the parental origin of the X chromosome. Although
there have been some suggestions that inactivation may not always
occur randomly, the evidence has not been compelling. On the basis
of enzyme phenotype in small numbers of blood samples from interspecies hybrids, it has been suggested that the paternally derived
X chromosome of marsupials is inactivated preferentially; on the
other hand, studies of other tissues have revealed that paternal
alleles are expressed (Cooper 1971; Cooper, Johnston, Murtagh,
Sharman, VandeBerg, and Poole 1974; Cooper, Johnston, Murtagh and
VandeBerg 1975). Observations compatible with preferential expression of the maternal allele in the mule, the interspecies hybrid
between female horse and male donkey (Hamerton, Richardson, Gee,
Allen, and Short 1971), proved to be the result of a relative
selective advantage for cells with an active horse X chromosome
(Hook and Brustman 1971). Similarly, the nonrandom pattern of X-
inactivation observed for structurally abnormal X chromosomes is
now known to result from selection rather than X inactivation
(Leisti, Kaback, and Rimoin 1975; Russell and Cacheiro 1978). It
seems quite certain, at least in eutherian mammals, that X inactivation occurs randomly in the cells of the fetus; however, there has
been recent evidence suggesting that this may not be true in fetal
membranes.

The first evidence for preferential activity of the maternally
derived X chromosome came from cytological observations of embryonic
membranes of mice. Tagaki and Sasaki (1975), using Cattanach's
translocation to mark the parental origin of the allocyclic X

379

chromosome, showed unbalanced mosaicism in the chorion and endoderm
of the yolk sac. Similar observations have been reported for the
rat (Wake, Tagaki, and Sasaki 1976; Takagi 1978). Although it is
not clear that the allocyclic behavior observed by Tagaki and colleagues can be equated with X inactivation, West, Frels, Chapman,
and Papaioannou (1977) and West, Papaioannou, Frels, and Chapman
(1978) have provided evidence that the paternal allele is indeed
excluded. Using an electrophoretic variant of phosphoglycerate
kinase (PGK) to study the expression of two X chromosomes in mice
heterozygous for the variant, they observed preferential expression
of the maternally derived PGK allele in the yolk sacs of heterozygous conceptuses, irrespective of maternal genotype or intrauterine
environment.

     To determine if these observations extend beyond rodents and
are true for human populations, we have undertaken a study of human
extraembryonic membranes, using, as a probe, the common electrophoretic variants of glucose-6-phosphate dehydrogenase (G6PD). We
began our exploration using full-term placentae for the following
reasons. (1) The sex of the newborn could be easily determined;
(2) cord blood for each newborn was available, having been collected
routinely at the time of delivery; and (3) maternal blood specimens
were available (with the mother's informed consent) for comparison
with her infant's G6PD type. Unfortunately, the yolk sac is only
a remnant and not easily found. Therefore, we have analyzed chorion, both the smooth membraneous portion overlying the amnion
(referred to as chorion) and the villous portion (referred to as
villi). The amnion, which is derived from the inner cell mass, was
sampled for comparison with the extraembryonic membranes (chorion
and villi), as shown in Figure 1.

     At this time, we have studied 71 newborns and placentae and
have found no compelling evidence for nonrandom inactivation in
full-term placentae. However, studies of appropriate control infants have indicated that contamination with maternal cells occurs
to a significant extent in the chorion, and that G6PD activity in
the amnion and membraneous chorion is very low.

                              METHODS

Subjects: Placentae heterozygous for G6PD$_A$ were from Negro
newborn females at the Johns Hopkins Hospital. Placental tissue
from Caucasian newborns, presumably of the G6PD$_B$ phenotype, was
obtained in a similar manner, as a control for the existence of
embryonic enzymes electrophoretically similar to the A variant.
Placental specimens were also obtained from Negro males as a further
control for contamination with maternal cells. In each case, cord
blood obtained at delivery was also analyzed; in some cases,
maternal venous blood was obtained.

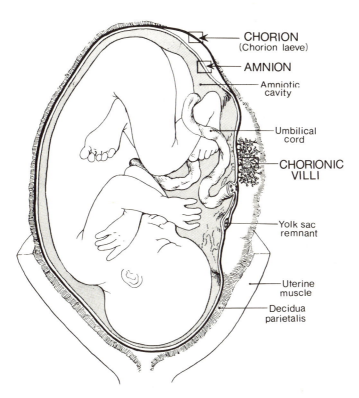

FIGURE 1. Relationship of fetus and extraembryonic membranes in utero, showing sites from which specimens were taken for enzyme analysis.

Samples of approximately 10 mm diameter from the villous portion of the chorion, and specimens of amnion and non-villous chorion (chorion laeve) (Fig. 1), were thoroughly rinsed with saline to remove contaminating blood. In the case of specimens of chorionic villi, the villi were dissected under a microscope and separated from other contaminating material. All solid specimens were prepared for electrophoresis by homogenization in water containing 1 mgm/ml of TPN, followed by lysis in an ultrasonic cleaner. The lysates were spun at 40 K x g for 30 min at 4°C, and the supernatant was used as enzyme extract. Blood specimens were prepared as previously described (Migeon and Kennedy 1975).

Electrophoresis. All samples were analyzed for G6PD on the day they were obtained. Lysates were then stored at −20°C for studies of phosphoglucomutase (PGM) and lactate dehydrogenase (LDH) when indicated. Electrophoresis of G6PD, LDH, and PGM were performed on cellulose acetate gels. For G6PD, we used the method previously described (Migeon and Kennedy 1975), using tris-glycine EDTA buffer, pH 9.2, at 340 V, 24 min. For LDH, we used tris-barbital-sodium barbital, pH 8.8 (Gelman), 180 V, 20 min, and stained with LDH isozyme substrate (Gelman). PGM electrophoresis was carried out according to the method of Sonneborn (1972).

RESULTS AND DISCUSSION

Ten specimens derived from newborns of Caucasian origin had exclusively the G6PD$_B$ phenotype in cord blood, chorionic villi, and non-villous chorion, providing no evidence for novel forms of G6PD (Table 1). We were unable to observe any G6PD isozymes in specimens of amnion in any of the placentae analyzed, even in specimens that had considerable LDH activity (Fig. 2.)

TABLE 1. G6PD phenotype of full-term placentae and newborn cord blood

Sample (No.)	G6PD type	Number of specimens			Discrepancy
		cord blood	villi	chorion *(both posts?)*	
White ♂ & ♀ (10)	B	10	10	10	0
	A	0	0	0	
	AB	0	0	0	
Black ♀ (35)	B	14	14	16	14
16 AB	A	4	4	5	
1 BB	AB	16	16	12	
8/17 only show Xⁿ in chorion	BB´	1	1	0	
Black ♂ (26)	B	19	19	15	6
	A	7	7	5	
	AB	0	0	6	

Of the 35 black newborn females studied (Table 1), 16 were heterozygous for the AB variants, and one was heterozygous for B and a new variant that migrated slightly slower than B, which we call B´ (Fig. 3). In 8 of the 17 heterozygous females (#4, 19, 30, 43, 66, 72, 107, and 114), one allele was excluded in the chorion. However, because this was not the case in all heterozygous chorions, we decided to look at specimens from nonheterozygotes to see if there were other exceptions. Among females of homozygous $G6PD_B$ or $G6PD_A$ genotype, we noted other kinds of discrepancies. Although the G6PD phenotype of the chorionic villi was always identical to that of the cord blood, the non-villous chorion (chorion laeve) sometimes had two bands. In all, there were 14 discrepancies between chorion and cord blood among the Negro females (Table 1). We therefore carried out an analysis of specimens from Negro males. Among these, there were 6 specimens of chorion that had two G6PD isozymes (Fig. 4). The presence of the heterozygous phenotype in specimens of male origin indicated to us that the chorion was most likely contaminated with maternal cells. Examination of the maternal blood in 13 cases revealed that, with two exceptions*, the chorion was identical in G6PD type to that of the mother's red cells (Table 2).

The studies of the phosphoglucomutase phenotype in these specimens confirmed our observations on G6PD by showing that the chorionic villi contained only fetal PGM isozymes, whereas the chorion contained a mixture of maternal and fetal types (Fig. 5).

Because of the stability of the $G6PD_A$ isozyme observed in all specimens of chorion, we believe the contamination is not attributable to blood cells, where the A^- variant is usually unstable; more likely, the contaminating maternal cells are of decidual origin (Fig. 1). It seems therefore that, like the amnion, the membraneous chorion has no measurable G6PD activity of fetal origin; the isozymes we observed were entirely attributable to the contaminating maternal cells. Examination of a few specimens at 16 weeks' gestation have indicated that the chorion is less likely to have maternal contamination at that time, but still has no measurable G6PD activity of fetal origin.

Table 3 compares the G6PD phenotype of cord blood from each of 17 heterozygotes with that of the chorionic villi with regard to intensity of the two bands. In 13 of these females, the

---

* In case #27, the mother was B, the son was A^+, the chorion was AB. The most likely explanation is that the maternal red cells excluded the allele transmitted, via oocyte, to her son; yet, the allele is expressed in maternal decidual cells contaminating the chorion. In the case of #51, whose mother's blood was BB´, only the B was expressed in the chorion.

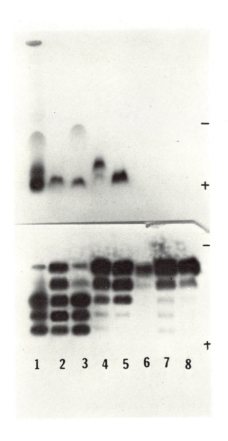
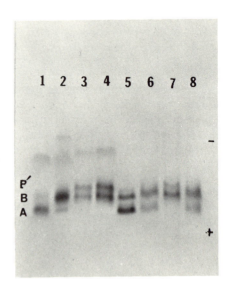

FIGURE 2   FIGURE 3

FIGURE 2. Cellulose acetate electrophoresis of G6PD (top) and LDH
        (bottom) from specimens of newborn villi (slot 2), chorion
        (slot 4), and amnion (slots 6-8).
        Note that the amnion does not express G6PD, although it has
        abundant LDH activity.

FIGURE 3. G6PD electrophoresis, PL-64, female.
        Slot 1, control AB blood; slot 2, maternal (A⁻B) blood; slots
        3 and 4, newborn cord blood (BB´); slot 5, fibroblast AB
        control; slots 6 and 8, chorion (AB); slot 7, chorionic villi
        (BB´). Note identity of phenotypes of maternal blood and
        chorion, and of newborn cord blood and villi. In villi, the
        maternally derived $G6PD_B$ allele is expressed with greater
        intensity than the paternal $G6PD_B´$ allele.

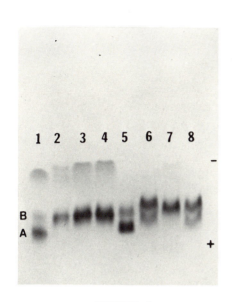 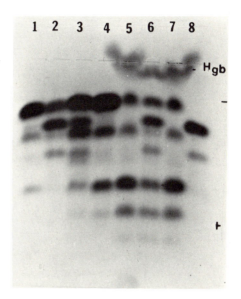

FIGURE 4   FIGURE 5

FIGURE 4. G6PD electrophoresis, PL-74, male.
Slot 1, control blood, G6PD$_{AB}$; slots 2-4, newborn cord blood;
slot 5, fibroblast AB control; slot 6 and 8, chorion, slot 7,
chorionic villi. Note the presence of two bands in chorion
(6 and 8).

FIGURE 5. PGM phenotype of newborn, maternal and membrane specimens.
Skin fibroblast controls: PGM 1-1 (slot 1), 1-2 (slot 2) and
2-2 (slot 8). Note that the isozyme pattern of the (chorionic)
villi (slot 4) is identical to that of the fetus (cord blood,
slots 5 and 7). On the other hand, the chorion (slot 3) is
a mixture of maternal (1-2) and fetal (1-1) types.

TABLE 2. Comparison of G6PD phenotype of newborn, membranes, and maternal specimens

Reference No. and sex of newborn	Newborn blood	Placenta		Mother's blood
		Villi	Chorion	
19 ♀	A⁻B	AB	A	A⁻
26 ♀	B	B	AB	AB
30 ♀	A⁻B	AB	B	B
62 ♀	AB	AB	AB	AB
63 ♀	B	B	B	B
64 ♀	BB´	BB´	AB	A⁻B
65 ♀	A⁻B	AB	AB	A⁻B
27 ♂	A	A	AB	B
69 ♂	B	B	AB	A⁻B
73 ♂	B	B	B	B
74 ♂	B	B	AB	A⁻B
97 ♂	A⁻	A	AB	A⁻B
51 ♂	B	B	B	BB´

In 11/13 cases chorion phenotype is same as maternal blood.

intensity of the two isozymes in chorionic villi was equal or approximately equal, ranging from 1 : 1 to 1.3 : 1. In the other 4 females, the ratio ranged from 2 : 1 to 3 : 1. Comparison with cord blood phenotypes reveal more variability in band intensity in the blood specimens, reflecting the instability of the A⁻ variant in that tissue. However, similar comparisons, excluding samples with the A⁻ variant, indicate no greater variation in villi than in cord blood (Table 3).

In 12 heterozygotes, primarily those from nonheterozygous mothers, we were able to determine the maternal allele (X^m, Table 3). In 3 of these (#30, 64, 114), there was significant deviation from equality of the two bands in villi, and in each case the skewing favored the maternal allele (Table 4; Fig. 3).

The excess of enzyme of the maternal type in these three specimens may be attributable to maternal cell contaminants, or may represent a disproportionate number of the infants' cells expressing the maternal allele. However, the skewing is neither invariable nor of sufficient magnitude to indicate preferential expression of the maternal X in chorionic villi of the full-term placenta.

How can we reconcile our findings with the substantial evidence for nonrandom patterns observed in rodents? Conceivably, evidence of differential expression early in development has been masked by subsequent events. The chorionic villi originating from the cytotrophoblast are intimately associated with vascular mesoderm of capillaries, difficult to eliminate even with careful dissection. Yet, one suspects that contamination of this kind would not completely obscure a nonrandom pattern, as West *et al.* (1977) noted significant skewing despite substantial contamination from yolk-sac mesoderm where both alleles were randomly expressed. More important perhaps is that the activity of glucose-6-phosphate dehydrogenase in the fetal membranes at term is relatively low. Therefore, it may be that the subtle skewing in favor of the maternal allele, observed in three heterozygotes where the X^m allele was known, reflects an underlying nonrandom pattern. For this reason, we will continue these studies in younger specimens to determine if preferential expression of the maternal X chromosome is a general characteristic of mammalian fetal membranes rather than a peculiarity of rodents.

This work was supported by NIH grant HD 05465.

TABLE 3. Comparison of G6PD phenotype of chorionic villi and cord blood from female newborns heterozygous for G6PD variants

Reference No.	Type of G6PD$_A$*	Cord blood†	Villi†	Maternal G6PD phenotype		X^{m}‡
				Maternal blood	Inferred from chorion	
38	A⁺	B = A	B ≤ A		AB	
50	A⁺	B ≧ A	B ≥ A		AB	
54	A⁺	B ≧ A	B ≦ A		AB	
62	A⁺	B = A	B ≦ A	A⁺B	AB	
64		B = B′	(B) > B′	A⁻B	AB	B
6	A⁻	B >>> A	B > A		AB	
65	A⁻	B >>> A	(B) = A	A⁺B	AB	B
105	A⁻	B >>> A	(B) ≧ A	A⁺B	AB	B
108	A⁻	B >>> A	(B) ≧ A	A⁺B	AB	B
4	A⁺	B > A	(B) ≧ A		B	B
43	A⁺	B ≦ A	(B) = A		B	B
72	A⁺	B < A	(B) = A		B	B

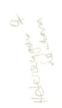

(handwritten marginal notes:) Heterozygous pattern   In chorion villi   X^{m} > X^{p}

107	A$^+$	B = A (circled)	B	B
114	A$^+$	B = A	A	A
19	A$^-$	B >>> A	A	A$^-$
30	A$^-$	B >>> A	B	B
66	A$^-$	B >>> A (circled)	B	B

* Based on relative intensity of G6PD$_A$ in cord blood.

†

Symbols	Ratio B : A
B = A	1 : 1
B ≥ A	1.3 : 1
B > A	2 : 1
B >> A	3 : 1
B >>> A	4 : 1

‡ G6PD specified by the maternally derived X chromosome in the newborn female.

Cases where X^m is known (ignoring A$^-$ gene which is low in blood)

[cord blood (fetal origin)] [chorionic villus (hyp. oldest)] [expression of X^m in villus = X^m in cord blood]

#64	$X^m = X^p$	$X^m ≥ X^p$	$X^m > X^p$
114	$X^m ≥ X^p$	$X^m > X^p$	+
72	$X^m ≤ X^p$	$X^m = X^p$	+
43	$X^m ≤ X^p$	$X^m ≥ X^p$	(+?)
107	$X^m = X^p$	$X^m ≥ X^p$	(+?)
ct	$X^m > X^p$	$X^m > X^p$	(−)

b/c cord blood may not be a good control (stem cell problems)

TABLE 4. Phenotype of chorionic villi as a function of the X^m allele*

X^m	G6PD phenotype of villi[†]						
	B>>A	B>A	B≥A	B=A	B≤A	B<A	B<<A
A				1		1	
B	1	1‡	5	3			

* Data from Table 3.

[†] For symbolism, see footnote to Table 3.

‡ Actually B > B´.

REFERENCES

Cooper, D. W. 1971. Directed genetic change model for X chromosome inactivation in eutherian mammals. Nature 230: 292-204.

Cooper, D. W., P. G. Johnston, C. E. Murtagh, G. B. Sharman, J. L. VandeBerg, and W. E. Poole. 1974. Sex-linked isozymes and sex chromosome evolution and inactivation in kangaroos. In, Proc. Third Intl. Isozyme Conf., Yale University, Academic Press, pp. 550-573.

Cooper, D. W., P. G. Johnston, C. E. Murtagh, and J. L. VandeBerg. 1975. In, The Eukaryote Chromosome, W. J. Peacock and R. D. Brock, Eds. National University Press, Canberra, Australia, pp. 381-393.

Hamerton, J. L., B. J. Richardson, P. A. Gee, W. R. Allen and R. V. Short. 1971. Nonrandom X chromosome expression in female mules and hinnies. Nature 232: 312-315.

Hook, E. B. and L. D. Brustman. 1971. Evidence for selective differences between cells with an active horse X chromosome and cells with an active donkey X chromosome in the female mule. Nature 232: 349-350.

Leisti, J. T., M. M. Kaback and D. L. Rimoin. 1975. Human X-autosome translocations: Differential inactivation of the X chromosome in a kindred with an X-9 translocation. Am. J. Hum. Genet. 27: 441-453.

Lyon, M. F.   1961.   Gene action in the X chromosome of the mouse.
Nature 190: 372-373.

Lyon, M. F.   1972.   X chromosome inactivation and developmental
patterns in mammals.   Biol. Rev. 47: 1-35.

Migeon, B. R. and J. F. Kennedy.   1975.   Evidence for the inactivation of an X chromosome early in the development of the human fetus.
Amer. J. Hum. Genet. 27: 233.

Russell, L. B. and N. L. A. Cacheiro.   1978.   Cell selection in
X-autosome translocation.   In, Genetic Mosaics and Chimeras in
Mammals, Liane B. Russell, Ed.   Plenum Press, New York and London.

Sonneborn, H. H.   1972.   Comment on the determination of isoenzyme
polymorphism (ADAAK, 6PGD, PGM) by cellulose acetate electrophoresis.   Humangenetik 17: 49-55.

Takagi, N.   1978.   Preferential inactivation of the paternally
derived X chromosome in mice.   In, Genetic Mosaics and Chimeras in
Mammals, Liane B. Russell, Ed.   Plenum Press, New York and London.

Takagi, N. and M. Sasaki.   1975.   Preferential inactivation of the
paternally derived X chromosome in the extraembryonic membrane of
the mouse.   Nature 256: 640-642.

Wake, N., N. Takagi, and M. Sasaki.   1976.   Nonrandom inactivation
of X chromosome in the rat yolk sac.   Nature 262: 580-581.

West, J. D., W. I. Frels, V. Chapman and V. Papaioannou.   1977.
Preferential expression of the maternally derived X chromosome in
the mouse yolk sac.   Cell 12: 873-882.

West, J. D., V. E. Papaioannou, W. I. Frels and V. M. Chapman.
1978.   Preferential expression of the maternally derived X chromosome in extraembryonic tissues of the mouse.   In, Genetic Mosaics
and Chimeras in Mammals, Liane B. Russell, Ed.   Plenum Press, New
York and London.

THE USE OF MOUSE X-AUTOSOME TRANSLOCATIONS IN THE STUDY OF X-INACTIVATION PATHWAYS AND NONRANDOMNESS

Liane B. Russell and Nestor L. A. Cacheiro

Biology Division, Oak Ridge National Laboratory, Oak Ridge, Tennessee 37830

Rearrangements between mammalian X chromosomes and autosomes are valuable tools in the study of X inactivation, since they provide a karyotype in which the physical continuity of the X chromosome is interrupted. In reciprocal X-autosome translocations, T(X;A)'s, there are three chromosomes within each cell of a heterozygote — instead of the usual two — that contain X-chromosome material. This circumstance may be put to use in addressing questions of X-differentiation mechanisms and randomness.

In utilizing translocations for these purposes, it is necessary to be able to identify individual cells with regard to the state of the X-chromosomal material within them. No X-linked variants are presently known that will serve as cell markers. Cytological analysis, on the other hand, gives direct evidence of the status of the X-chromosomal material in its various locations within individual cells. Specifically, banding techniques permit identification of all mouse chromosomes (Nesbitt and Francke 1973); and refinements in the autoradiography of mouse nuclei (Nesbitt and Gartler 1970) allow identification of the asynchronously replicating X chromosome, which is assumed to be the inactive one (Ray, Gee, and Richardson 1972).

The direct identification of chromosomes by banding and replication stage also serves to quantitate the two alternative types of cells expected to exist in an XX mammal and thus to shed some light on questions of randomness. According to the classical inactive-X-chromosome hypothesis, there should be random and complete inactivation (Lyon 1961). Since 1961, nonrandomness has been established for marsupials (Cooper, Johnston, Murtagh, and VandeBerg 1975) and

393

for the extraembryonic membranes of placental mammals (Takagi 1978; West, Papaioannou, Frels, and Chapman 1978). But examples of non-randomness are also found in eutherian females (see Discussion). Where these cases involve rearranged X chromosomes, a likely explanation is cell selection. In the case of T(X;A)'s, for example, some of the autosomal material attached to an X also is subject to inactivation (Russell and Bangham 1961; Russell 1961; Cattanach 1961; Russell and Montgomery 1969, 1970) and thus becomes "functionally hemizygous" (Russell 1964) when the normal X is the active one. The identification of individual cells in each of a number of T(X;A)'s at different stages of development can provide evidence on whether cell selection plays a part in nonrandomness, and, if so, on when and where such selection occurs.

The autoradiographic studies with mouse T(X;A)'s described in this paper have provided evidence for tissue-specific cell selection governed by certain chromosomal regions. The results also support a single-inactivation-center model of X differentiation for the mouse. The various translocations used involve eight different breakpoint locations in the X, six in chromosome 7 (Ch 7), two in Ch 4, and one in Ch 16. It is therefore likely that the picture we have obtained is a broad one.

MATERIALS AND METHODS

Eight independent mouse X-autosome translocations were used in this study. Among these are six reciprocal translocations that arose at Oak Ridge; a seventh reciprocal translocation, Searle's *T(X;16)16H*, abbreviated T16H (Lyon, Searle, and Ford 1964; Ohno and Lyon 1965); and the insertional *flecked* translocation, *T(X;7)1Ct* (Cattanach 1961; Ohno and Cattanach 1962), to be abbreviated T1Ct. (T1Ct-Type-I females carry a balanced complement, i.e., the inserted X and a correspondingly deleted Ch 7; while T1Ct-Type-II females have two normal autosomes and are thus unbalanced.)

Among the six Oak Ridge translocations, four involve Ch 7, and these are designated *T(X;7)2Rl*, *T(X;7)3Rl*, *T(X;7)5Rl and T(X;7)6Rl*. Two involve Ch 4 and are designated *T(X;4)1Rl* and *T(X;4)7Rl**. The abbreviated nomenclature R1, R2, R3, R5, R6, R7 will be used. The derivation, phenotypic properties, and some of the breakpoint locations have been described elsewhere (Russell and Montgomery 1969, 1970). All of the Oak Ridge translocations have been studied cytologically in banded mitotic chromosomes, as well as in diakinesis (Cacheiro, unpublished). The combined genetic and cytological

---

* In earlier publications, we identified these translocations by linkage group — instead of chromosome — as T(X;1)'s and T(X;8)'s, respectively.

evidence clearly points to the translocations being reciprocal.
In addition, visualizations of the synaptonemal complex axes for
two of the translocations, R2 and R6, reveal almost classical
pachytene-cross formations (Moses, Russell, and Cacheiro 1977).
The six Oak Ridge T(X;A)'s as well as T16H and T1Ct are shown in
Fig. 1. It should be noted that, in some of the translocations
(R1, R5, R6, T1Ct, T16H), the long translocation product has an X
centromere and proximal portion; while in others (R2, R3, R7), the
long translocation product has an autosomal centromere and proximal
portion.

      Short-term cell cultures were prepared from the kidney of adult
females, from the kidney of 18-day fetuses, or from minced skin and
connective tissue of 18-day fetuses. By using autosomal markers
closely linked to the breakpoint (b in R1, c in R3, p in R6), most
fetal translocation females could be identified by eye color. Cells
were cultured in large Leighton tubes in improved 199 medium at 37°
C. On the fifth day of culture, cells were given a 20-minute pulse
of ^{3}H-thymidine; colchicine was added 7 hours after the pulse, and
the cells were harvested 4 hours later. This technique, developed
by Nesbitt and Gartler (1970), yields cells labeled early in the S
period, with late-replicating chromosomes differentially unlabeled.
Quinacrine-mustard staining was used to identify chromosomes by
their banding patterns, and photographic records were obtained.
Slides were then coated with Kodak Nuclear Track Emulsion, NTB$_2$,
exposed for a week at 4°C, developed and stained with Giemsa.

      Cells that had incorporated an adequate amount of ^{3}H-thymidine
were analyzed as to the amount and distribution of label in the X,
the translocation products, and Chromosomes 19 (the smallest pair
of autosomes). The long and short translocation product will be
referred to as XT$^\ell$ and xt^s, respectively, and the intact X as X^n.
(In the case of T1Ct, XT$^\ell$ is, of course, an X chromosome with an
autosomal insertion.)

                            RESULTS

Distribution of cells from adult kidney

      From the kidney cultures of 22 adult females (2 to 5 from each
translocation type), altogether 4515 cells were screened, of which
1856 had adequate incorporation of ^{3}H-thymidine. Among 1386 of the
latter (omitting for the purpose of this calculation three preparations in which too long a pulse was given) the overall frequencies
of cells with one differentially unlabeled chromosome, with two unlabeled chromosomes, and with none unlabeled (i.e., with substantial numbers of grains on all chromosomes) were 85.9, 4.0, and
10.2%, respectively. (For similar categories, Nesbitt and Gartler
[1970] report about 55%, 17%, and 28%, respectively.) The last

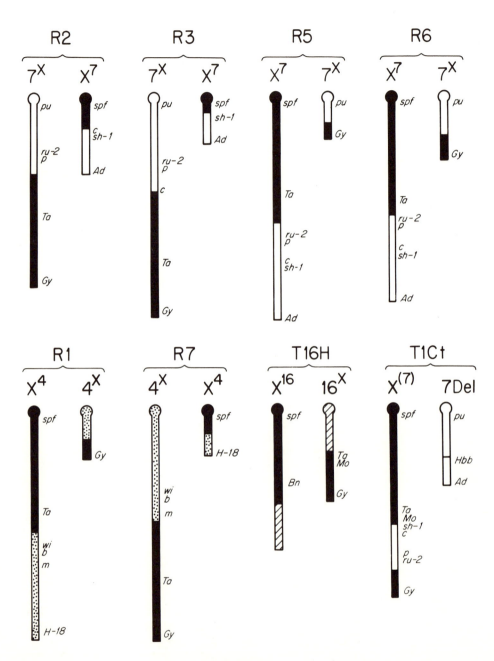

FIGURE 1

FIGURE 1. Diagrammatic representation of the eight X-autosome
   translocations employed in the autoradiographic study. The
   ratios of chromosomal lengths and the breakpoint positions
   are based on our cytological measurements and on cytological
   information published for T16H (Eicher, Nesbitt, and Francke
   1972; Nesbitt and Francke 1972) and T1Ct (Francke and Nesbitt
   1971; Kouri, Miller, Miller, Dev, Grewal, and Hutton 1971;
   Nesbitt and Francke 1972; Eicher and Washburn 1978). X chromosome material is shown in black, Ch 7 in white, Ch 4 stippled,
   Ch 16 cross-hatched. The positions of several pertinent X and
   autosomal markers is approximate (Russell and Montgomery 1970
   and unpublished; Eicher 1970).

←——————————————————————————

category is assumed to have incorporated ^{3}H-thymidine in mid-S,
instead of early S. Cells with one differentially unlabeled chromosome were designated "informative." In all 1415 such cells, the
unlabeled chromosome was either the X or the long translocation
product. An "unlabeled" (presumed inactive) X, designated as $X^n=0$,
had no more than 3 grains overlying it, and these were generally
near the distal end. On the other hand, an "unlabeled" XT^ℓ, designated $XT^\ell=0$, virtually always had substantial numbers of grains
toward that end of the autosomal segment that was most distant from
the X portion (regardless of whether this was the telomeric or
centromeric end). Fig. 2 shows a cell before and after development
of the autoradiograph.

     Results for individual translocations are listed in Table 1.
The last two columns show the frequencies, among informative cells
only, of cells in which the normal X was unlabeled. It may be noted
that this does not differ significantly from 50% in the two
$T(X;4)$'s, R1 and R7, and in two T1Ct-Type-II females. On the other
hand, the relative proportions of $X^n=0$ and $XT^\ell=0$ cells depart significantly from a 50:50 ratio in the case of R2, R3, R5, R6, and
T1Ct-Type-I, in all of which there is a preponderance of cells with
the normal X unlabeled (inactive). In T16H, all cells were of the
$X^n=0$ type.

Distribution of cells from fetal tissues

     Two translocations (R6 and R3) showing very nonrandom, and
another (R1) showing random distribution of cells in cultures from
adult kidney were chosen for further labeling experiments, using
18-day fetal tissues. The fetal kidney was cultured separately
from other tissues (mainly skin and muscle), which were macerated
and mixed up prior to culturing. Results are shown in Table 2.

TABLE 1. Results of ^{3}H-thymidine labeling in early S period of adult kidney cells from female X-autosome translocation heterozygotes in the mouse.

Translocation Type	Symbol	Females (no.)	Labeled cells (no.)	All chromosomes labeled (%)	$X^n=0$ and $XT^\ell=0$ (%)	One chrom. unlabeled: Informative cells (no.)	Cells with $X^n=0$ Individual (%)*	Average (%)†
T(X;4)	R1	2	199	8.0	5.5	172	35.0, 54.3	44.7
	R7	2	83	9.6	9.6	67	42.9, 45.0	43.9
	R2	2	196	4.1‡	1.0‡	134	56.7, 63.4	60.1
	R3	5	539	12.8‡	4.1‡	393	65.8, 73.0, 78.2, 86.9, 89.3	78.6
T(X;7)	R5	2	285	7.1‡	9.5‡	167	70.1, 88.6	79.4
	R6	2	69	13.0	5.8	56	98.2	98.2
	TCt-I	2	124	12.9	0.8	107	96.2, 96.4	96.3
	TCt-II	4	270	10.7	1.5	237	42.6, 54.2, 86.4, 88.2	67.9
T(X;16)	T16H	1	91	6.6	3.3	82	100.00	100.0
Total		22	1856	10.2‡	4.0‡	1415		

*Based on "informative" cells. In all such cells, the unlabeled chromosome was either X^n or XT^ℓ.

†Unweighted average of individual percentages

‡Excludes results from preparations in which, through a technical error, too long a ^{3}H-thymidine pulse was given, yielding too many cells with all chromosomes labeled

TABLE 2. Results of ^{3}H-thymidine labeling in early S period of cells derived from 18-day female fetuses heterozygous for reciprocal X-autosome translocations

Translocation	Tissue	Fetal females (no.)	Labeled cells (no.)	All chromosomes labeled (%)	$X^n=0$ and $XT^\ell=0$ (%)	One chrom. unlabeled: Informative cells (no.)	Cells with $X^n=0$ Individual (%)*	Average (%)†
R1	Non-kidney	2	88	22.7	1.1	67	47.6, 58.7	53.1
R3	Non-kidney	1	55	—‡	—‡	20	55.0	55.0
R6	Non-kidney	3	189	25.4	2.1	137	53.2, 51.4, 60.4	58.0
R6	Kidney	3	98	15.3	3.1	80	(33.3)§, 65.2, 72.2	68.7

* Based on "informative" cells, i.e., those with either $X^n=0$ or $XT^\ell=0$

† Unweighted average of individual percentages

‡ Percentages meaningless because too long a pulse was given in this preparation

§ Based on 3 cells only; not included in average

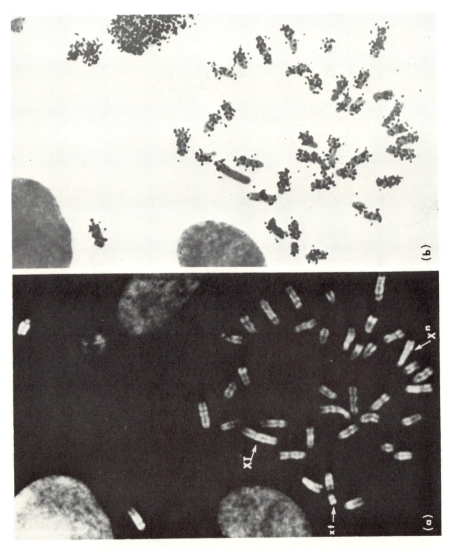

FIGURE 2

FIGURE 2. Metaphase spread from kidney of adult R6, (a) before
   and (b) after development of autoradiogram. The long translocation product is allocyclic. Note that even though XT^ℓ is
   selectively unlabeled, a number of grains are found overlying
   the most distal end of its autosomal segment.

←————————————————

Of 806 cells screened, 430 (53.3%) had adequate incorporation
of ^3H-thymidine. This frequency is not too dissimilar from the 42%
found by Nesbitt and Gartler (1970). Among the labeled cells, 75.7%
had one differentially unlabeled chromosome, 2.1% had two, and the
remaining 22.1% showed substantial numbers of grains on all chromosomes. These relative proportions are roughly similar to those
found in adult kidney (see above).

It appears that, in the fetal non-kidney tissue of all three
translocations, $X^n=0$ and $XT^\ell=0$ cells are present in approximately
equal numbers. In the case of R6, which has predominantly $X^n=0$
cells in adult kidney, fetal kidney gives a very significantly less
lopsided distribution: 68.7% of cells are $X^n=0$, instead of 98.2%
(P<0.0001). This proportion is still significantly different from
50% (P<0.001), but is barely significantly different from the proportion of $X^n=0$ cells in fetal non-kidney tissue (P = 0.05). That
is, the nonrandomness that exists in adult kidney is not found in
fetal non-kidney; and fetal kidney appears to be intermediate between these two conditions (Fig. 3).

The small translocation product, xt^s

In cells derived from adult kidney cultures (Table 1), it
appeared visually that no chromosome, besides the X^n or XT^ℓ, was
differentially unlabeled (i.e., inactive). However, in order to
obtain more quantitative data on the status of the short translocation product, xt^s, we counted grains over this chromosome, as well
as over each member of the shortest pair of intact autosomes, Ch 19,
in the same cell. Table 3 shows mean grain counts in various translocations, both for cells in which $X^n=0$ and for cells in which
$XT^\ell=0$.

Because of different absolute amounts of ^3H-thymidine incorporation in different samples, one can compare only relative counts,
within translocations. In each of the six stocks, the ratio of xt^s
to Ch 19 grain counts was found to be very nearly the same in the
group of cells with X inactive and the group with XT^ℓ inactive. --
The differences between translocations in the xt^s/Ch 19 ratio are
roughly related to the different lengths of the xt^s chromosome.

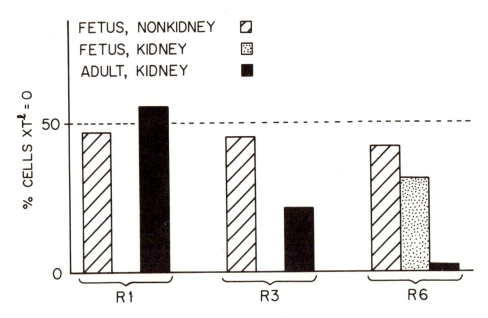

FIGURE 3. Percentages of cells with $XT^{\ell}=0$ in various tissues of
    three reciprocal translocations. Although the three translo-
    cations differ markedly with respect to cell distribution in
    adult kidney, all of them yield not far from 50% cells of type
    $XT^{\ell}=0$ in fetal non-kidney.

DISCUSSION

Only one portion of the severed X is allocyclic

In virtually all of the cells labeled in early S, only one
chromosome per cell was differentially unlabeled and therefore presumed inactive. Overall, only 4% of early-S cells were found to
contain two unlabeled chromosomes, namely X^n and XT^{ℓ}. It should be
noted that we never found both XT^{ℓ} and xt^s to be unlabeled in the
same cell. In view of the facts that cells with $X^n=0$ *and* $XT^{\ell}=0$ (a)
occur with similar frequencies in all the stocks, (b) would be functionally almost nullosomic for X-linked loci, and (c) are often
lightly labeled overall, as also found by Nesbitt and Gartler
(1970), we conclude that they are artifacts of the method. In
further support of this conclusion is the fact that, in seven of

TABLE 3. Mean grain counts over the short translocation product and the shortest autosomes in cells in which either the normal X (X^n) or the long translocation product (XT^ℓ) is allocyclic.

Translocation	$X^n = 0$				$XT^\ell = 0$			
	a	b	c	b/c	d	e	f	e/f
	No. cells*	Average no. grains over			No. cells*	Average no. grains over		
		xt^s	Ch19†			xt^s	Ch19†	
R1	54	5.2	10.5	0.5	53	4.9	8.9	0.6
R7	13	5.7	7.1	0.8	15	6.4	6.3	1.0
R2	46	7.7	6.8	1.1	26	6.9	7.1	1.0
R3	129	8.1	8.9	0.9	33	8.6	10.0	0.9
R5	58	3.4	7.6	0.5	7	3.0	8.0	0.4
R6	17	5.4	7.2	0.8	3	6.3	9.0	0.7

* Each cell supplied both xt^s and Ch 19 counts

† Average of the two Ch 19's in each cell

the stocks, there were, in addition to these few cells, also two clear alternative groups of cells having a single allocyclic chromosome, namely X^n or XT^ℓ.

The cell-distribution results provide an indication that, in the case of mouse reciprocal translocations, one of the translocation products is not subject to alternate states. The grain counts carried out for xt^s and Ch 19 add more precision to this conclusion. If both portions of the severed X were subject to inactivation, one would expect xt^s, or at least its X-chromosomal portion, to be unlabeled when XT^ℓ is unlabeled, and thus the xt^s grain count to be lower in $XT^\ell=0$ cells than in $X^n=0$ cells. Actually, for each reciprocal translocation, the xt^s/Ch 19 ratio is very nearly the same in $XT^\ell=0$ and $X^n=0$ cells. This is true in spite of the fact that different X-chromosome breakpoints are involved in the different translocations, and that the xt^s in some of the cases (R2, R3, R7) is as long as, or longer than, Ch 19.

The genetic evidence that only one of the translocation products may be subject to inactivation (Russell 1963) has heretofore rested on the finding that c^+, which in R3, R5, and R6 is inactivated with different frequencies, roughly related to distance from breakpoint, is fully active in R2, even though this locus lies close to the breakpoint. Bernstine (unpublished) has recently obtained evidence that *Mod-2*, 1 cM distal to the *c*-locus, also is not inactivated in R2, whereas it is clearly inactivated in other reciprocal T(X;7)'s.

The X-differentiation process

There is now abundant evidence that in normal XX eutherian mammals, both X's are active in preblastocyst stages, and that the process of X differentiation in the embryo proper involves one X becoming inactive (Chapman, West, and Adler 1978; Kratzer and Gartler 1978; Monk 1978; Epstein, Travis, Tucker, and Smith 1978). For the purpose of formalizing alternate schemes for differential X-chromosome behavior, it seems necessary to consider two separate events: the selection of one X to remain active; and the process by which the other X (or X's) and contiguous autosomal material are inactivated.

The question of whether the process of "choice" focuses on the X that is to remain active or on the one that will become inactive entered into the earliest thinking on X differentiation. Thus, the emphasis was either on the "inactivation of one X" (Lyon 1961) or, alternatively, on the single active X (Russell 1961). Subsequent reports of individuals with supernumerary X's in which all but one were heteropyknotic (reviewed by Lyon 1968) lent weight to the early statement that "genic balance requires the action of *one* X ...so that only any additional X's present assume the properties characteristic of heterochromatin" (Russell 1961). Various mechanisms have subsequently been proposed for the way in which the one active X is established, e.g., attachment of an episome into a specific receptor locus on one X at random, with subsequent destruction of additional episomes (Grumbach, Morishima, and Taylor 1963); a product made by one or more pairs of autosomes sufficient to keep only one X in the autosomal rhythm (Russell 1964); only one X-attachment site on the nuclear membrane (Comings 1968); or an autosomal "sensitive site" which becomes inactivated by passage through the paternal germ line so that only one dose of an "informational entity" is available to attach randomly to the receptor site of one X (Brown and Chandra 1973). Recent evidence (Kaufman, Guc-Cubrilla, and Lyon 1978; Martin, Epstein, and Martin 1978) indicates that the mechanism proposed by Brown and Chandra is not essential for initiation of X inactivation.

Regardless of the mechanism by which one X is chosen to remain active, one must also consider the subsequent step, namely the process by which inactivation of the other X (or X's) occurs. Since the physical continuity of X-chromosomal material is interrupted in X-autosome translocations, evidence from such rearrangements has been useful in deriving hypotheses of inactivation, including a single inactivation center in mouse (Russell and Montgomery 1965, 1970) and man (Therman and Pätau 1974); or two or more inactivator units, each with its own polarity (Cattanach 1970, 1975; Eicher 1970). Another alternative to be considered for T(X;A)'s is that interaction of at least two factors in *cis* position is needed to produce inactivation; or (formally equivalent), that some minimal length of X material is required.

The results reported in this paper produced no support for the occurrence of inactivation in both translocation products. Allocycly affected only one chromosome, as shown by the absence of label in X^n *or* XT^ℓ, as well as by the fact that grain counts in the other translocation product (xt^s) were the same in $X^n=0$ and $XT^\ell=0$ cells. These results argue strongly against a memory system (i.e., correlation of X portions derived from the same parent), and even against the incomplete memory system that has been proposed by Eicher (1970). It may be noted that Eicher's conclusion was based on identification of T16H heteropyknotic chromosomes by their size (Ohno and Lyon 1965), prior to the availability of more accurate means of identifying allocyclic chromosomes by banding and autoradiography. In the present experiment, no T16H cells were found in which both translocation products were unlabeled.

Cells in which *two* chromosomes were found to be relatively unlabeled occurred with low frequencies in all translocation stocks, but these chromosomes were never the two translocation products, and, as discussed above, such cells are considered to be artifactual and noninformative. What may be equivalent cells have been reported for a minority of human balanced X-autosome translocations (summarized by Leisti, Kaback, and Rimoin 1975) where both X^n and X^t appeared to be late replicating in some cells.

The present finding in the mouse translocations (except T16H, for which see below) of alternative states of X^n and XT^ℓ *only*, and the fact that contiguous autosomal material in XT^ℓ is inactivated in these translocations, are most easily explained by a single inactivation center located somewhere between the R2 and R6 breakpoints and having polarity in both directions (Russell and Montgomery 1965, 1970). Multiple inactivator units can also account for the results, but only under the special conditions that X-chromosome breakage in every one of the translocations has occurred within a unit that has polarity toward the attached autosomal material and that, in the case of T1Ct, it occurred at the junction of two units with facing polarities and destroyed both terminators (Eicher 1970).

The argument that there are two or more inactivation centers (Cattanach 1970, 1975; Eicher 1970) is based partly on phenotypes resulting from inactivation in the inserted autosomal piece in T1Ct, and partly on the cytological pattern of the insertion-bearing X. However, until more is known concerning the relationship between distributions of cellular genotypes and "units of phenotype" for each of the markers on which the phenotypic observations were based, it is not inconceivable that something like the threshold effect proposed by Falconer and Isaacson (1972), illustrated in Fig. 4A below, may be operating. The cytological argument that has been made for two or more inactivator units (Cattanach 1975) states that both parts of the insertion-bearing X "appear to be inactivated" and offers as evidence observations on heteropyknosis (Ohno and Cattanach 1962) and on absence of grains over the entire X^t when labeling is done in early S (Nesbitt and Gartler 1970). However, Nesbitt and Gartler often found some grains in the relatively unlabeled (late replicating) chromosomes, particularly over the distal part; and heteropyknosis in prophase is not a precise enough measure for specific chromosomal regions.

If it can be established that one of the recently identified X-linked biochemical markers is located in xt^s of one of the reciprocal translocations, gene-dosage determinations could provide the means for settling the question of single versus multiple inactivation centers. It may be noted that T1Ct does not furnish a critical test system for this purpose, since, in an insertional translocation, even a single inactivation center could *a priori* affect both

X portions, unless there is incontrovertible evidence for inter-
ruption of inactivation within the autosomal insertion.

The other inactivation process to be examined is interaction
of two factors in *cis* position. At first glance, this may appear
like an attractive hypothesis to explain T16H and several human
balanced T(X;A)'s (summarized by Leisti *et al*. 1975) in which neither translocation product is ever inactivated. One consequence
of the *cis*-interaction hypothesis is that — once the conditions
of inactivation are met — any further variation in X-breakpoint
position should have no influence over degree of inactivation in
the attached autosomal material. To test this, one ideally needs
two translocations with the same autosomal breakpoint but with
different X breakpoints. Such a pair is not yet available, but R2
and R3 approach these conditions, as do R5 and R6. In each comparison, one finds greatly different effects on inactivation of
the same autosomal loci (Russell and Montgomery 1970). The inac-
tivation-center hypothesis, on the other hand, leads to the expectation that X-breakpoint location does influence degree of autosomal inactivation. Because of this fact, and because of the conclusion (see below) that nonrandomness in the T(X;A)'s results from
cell selection, we feel that T16H and the various human cases are
better explained by extreme selection than by a severing of *cis*
interaction of two factors needed for inactivation.

On the basis of the various considerations, a single inactivation center in the mouse seems to us to be the hypothesis most consistent with present and past observations. The single-inactivation-center hypothesis can be further simplified if one assumes
that this center is synonymous with a site on the X that acts as
receptor for the message to remain active (see above). When this
message is not received, inactivation then proceeds in both directions along the X and for some distance into any contiguous autosomal material.

Nonrandomness

Departures from randomness in the behavior of the two X's were
clearly found in the results of the present experiments. In Fig.
4, we illustrate some of the explanations that have been proposed
for such departures observed in the past.

Nonrandomness may be apparent, rather than real, in cases
where the overall phenotype is, in fact, not representative of the
existing cellular distribution. Thus, the unit of phenotype (e.g.,
a hair), may require a certain proportion of variant cells before
it expresses the variant phenotype (Fig. 4A). An elegant demonstration of such a "threshold effect" was brought by Falconer and

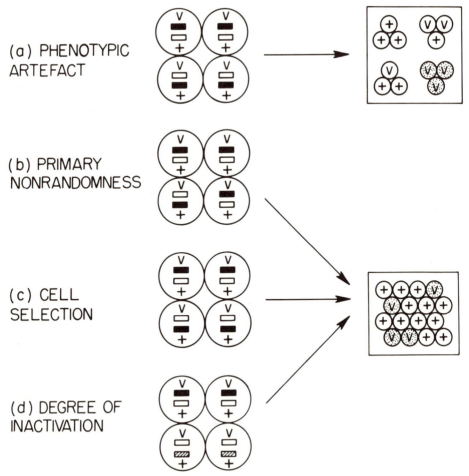

FIGURE 4. Possible causes of departures from randomness in ob-
    served phenotypes for X-linked genes. The middle column shows
    cell proportions at time of X differentiation under different
    hypotheses: +, wild-type allele; v, variant; ■, inactiva-
    ted; ⊏⊐, active; ▨ variable inactivation (see text).
    The final cell distribution is shown on the right with expres-
    sion of the + phenotype indicated by open circles.
    By pathway (a), though cells with + or v active are overall
    equal in number in the final cell distribution, the unit of
    phenotype (shown as a grouping of cells) expresses the + pheno-
    type even when some v cells (fewer than a certain proportion)
    are present. Alternative pathways (b), (c), and (d) all
    result in more of one cell type (here, +) than of the other
    in the final distribution: pathway (b) directly, because of
    nonrandomness in the differentiation process; pathway (c)
    secondarily, because of selection favoring + cells; pathway
    (d) because + is not invariably inactive.

Isaacson (1972). In the present experiment, however, classification was done on the cellular level, and this type of explanation
is thus not applicable.

There are two possible ways in which primary randomness of X
differentiation can be translated into subsequent nonrandomness in
the expression of X-linked genes. One proposed mechanism is that
of "incomplete inactivation" (Fig. 4D), including, for example,
the possibility that, when an X is differentiated to be inactive,
this inactivity does not regularly encompass the entire chromosome
(Russell 1963; Cattanach, Pollard, and Perez 1969), or the possibility that reactivation may occur following initial inactivation (Cattanach 1974). Within autosomal material attached to X-chromosome material, it has been documented that, for a given reciprocal
translocation, frequency of inactivation of different loci is correlated with proximity to the breakpoint, and, overall, to proximity to a postulated inactivation center in the X (Russell and Montgomery 1965, 1970). The strength of this spreading effect appeared
to be governed by alleles at the *Xce* (X controlling element) locus
(Cattanach and Isaacson 1967; Cattanach, Pollard, and Perez 1969;
Cattanach 1975). However, a test of the postulate that allelic
differences at *Xce* affect degree of inactivation within X-chromosome material, as well as within translocated autosomal material,
resulted in negative findings (Cattanach and Williams 1972). As
an alternative, these authors favored an explanation of primary
nonrandomness (Fig. 4B), based on their conclusion that one modify-
ing factor (presumably *Xce*) appeared to be involved in the differential effects of intact X chromosomes, derived from different
sources, on the expression of X-linked genes (Cattanach, Pollard,
and Perez 1969; Grahn, Fry, and Hamilton 1969; Russell 1971; Falconer and Isaacson 1972; Krzanowska and Wabik 1973; Ohno, Christian,
Attardi, and Kan 1973).

While the existence of primary nonrandomness has so far been
only inferred for the animal proper — having been clearly established only in the case of fetal membranes (Takagi 1978; West *et
al*. 1978) — secondary nonrandomness, resulting from selection
(Fig. 4C), has been demonstrated in a more direct manner. Selection working differentially on the cellular phenotypes produced by
intact horse or donkey X chromosomes was found to explain nonrandomness in female mules (Hamerton, Richardson, Gee, Allen, and
Short 1971) and was found to be tissue specific (Hook and Brustman
1971). Migeon (1978) has presented evidence for tissue-specific
selection in women heterozygous for X-linked genes. She has also
demonstrated transfer of gene products between cells, a process
which could masquerade as selection. Falconer and Isaacson have
pointed out that even a small selective differential (e.g., only
one fewer cell division of one cell type) can cause a big difference in distribution. Because of this, they feel there might be
many loci on the X capable of causing secondary nonrandomness.

For X chromosomes that have been juxtaposed with autosomal
material, there have been reports of apparently random inactivation (Russell and Montgomery 1970; Cattanach and Isaacson 1967;
Nesbitt and Gartler 1970), and others of nonrandomness (Lyon et al.
1964 for the mouse; Gustavsson, Fraccaro, Tiepolo, and Lindsten
1968 for a cow; Therman and Pätau 1974, and Leisti et al. 1975,
summarizing human cases). While nonrandomness is virtually always
in the direction that would be expected if there is selection
against "functional hemizygosity" (Russell 1964) of autosomal loci
(i.e., with X^n late replicating), the opposite situation (X^t predominantly inactive) has recently been demonstrated also (Cacheiro,
Russell, and Bangham 1978).

The present autoradiographic results indicate that, in adult
kidney cells, there is nonrandomness not only in T16H, but also
in T1Ct-Type-I, and in four different $T(X;7)$'s. On the other hand,
cells from two different $T(X;4)$'s and two T1Ct-Type-II* females
were evenly distributed between $X^n=0$ and $XT^{\ell}=0$.

This array of results may be interpreted on the assumption
that a region of Ch 7 contains genetic material critical for growth
or maintenance of kidney cells, so that cells in which this region
is made functionally hemizygous by the various $T(X;7)$ rearrangements (including T1Ct-Type-I but not Type-II) are selected against.
(It should be noted that such selection could have occurred in
vitro since the labeling studies were carried out after cells had
been in culture for about 5 days. Hamerton et al. [1971] found
that in vitro paralleled in vivo selection in mules and hinnies.)

That the action of the postulated gene(s) is probably needed
specifically in a certain tissue at a certain level of maturity is
indicated by the finding that, in fetal non-kidney cells of R6 and
R3, the frequencies of the two types of cells ($X^n=0$ and $XT^{\ell}=0$) are
about equal. Further, the selective process is apparently not complete in 18-day fetal kidney of R6. In the $T(X;4)$'s, as well as in
T1Ct-Type-II females, the critical Ch 7 genetic material is present
in double dose in all cells, accounting for the approximately equal
numbers of $X^n=0$ and $XT^{\ell}=0$ cells. This observed $T(X;4)$ randomness
suggests that it is not autosomal functional hemizygosity, in
general, that is being selected against. We have earlier proposed
that inactivation of "critical" autosomal genes may be responsible
for the relatively poor survival and productivity of $T(X;A)$ females
and for the dearth of $T(X;A)$'s in general (Russell and Montgomery
1969). The present autoradiographic results provide a specific
example of such a process. It seems probable that some tissue(s)

---

* The other two, atypical, fd-II females came from a line that is
  now extinct and cannot be re-tested.

could be found in which T(X;4)'s, too, would have nonrandom distribution of cells. In general, therefore, it is not proper to base any conclusions of randomness in a given T(X;A) on studies with only one cell type at one age.

If nonrandomness is due to functional genetic imbalance, this could be the result of excessive X material, deficient autosomal material, or both. The segment of X chromosome that is active in excess is roughly similar for R1 [a $T(X;4)$], R5, and R6 [$T(X;7)$'s]; and similar for R7 [a $T(X;4)$] and R3 [a $T(X;7)$] (Fig. 1). It is, however, very dissimilar for R5 and R6 on the one hand, and R2 and R3 on the other [all $T(X;7)$'s]. Yet all $T(X;7)$'s behave nonrandomly, while both $T(X;4)$'s are random. Therefore, we conclude that it is deficient autosomal function, rather than excessive X function, that is responsible for the secondary nonrandomness we have documented.

SUMMARY

By means of autoradiographic study of an array of mouse X-autosome translocations with different breakpoints, we have demonstrated that, in each case, only one translocation product is subject to allocyclic behavior, and that there is thus no memory system. This finding, in conjunction with earlier evidence that degree of inactivation of translocated autosomal loci is influenced by breakpoint position, is most easily interpreted by assuming a single inactivation center, with polarity in both directions. Other interpretations require special assumptions.

In short-term cultures from adult kidney of five T(X;7)'s there is nonrandomness in X-chromosome allocycly, with X^n predominantly (but not exclusively) inactive. This nonrandomness is not observed in two T(X;4)'s, nor does it occur in some fetal tissues of the T(X;7)'s. We propose that a region of Chromosome 7 contains genetic material critical for growth or maintenance of kidney cells, and that inactivation of this region in T(X;7)'s results in tissue-specific selection. Translocations in which X^n exclusively is inactive are presumably extreme examples of selection resulting from autosomal inactivation.

This research sponsored by the Division of Biomedical and Environmental Research, U. S. Department of Energy under contract W-7405-eng-26 with the Union Carbide Corporation.

REFERENCES

Brown, S. W. and H. S. Chandra. 1973. Inactivation system of the mammalian X chromosome. Proc. Nat. Acad. Sci. USA 70: 195-199.

Cacheiro, N. L. A., L. B. Russell, and J. W. Bangham. 1978. A new mouse X-autosome translocation with nonrandom inactivation. Genetics 88: s13-s14.

Cattanach, B. M. 1961. A chemically-induced variegated-type position effect in the mouse. Zeitschrift für Vererbungslehre 92: 165-182.

Cattanach, B. M. 1970. Controlling elements in the mouse X-chromosome. III. Influence upon both parts of an X divided by rearrangement. Genet. Res., Camb. 16: 293-301.

Cattanach, B. M. 1974. Position effect variegation in the mouse. Genet. Res., Camb. 23: 291-306.

Cattanach, B. M. 1975. Control of chromosome inactivation. Ann. Rev. of Genetics 9: 1-18.

Cattanach, B. M. and J. H. Isaacson. 1967. Controlling elements in the mouse X chromosome. Genetics 57: 331-346.

Cattanach, B. M., C. E. Pollard, and J. N. Perez. 1969. Controlling elements in the mouse X-chromosome. I. Interaction with the X-linked genes. Genet. Res., Camb. 14: 223-235.

Cattanach, B. M. and C. E. Williams. 1972. Evidence of non-random X-chromosome activity in the mouse. Genet. Res., Camb. 19: 229-240.

Chapman, V. M., J. D. West, and D. A. Adler. 1978. Bimodal distribution of α-galactosidase activities in mouse embryos. In, Genetic Moaaics and Chimeras in Mammals, Liane B. Russell, Ed. Plenum Press, New York and London.

Comings, D. F. 1968. On the rationale for an ordered arrangement of chromatin in the interphase nucleus. J. Hum. Genet. 20: 440-460.

Cooper, D. W., P. G. Johnston, C. E. Murtagh, and J. L. VandeBerg. 1975. Sex chromosome evolution and activity in mammals, particularly kangaroos. In, Eukaryote Chromosome, W. J. Peacock and R. D. Brock, Eds. Australian Natl. University Press, Canberra, pp. 381-393.

Eicher, E. M. 1970. X-autosome translocations in the mouse: total inactivation versus partial inactivation of the X chromosome. Adv. in Genet. 15: 175-259.

Eicher, E. M., M. N. Nesbitt, and U. Francke. 1972. Cytological identification of the chromosomes involved in Searle's translocation and the location of the centromere in the X chromosome of the mouse. Genetics 71: 643-648.

Eicher, E. M. and L. L. Washburn. 1978. Assignment of genes to regions of mouse chromosomes. Proc. Natl. Acad. Sci. USA 75: 946-950.

Epstein, C. J., B. Travis, G. Tucker, and S. Smith. 1978. The direct demonstration of an X-chromosome dosage effect prior to inactivation. In, Genetic Mosaics and Chimeras in Mammals, Liane B. Russell, Ed. Plenum Press, New York and London.

Falconer, D. S. and J. H. Isaacson. 1972. Sex-linked variegation modified by selection in brindled mice. Genet. Res., Camb. 20: 291-316.

Francke, U. and M. N. Nesbitt. 1971. Cattanach's translocation: cytological characterization by quinacrine mustard staining. Proc. Natl. Acad. Sci. USA 68: 2918-2920.

Grahn, D., R. J. M. Fry, and K. F. Hamilton. 1969. Genetic and pathologic analysis of the sex-linked allelic series, mottled, in the mouse. Genetics 61: s22-s23.

Grumbach, M. M., A. Morishima, and J. H. Taylor. 1963. Human sex chromosome abnormalities in relation to DNA replication and hetero-chromatization. Proc. Natl. Acad. Sci. USA 49: 581-589.

Gustavsson, I., M. Fraccaro, L. Tiepolo, and J. Lindsten. 1968. Presumptive X-autosome translocation in a cow: preferential inac-tivation of the normal X chromosome. Nature 218: 183-184.

Hamerton, J. L., B. J. Richardson, P. A. Gee, W. R. Allen, and R. V. Short. 1971. Non-random X-chromosome expression in female mules and hinnies. Nature 232: 312-315.

Hook, E. B. and L. D. Brustman. 1971. Evidence for selective differences between cells with an active horse X chromosome and cells with an active donkey X chromosome in the female mule. Nature 232: 349-350.

Kaufman, M. H., M. Guc-Cubrillo, and M. F. Lyon. 1978. X chromo-some inactivation in diploid parthenogenetic mouse embryos. Nature 271: 547-549.

Kouri, R. E., D. A. Miller, O. J. Miller, V. G. Dev, M. S. Grewal, and J. J. Hutton. 1971. Identification by quinacrine fluorescence of the chromosome carrying mouse Linkage Group I in the Cattanach translocation. Genetics 69: 129–132.

Kratzer, P. G. and S. M. Gartler. 1978. HGPRT expression in early mouse development. In, Genetic Mosaics and Chimeras in Mammals, Liane B. Russell, Ed. Plenum Press, New York and London.

Krzanowska, H. and B. Wabik. 1973. Expression of the sex-linked gene Ms (Mosaic) in mice selected for different levels of variegation. Genetics 74: s146.

Leisti, J. T., M. M. Kaback, and D. L. Rimoin. 1975. Human X-autosome translocations: differential inactivation of the X chromosome in a kindred with an X-9 translocation. Am. J. Hum. Genet. 27: 441–453.

Lyon, M. F. 1961. Gene action in the X-chromosome of the mouse (Mus musculus L.). Nature 190: 372–373.

Lyon, M. F. 1968. Chromosomal and subchromosomal inactivation. Ann. Rev. Genet. 2: 31–52.

Lyon, M. F., A. G. Searle, and C. E. Ford. 1964. A mouse translocation suppressing sex-linked variegation. Cytogenetics 3: 306–323.

Martin, G. R., C. J. Epstein, and D. W. Martin, Jr. 1978. Use of teratocarcinoma stem cells as a model system for the study of X-chromosome inactivation in vitro. In, Genetic Mosaics and Chimeras in Mammals, Liane B. Russell, Ed. Plenum Press, New York and London.

Migeon, B. R. 1978. Selection and cell communication as determinants of female phenotype. In, Genetic Mosaics and Chimeras in Mammals, Liane B. Russell, Ed. Plenum Press, New York and London.

Monk, Marilyn. 1978. Biochemical studies on X-chromosome activity in preimplantation mouse embryos. In, Genetic Mosaics and Chimeras in Mammals, Liane B. Russell, Ed. Plenum Press, New York and London.

Moses, M., L. B. Russell, and N. L. A. Cacheiro. 1977. Mouse chromosome translocations: visualization and analysis by electron microscopy of the synaptonemal complex. Science 196: 892–899.

Nesbitt, M. N. and U. Francke. 1973. A system of nomenclature for band patterns of mouse chromosomes. Chromosoma 41: 145–158.

Nesbitt, M. N. and S. M. Gartler. 1970. Replication of the mouse sex chromosomes early in the S period. Cytogenetics 9: 212-221.

Ohno, S. and B. M. Cattanach. 1962. Cytological study of an X-autosome translocation in *Mus musculus*. Cytogenetics 1: 129-140.

Ohno, S., L. Christian, B. J. Attardi, and J. Kan. 1973. Modification of expression of the *Testicular feminization* (*Tfm*) gene of the mouse by a "Controlling Element" gene. Nature New Biol. 245: 92-93.

Ohno, S. and M. F. Lyon. 1965. Cytological study of Searle's X-autosome translocation in *Mus musculus*. Chromosoma 16: 90-100

Ray, M., P. A. Gee, B. J. Richardson, and J. L. Hamerton. 1972. G6PD expression and X chromosome late replication in fibroblast clones from a female mule. Nature 237: 396-397.

Russell, L. B. 1961. Genetics of mammalian sex chromosomes. Science 133: 1795-1803.

Russell, L. B. 1963. Mammalian X-chromosome action: inactivation limited in spread and in region of origin. Science 140: 976-978.

Russell, L. B. 1964. Genetic and functional mosaicism in the mouse. In, The Role of Chromosomes in Development, Michael Locke, Ed. Academic Press, New York, pp. 153-181.

Russell, L. B. 1971. Attempts to demonstrate different inactivating states for normal mouse X chromosomes. Genetics 68: 55-56.

Russell, L. B. and J. W. Bangham. 1961. Variegated-type position effects in the mouse. Genetics 46: 509-525.

Russell, L. B. and C. S. Montgomery. 1965. The use of X-autosome translocations in locating the X-chromosome inactivation center. Genetics 52: 470-471.

Russell, L. B. and C. S. Montgomery. 1969. Comparative studies on X-autosome translocations in the mouse. I. Origin, viability, fertility, and weight of five T(X;1)'s. Genetics 63: 103-120.

Russell, L. B. and C. S. Montgomery. 1970. Comparative studies on X-autosome translocations in the mouse. II. Inactivation of autosomal loci, segregation, and mapping of autosomal breakpoints in five T(X;1)'s. Genetics 64: 281-312.

Takagi, N. 1978. Preferential inactivation of the paternally derived X chromosome in mice. In, Genetic Mosaics and Chimeras in Mammals, Liane B. Russell, Ed. Plenum Press, New York and London.

Therman, E. and K. Pätau. 1974. Abnormal X chromosomes in man: Origin, behavior and effects. Humangenetik 25: 1-16.

West, J. D., V. E. Papaioannou, W. I. Frels, and V. M. Chapman. 1978. Preferential expression of the maternally derived X chromosome in extraembryonic tissues of the mouse. In, Genetic Mosaics and Chimeras in Mammals, Liane B. Russell, Ed. Plenum Press, New York and London.

SELECTION AND CELL COMMUNICATION AS DETERMINANTS OF FEMALE PHENOTYPE

Barbara R. Migeon

Department of Pediatrics, Johns Hopkins University
School of Medicine, Baltimore, Maryland 21205

As a consequence of X-chromosome inactivation, one X chromosome becomes the sole determinant of the X-specified characteristics of the cell, leading to potential cellular mosaicism in females. If there were no differences between the maternal and paternal alleles at any X-linked locus, there would be no cellular mosaicism. However, unlike the relatively homogeneous laboratory mouse populations, the human population is very heterogeneous, largely attributable to heterozygosity at many loci. Based on estimates by Harris and Hopkinson (1972), it seems certain that most women are heterozygous at one and probably more than ten X-linked loci. Therefore, with respect to her X-linked genes, the phenotype of the female is determined by the nature of her individual heterozygosity, the effect of random inactivation on the proportions of cells of the two types in each tissue, and the result of selection following inactivation.

There is considerable evidence that inactivation is random with respect to the parental origin of the X chromosome, but that selection favoring one cell population occurs subsequently. Due to X inactivation, cells which are genetically identical may be phenotypically dissimilar as a result of differences in the nature of maternal and paternal alleles at various X-linked loci. Some of these heterozygous alleles may influence the proliferation of embryonic cells. In the developing embryo, competition between the two cell populations that result from X inactivation is not only conceivable but likely, and may play a significant role in determining female phenotype.

EVIDENCE THAT SELECTION OCCURS IN SOMATIC CELLS

There is little doubt that selection occurs in the somatic cells of female embryos carrying X chromosomes with altered morphology. Invariably, when an X chromosome carries a significant deletion, it is inactivated. This is expected because cells having inactivated the normal X chromosome lack an essential portion of the X (the deleted segment) and consequently are inviable or have a severe proliferative disadvantage (Gartler and Sparks 1963). On the other hand, in the case of X chromosomes involved in balanced translocations with autosomes, the normal X is the one that is usually turned off; inactivation in the X-chromosome portion of the translocation chromosome is known to turn off genes in adjacent autosomal segments (Russell 1961; Russell and Montgomery 1969; Cattanach 1970; Leisti, Kaback, and Rimoin 1975), resulting in effective monosomy at autosomal loci that is at the least detrimental, and more likely lethal, to the cell in which it occurs. Therefore, the best explanation for nonrandom inactivation patterns observed with morphologically variant X chromosomes is cell death rather than preferential inactivation. Selection of this intensity implies an extensive cell loss in the embryo; yet, losses of this magnitude are known to occur during the development of monozygotic twins, while mice of normal size have been derived from partial blastocysts.

Further evidence that cells with unbalanced karyotypes are disfavored is that the frequency of cells with abnormal karyotype decreases in individuals mosaic for X-chromosome aneuploidy as the individual ages (Eller, Frankenburg, Puck, and Robinson 1971). Recently, Russell and Cacheiro (1978) have observed a nonrandom pattern of inactivation in kidneys of mice carrying balanced X-autosome translocations; the skewing presumably results from selection against those cells in which an autosomal locus important to kidney cells has been inactivated by neighboring X material.

Selection has been implicated as an explanation for the paucity of enzyme-deficient red blood cells in heterozygotes for the Lesch-Nyhan mutation [X-linked deficiency of hypoxanthine-guanine phosphoribosyltransferase (HGPRT)]. Although mosaicism with regard to HGPRT activity is expected in these heterozygotes, few if any enzyme-deficient cells have been detected among their red blood cells. Studies of females simultaneously heterozygous for two X-linked genes, HGPRT and glucose-6-phosphate dehydrogenase (G6PD), disclosed that the blood cells of such individuals expressed only the G6PD allele that was coupled with the wild-type HGPRT allele (Nyhan, Bakay, Connor, Marks, and Keele 1970; also, Fig. 1). The population of cells having the mutant HGPRT allele on the active X chromosome had been excluded. The reason for the proliferative disadvantage of HGPRT-deficient erythrocytes is not apparent, but presumably the ability to utilize preformed purines is beneficial.

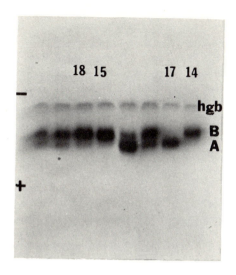

FIGURE 1. G6PD phenotype of erythrocytes from Lesch-Nyhan hetero-
    zygotes in the C. T. family (see pedigree in Fig. 6).
    Individuals IV-18, III-15, and III-14 are heterozygous both
    for HGPRT deficiency and for G6PD$_A$, yet express little if any
    G6PD$_A$, the allele coupled with the mutant HGPRT allele. A
    small amount of G6PD$_A$ is seen in IV-18, who is 8 years old.

What *is* clear is that selection is directed against cells having a
severe enzyme deficit: in the case of females heterozygous for
mutations leading to only partial deficiency of HGPRT, red cells
of mutant type are not disfavored (Johnson, Gordon, and Emmerson
1976). Selection against HGPRT-deficient red cells in Lesch-Nyhan
heterozygotes, although always substantial, does not invariably
result in complete elimination of the cells of mutant phenotype;
some young heterozygotes have minor populations of the disfavored
cell (Fig. 1). Selection of this kind is not confined to red cells
but also occurs in lymphocytes of the heterozygote, where the absence of mosaicism has been noted (Dancis, Berman, Jansen, and
Balis 1968). Albertini and DeMars (1974) observed a small population (less than 10%) of enzyme-deficient lymphocytes in adolescent
girls, but not in their mother. The presence of rare cells of
mutant type in some heterozygotes, especially the younger ones,
suggests that the selection may be an ongoing event leading to
gradual elimination of the disfavored cells.

EVIDENCE THAT SELECTION IS TISSUE SPECIFIC

In contrast to blood cells, HGPRT-deficient skin fibroblasts
from heterozygotes for the Lesch-Nyhan mutation are not at a proliferative disadvantage. Cloning efficiencies for mutant and wild-
type cells are similar, at least in the culture medium used for
these studies (Migeon 1971). Analysis of skin fibroblast clones
from heterozygotes also reveals no evidence of an *in vivo* proliferative advantage for either allele; among 4,000 clones from 21
heterozygotes, approximately half were of the mutant type, as
determined by autoradiographic analysis of HGPRT phenotype (Migeon
1971; see Fig. 2, this paper).

Between individual heterozygotes, however, there is considerable variability in HGPRT phenotype. Some have a small population
of enzyme-deficient fibroblasts while others have relatively few
clones of normal type (Fig. 3). Although sampling may explain some
of the variability, the results of duplicate studies from the same
specimen (Migeon 1971; Table 1, this paper) or from replicate
biopsies (Table 1) are remarkably reproducible. The variability
among heterozygotes is reflected in the wide range of enzyme activity that characterizes uncloned skin fibroblasts (Migeon 1971;
Fujimoto and Seegmiller 1970; Fig. 3).

Among heterozygotes, the population of HGPRT-deficient skin
fibroblasts is usually greater than 10% (Migeon 1971; Felix and
DeMars 1971). However, because it is expected that some heterozygous females have only rare cells of mutant phenotype, we have
devised a means for increasing the sensitivity of heterozygote
detection by using nutrient media which favor the growth of mutant

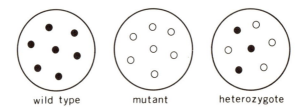

wild type   mutant   heterozygote

● Clones, labeled with ^{3}H Hypoxanthine
○ Clones, unlabeled

FIGURE 2. X-linked HGPRT deficiency: detection of heterozygotes
    by autoradiographic studies of labeled hypoxanthine incorpora-
    tion in skin fibroblast clones.

TABLE 1. Frequency of HGPRT-deficient clones in replicate biopsy
specimens from heterozygotes, determined by autoradiography of
skin fibroblast clones.

Specimen ref. no.[*]	Clonal data		
	No. analyzed	Efficiency[‡]	% HGPRT⁻ clones
11 a	78	0.24	67.9
b	223	0.60	51.6
13 a	28	0.40	28.6
b	112	0.42	50.0
20 a	202	0.55	55.5
b	88	0.17	46.6
c	125	0.33	43.2
d	110	0.30	50.0
24 a	202	0.67	31.7
b	122	0.37	30.4
c	166	0.49	44.6
d	128	0.47	29.7
26 a	291	0.59	24.3
b	241 (121)[†]	0.32 (0.36)	77.6 (71.1)
c	323	0.42	33.4
d	347	0.43	31.7
76 a	140	0.50	45.0
b	213	0.30	18.7
81 a	70	0.17	32.8
b	210 (63)[†]	0.31 (0.09)	30.0 (25.4)
121 a	56	0.47	0.0[§]
b	154	0.43	0.0

[*] Including site of biopsy. A, one upper extremity; b, the other.
c, one lower extremity; d, the other.

[†] Repeat analysis from same specimen.

[‡] Clones obtained/cells plated.

[§] Heterozygous, but with rare cells of mutant type.

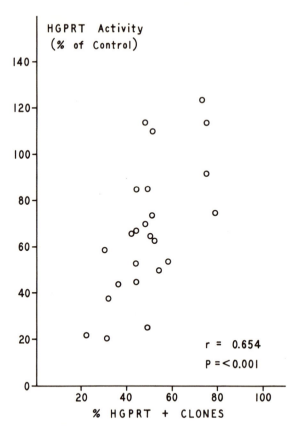

FIGURE 3. Scattergram showing a linear correlation between the percentage of HGPRT⁺ clones in heterozygotes and the HGPRT activity of the uncloned fibroblasts from which the clones were derived. HGPRT activity has been assayed by measuring the incorporation of ³H hypoxanthine by intact cells and is expressed as percent of control incorporation. [Reproduced by permission (Migeon 1971)]

cells (Migeon 1970; Felix and DeMars 1971). In contrast to cells with normal HGPRT activity, those lacking this enzyme can proliferate in the presence of $6 \times 10^{-5}M$ 6-thioguanine (6TG) (Fig. 4).

Using the ability of HGPRT-deficient cells to proliferate in 6TG as an assay, we have detected two heterozygotes who have very few skin fibroblasts of mutant phenotype. The first obligate heterozygote has a grandson affected with the Lesch-Nyhan syndrome, as well as three heterozygous daughters (Fig. 5). We did not observe any HGPRT-deficient clones by autoradiography; however,

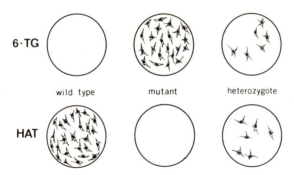

FIGURE 4. X-linked HGPRT deficiency: detection of heterozygotes
by selective medium.
Cell proliferation is influenced by genotype and environment
(nutrient medium). Medium containing the purine analogue 6TG
favors the growth of HGPRT-deficient cells; HAT medium
selects for normal cells (Szylbalski, Szybalska, and Ragni
1962).

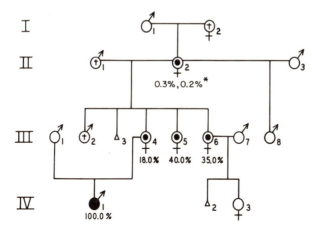

FIGURE 5. Pedigree of D.C. family segregating the Lesch-Nyhan
mutation, showing percent of HGPRT-deficient cells among skin
fibroblasts of the affected male (IV-1), his heterozygous
mother (III-4) and aunts (III-5 and III-6), and in the two
speciments* from his heterozygous grandmother (II-2). The
number of clones obtained in 6TG is expressed as a percent of
clones obtained in nonselective medium. Percent of HGPRT-
clones by autoradiography: III-4, 29%; III-5, 29%; III-6,
38%; and II-2, 0% and 0%.

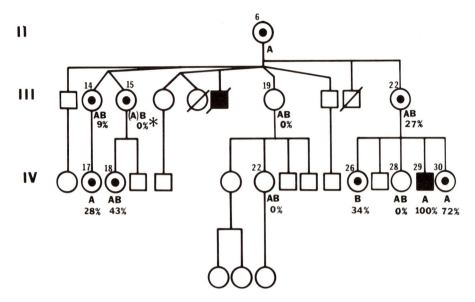

FIGURE 6. Partial pedigree of the C.T. family showing G6PD phenotype of skin fibroblasts and frequency of HGPRT-deficient skin
fibroblast clones in heterozygotes for Lesch-Nyhan disease.
■ affected males; ◉ heterozygotes; **A AB B** G6PD phenotypes in skin fibroblasts; * exceptional female, with rare
6TG-resistant clones of G6PD$_A$, HGPRT$^-$ phenotype.

6TG selection in cultures established from two independent skin
biopsies revealed the rare mutant cells in both specimens (Fig. 5;
Table 1, #121 a and b) (Migeon 1978).

Figure 6 shows the partial pedigree of the family in which we
found the second exceptional heterozygote (III-15). She is an
obligate heterozygote because her mother (II-6) and her daughter
(IV-18) were shown to be heterozygous by our studies. Examination
of skin fibroblast clones from this exceptional female did not
reveal the expected population of enzyme-deficient cells. However,
using 6TG selection and low cell densities, we obtained seven 6TG-
resistant clones; each of these was HGPRT deficient and of the
G6PD$_A$ phenotype, occurring with a frequency of 3×10^{-4}. It is
interesting to note that skin fibroblasts from her dizygotic twin
sister (III-14) are also predominantly of normal type (Fig. 2).
One would expect that the results of competition between the two
clonal populations might be more similar between sisters, who have
the same paternal X chromosome, than between mothers and daughters
who have different paternal X chromosomes.

The low frequency of HGPRT-deficient fibroblasts in these exceptional heterozygotes is most likely attributable to some proliferative advantage of the skin cells that have normal HGPRT activity. Selection, however, is probably not directed at the HGPRT locus, because HGPRT-deficient cells are not usually disfavored in skin. The paucity of HGPRT-deficient cells most likely is a consequence of selection against unknown genes coupled with the HGPRT$^-$ allele; the HGPRT$^+$ allele has been selected for the company it keeps.

Selective advantages of the wild-type alleles have been observed at other X-linked loci. Distribution of G6PD red blood cell phenotypes, in an unbiased sample of females heterozygous for the G6PD$_{Mediterranean}$ mutation (which leads to deficiency of the enzyme(is skewed in favor of cells expressing the normal enzyme phenotype (Rinaldi, Filippi, and Siniscalco 1976). It is conceivable, as suggested by Beutler (1964), that mutant red-cell precursors in the bone marrow have some proliferative disadvantage and that their numbers may thus be reduced. We have recently obtained evidence suggesting that the amelioration of clinical symptoms in heterozygotes at the Incontinentia Pigmenti locus may be attributable to selection against cells of the mutant type. In this case, the family under study was segregating G6PD variants as well as the Incontinentia Pigmenti mutation. Both mother and daughter are heterozygous for the mutation and are affected with a mild form of the disease. The daughter's erythrocytes and leukocytes excluded the maternal G6PD allele; and her fibroblasts had only a minor population of cells expressing the maternal G6PD allele, which is coupled with the mutant allele at the Incontinentia Pigmenti locus (Fig. 7).

The possibility that selection acting on the mosaic cell population might confer an advantage to heterozygotes has long been recognized (Gartler and Linder 1964; Beutler 1964). Such selection has, however, been considered not to play a significant role in embryogenesis, primarily because of the relatively low (1–3%) frequency of single phenotype in blood samples of obligate G6PD heterozygotes and in tissue specimens of these heterozygotes (Gartler 1976).

Why is there not more evidence for selective overgrowth of one population of cells in individuals heterozygous for X-linked variants? One problem is ascertainment. One needs informative mother-offspring pairs as well as suitable genetic markers; for example, exclusion at the G6PD locus is *apparent* only if the mother is heterozygous for the pertinent allele, but it may occur as well in females homozygous for G6PD alleles. Kirkman and Hendrickson (1963) found that 8 of 79 heterozygous mothers excluded the allele they transmitted to their sons. They attributed this discrepancy to the inability to accurately detect the relatively unstable and

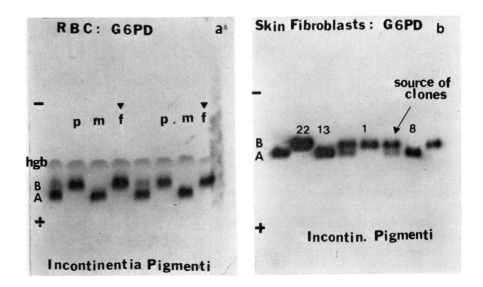

FIGURE 7. (a) G6PD phenotype of erythrocytes from a four-month-old
female (f) heterozygous for the Incontinentia Pigmenti mutation and affected with the disease, her mother (m), and her
father (p). Note that the infant does not express the maternal G6PD allele (G6PD$_A$). Her white blood cells also excluded
G6PD$_A$.
(b) G6PD phenotype of skin fibroblast clones 22, 13, 1, and 8
from the infant, revealing her heterozygosity at this locus.
Note faint G6PD$_A$ band in uncloned fibroblasts from which
clones were derived.

common G6PD$_A$-variant in maternal blood specimens, yet they had no
difficulty in detecting the variant in male samples, where it is
present by itself. Nance (1964) observed one of 30 heterozygotes
who essentially excluded the G6PD$_B$ allele from her red cells.
Using an assay sensitive enough to detect G6PD$_{A-}$ variants, we have
noted three examples of allelic exclusion in a small population
under study for other reasons. Among 15 maternal-fetal specimens
obtained from induced abortions, we found two cases where the fetal
tissue expressed a G6PD type not expressed in the maternal blood
(Migeon and Kennedy 1975). Among seven full-term males, we noted
one who was G6PD$_{A+}$ while his mother's white cells were G6PD$_B$
(Migeon and Do 1978). In these cases, the allelic exclusion has
taken place in *normal* females; the G6PD variant has no selective
value but serves only to indicate the population which has been
excluded. The basis for exclusion presumably is some other X-
linked locus heterozygous for an allele that is detrimental, at
least in blood cells.

EFFECT OF CELL COMMUNICATION

It is likely that selective overgrowth is prevented to a considerable extent by the transfer of gene products from one cell to
another in some tissues. This explains why the complete elimination of one clonal population in the heterozygous female is not
observed more frequently. The presence of rare mutant cells can
be obscured by contact-mediated communication of the pertinent
product from wild-type to mutant cells by "metabolic cooperation"
(Subak-Sharpe, Bürk, and Pitts 1966). In the case of the Lesch-
Nyhan mutation, it seems to be the enzyme product, inosinic acid,
which is transferred (Cox, Krauss, Balis, and Dancis 1970). This
is not merely a cell-culture phenomenon since HGPRT-deficient cells
are also masked in uncultured skin specimens from obligate heterozygotes (Frost, Weinstein, and Nyhan 1970). We have developed an
assay that quantitates the communication of nucleotides between
skin fibroblasts. The assay is based on inhibition of the recovery
of HGPRT-deficient clones in 6TG by increasing numbers of HGPRT
wild-type cells (Fig. 8) (Corsaro and Migeon 1975). The inhibition
is attributable to the transfer of the toxic enzyme product, 6-
thioguanylic acid, from normal to mutant cells. Using this assay,
we have found that contact feeding of this kind occurs extensively
and is a stable characteristic of the cells of all individuals
studied. This type of cell communication increases the difficulty
of detecting rare HGPRT-deficient cells in heterozygotes; and tests
must be carried out at low density to minimize cell contact.

Cell communication mediated through gap junctions (Gilula,
Reeves, and Steinbach 1972) undoubtedly influences the viability
of HGPRT-deficient cells. Erythrocytes and lymphocytes (unless
stimulated) do not establish these low-resistance junctions (Hülser
and Peters 1972; Oliveira-Castro, Barcinski, and Cukierman 1973).
Therefore, blood cells of mutant type maintain a severe enzyme
deficiency and are subject to selection, whereas cells of mutant
type in the skin bypass the enzyme deficiency via contact transfer
of nucleotides. Contact feeding eliminates differences between
mutant and normal cells and therefore any potential proliferative
advantage of the normal cell. Gap-junction-mediated communication
is not limited to transfer of nucleotides; it is likely that many
ions and molecules of less than 1,200 daltons are transferred from
one cell to another in this way (Simpson, Rose, and Loewenstein
1976; Corsaro and Migeon 1977).

Metabolic cooperation of another kind takes place in females
heterozygous for X-linked mutations involving lysosomal enzymes.
In this case, wild-type cells secrete the enzyme, making it available for uptake by cells expressing the mutation, and thereby cor-
recting the defect. Studies of clonal populations of skin fibroblasts from females heterozygous for the Hunter mutation (X-linked

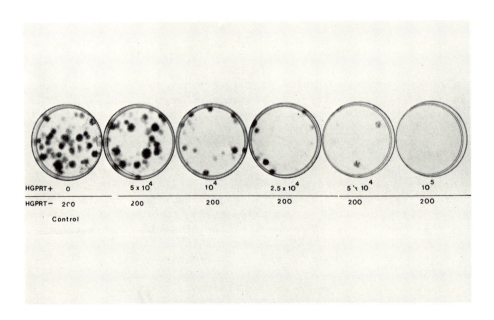

FIGURE 8. Contact-feeding assay based on the number of clones
        recoverable from mixed populations of HGPRT+ donor and HGPRT−
        recipient cells in 6TG medium. The number of 6TG^r clones
        obtained from these mixtures is compared with that in the
        control dish. [Reproduced by permission (Corsaro and Migeon
        1975)].

iduronate sulfatase deficiency)indicate that the presence of a
majority of cells with the Hunter phenotype may be obscured as a
result of correction by the minority population of normal type
cells in the mixture (Migeon, Sprenkle, Liebaers, Scott, and Neufeld 1977). Correction of this kind precludes selection against
cells of mutant phenotype.

CONCLUSIONS

     The ultimate phenotype of the female therefore results from
the interplay between selection and cell communication. As a consequence of random inactivation, one expects that expression of
mutant alleles among heterozygotes for X-linked genes would be
variable, and that the clinical phenotype of some heterozygotes
could be as severe as that of their affected sons. The fact that
only minimal abnormalities of purine metabolism have been noted
among carriers of the Lesch-Nyhan syndrome may indicate that even
a few cells with normal HGPRT activity can prevent manifestation

of the enzyme deficiency in the heterozygote. On the other hand, perhaps through metabolic cooperation, the enzyme product is made available to *all* cells in sufficient quantities to prevent clinical manifestations. Conceivably, the proliferation of cells expressing the normal allele is favored, not only in blood but in other non-communicating tissues as well. Advantages of this type, however, would result only if the pertinent locus were expressed in cells at the time they were undergoing proliferation and if the variant influenced the cell's ability to multiply. Although many mutations are neutral with respect to cell proliferation, some mutations are likely to confer a selective advantage, in the appropriate environment.

In any event, it seems likely that X inactivation occurs randomly and results in two populations of cells differing with regard to their X-chromosome phenotype. During embryogenesis, the overgrowth of one cell population may occur with elimination or diminution of the other. The outcome of the competition between the two cell populations may differ from one tissue to another because it depends on complicated interactions related to the nature of the variant alleles, the time of expression, and whether the pertinent gene product is transferred between cells. Cell communication masks the genotype, corrects the deficiency, and obviates the selective advantage of the wild-type cell.

The opportunity for females to carry two alleles at the same locus simultaneously must provide versatility not possible in the hemizygous male, masking or ameliorating the effect of the variant allele. Yet, the observations discussed here indicate that selection favoring one of the two cell populations produced by X inactivation plays a role in determining female phenotype by eliminating abnormal cells. It seems likely that cellular mosaicism during embryogenesis provides a unique adaptive advantage for the female; therefore, it is not only the variety of alleles in the female, but also the choice between the two alleles which contributes to her greater biological fitness.

This work was supported by NIH grant HD 05465.

REFERENCES

Albertini, R. J. and R. DeMars. 1974. Mosaicism of peripheral blood lymphocyte populations in females heterozygous for the Lesch-Nyhan mutation. Biochem. Genet. 11: 397-411.

Beutler, E. 1964. Gene inactivation: The distribution of gene products among populations of cells in heterozygous humans. Cold Spring Harbor Symposia on Quantitative Biology, Vol. 29, pp. 261-271.

Cattanach, B. M. 1970. Controlling elements in the mouse X chromosome. III. Influence upon both parts of an X divided by rearrangement. Genet. Res. 16: 293-301.

Corsaro, C. M. and B. R. Migeon. 1975. Quantitation of contact-feeding between somatic cells in culture. Exp. Cell Res. 95: 39-46.

Corsaro, C. M. and B. R. Migeon. 1977. Contact-mediated communication of ouabain resistance in mammalian cells in culture. Nature 268: 737-739.

Cox, R. P., M. R. Krauss, M. E. Balis, and J. Dancis. 1970. Evidence for transfer of enzyme product as the basis of metabolic cooperation between tissue culture fibroblasts of Lesch-Nyhan disease and normal cells. Proc. Natl. Acad. Sci. 67: 1573-1579.

Dancis, J., P. H. Berman, V. Jansen, and M. E. Balis. 1968. Absence of mosaicism in the lymphocyte in X-linked congenital hyperuricosuria. Life Sci. 7: 587-591.

Eller, E., W. Frankenburg, M. Puck, and A. Robinson. 1971. Prognosis in newborn infants with X-chromosomal abnormalities. Pediat. 47: 681-687.

Felix, J. S. and R. DeMars. 1971. Detection of females heterozygous for the Lesch-Nyhan mutation by 8-azuguanine resistant growth of cultured fibroblasts. J. Lab. Clin. Med. 27: 596-604.

Frost, P., G. D. Weinstin, and W. L. Nyhan. 1970. Diagnosis of Lesch-Nyhan syndrome by direct study of skin specimens. JAMA 212: 316-318.

Fujimoto, W. Y. and J. E. Seegmiller. 1970. Hypoxanthine-guanine phosphoribosyl transferase deficiency: Activity in normal, mutant and heterozygote-cultured human skin fibroblasts. Proc. Natl. Acad. Sci. 65: 577-584.

Gartler, S. M. 1976. X chromosome inactivation and selection in somatic cells. Federation Proceedings, 2191-2194.

Gartler, S. M. and D. Linder. 1964. Selection in mammalian mosaic cell populations. Cold Spring Harbor Symposia on Quantitative Biology 29: 253-259.

Gartler, S. M. and R. S. Sparks. 1963. The Lyon-Beutler hypothesis and isochromosome X patients with Turner's syndrome. Lancet ii: 411.

Gilula, N. B., O. R. Reeves, and A. Steinbach. 1972. Metabolic coupling, ionic coupling and cell contacts. Nature 235: 262-265.

Harris, H. and D. A. Hopkinson. 1972. Average heterozygosity per locus in man: An estimate based on the incidence of enzyme polymorphism. Ann. Hum. Genet. Lond. 36: 9-20.

Hülser, D. F. and J. H. Peters. 1972. Contact cooperation in stimulated lymphocytes. II. Electrophysiological investigations on intercellular communication. Exp. Cell Res. 74: 319-326.

Johnson, L. A., R. B. Gordon, and B. T. Emmerson. 1976. Two populations of heterozygote erythrocytes in moderate hypoxanthine guanine phosphoribosyltransferase deficiency. Nature 264: 172-174.

Kirkman, H. N. and E. M. Hendrickson. 1963. Sex-linked electrophoretic difference in glucose-6-phosphate dehydrogenase. Amer. J. of Hum. Genet. 15: 241-258.

Leisti, J. T., M. M. Kaback, and D. L. Rimoin. 1975. Human X-autosome translocations: Differential inactivation of the X chromosome in a kindred with an X-9 translocation. Amer. J. of Hum. Genet. 27: 441-453.

Migeon, B. R. 1970. X-linked HGPRT deficiency: Detection of heterozygotes by selective medium. Biochem. Genet. 4: 377-383.

Migeon, B. R. 1971. Studies of skin fibroblasts from 10 families with HGPRT deficiency, with reference to X-chromosomal inactivation. Amer. J. Hum. Genet. 23: 199-210.

Migeon, B. R. 1978. X-chromosome inactivation as a determinant of female phenotype. In, Genetic Mechanisms of Sexual Development, L. Vallet and I. Porter, Eds. Academic Press, New York. In press.

Migeon, B. R. and T. T. Do. 1978. Study of the placenta from newborns heterozygous for glucose-6-phosphate dehydrogenase in search of nonrandom X inactivation. In, Genetic Mosaics and Chimeras in Mammals, Liane B. Russell, Ed. Plenum Press, New York and London.

Migeon, B. R. and J. F. Kennedy. 1975. Evidence for the inactivation of an X chromosome early in the development of the human fetus. Amer. J. Hum. Genet. 27: 233.

Migeon, B. R., J. A. Sprenkle, I. Liebaers, J. F. Scott, and E. F. Neufeld. 1977. X-linked Hunter syndrome: The heterozygous phenotype in cell culture. Amer. J. Hum. Genet. 29: 448.

Nance, W. E. 1964. Genetic tests with a sex-linked marker: Glucose-6-phosphate dehydrogenase. Cold Spring Harbor Symposia on Quantitative Biology 29: 415-424.

Nyhan, W. L., B. Bakay, J. D. Connor, J. F. Marks, and D. K. Keele. 1970. Hemizygous expression of glucose-6-phosphate dehydrogenase in erythrocytes of heterozygotes for the Lesch-Nyhan syndrome. Proc. Natl. Acad. Sci. 65: 214-218.

Oliveira-Castro, G. M., M. A. Barcinski, and S. Cukierman. 1973. Intercellular communication in stimulated human lymphocytes. J. of Immunol. 111: 1616-1619.

Rinaldi, A., G. Filippi, and M. Siniscalco. 1976. Variability of red cell phenotypes between and within individuals in an unbiased sample of 77 certain heterozygotes for G6PD deficiency in sardinias. Amer. J. of Hum. Genet. 28: 496-505.

Russell, L. B. 1961. Genetics of mammalian sex chromosomes. Science 133: 1795-1803.

Russell, L. B. and N. L. A. Cacheiro. 1978. Cell selection in X-autosome translocation mosaics in genetic mosaics and chimeras in mammals. In, Genetic Mosaics and Chimeras in Mammals. Liane B. Russell, Ed. Plenum Press, New York and London.

Russell, L. B. and C. S. Montgomery. 1969. Comparative studies on X-autosome translocations in the mouse. I. Origin, viability, fertility, and weight of five T(X;1)'s. Genetics 63: 103-120.

Simpson, I., B. Rose, and W. R. Loewenstein. 1976. Size limit of molecules permeating the junctional membrane channels. Science 195: 294-296.

Subak-Sharpe, H., R. Bürk, and J. Pitts. 1966. Metabolic cooperation by cell-to-cell transfer between genetically different mammalian cells in tissue culture. Heredity 21: 342.

Szybalski, W., E. H. Szybalska, and G. Ragni. 1962. Genetic studies with human cell lines. In, National Cancer Institute Monograph 7: 75-89.

**Mathematical and Statistical
Analyses of Mosaic Patterns**

CLONAL GROWTH VERSUS CELL MINGLING

John D. West

Department of Zoology, University of Oxford, South
Parks Road, Oxford, OX1 3PS, England

INTRODUCTION

The variegated patterns seen in tissues of chimaeras and mosaics should tell us something about the developmental histories of these tissues. A number of ingenious approaches have been made to try to analyse these patterns, but there is still considerable controversy about the interpretation and relevance of this type of analysis (Mintz 1974; McLaren 1976; West 1978). Comparative analysis between different groups of animals or tissues, or between individuals of different ages, offers one of the more reliable approaches since this type of analysis is not dependent on precise numerical estimates. Even this approach, however, requires some caution and, in the past, a number of inappropriate comparisons have been made. It is essential to understand the contribution of the different elements to the total variegated pattern before a meaningful comparison can be made. The purpose of this article is to consider the organisation of variegated patterns seen in chimaeras and mosaics, and how the degrees of cell mixing and clonal growth in different groups of animals may be compared.

TWO TYPES OF OBSERVATION

Variegated patterns have been analysed in two main ways. One approach is to look at the overall distribution of the two cell populations in a whole tissue; the other is to examine a small region of a tissue in greater detail at the cellular level.*

---

* Although there may be more than two cell populations, this discussion will be restricted to two for the sake of simplicity.

Analysis of the whole coat of a large number of mouse chimaeras or mosaics gives us an overall picture of the distribution of the two melanocyte populations. The different populations of melanocytes tend to separate into zones or stripes, each of which is colonised predominantly, but not exclusively, by one population. (The article by Searle in this volume shows examples of melanocyte mosaicism caused by the p^{un} gene.) This type of observation has led to the interpretation of the pattern of stripes in terms of descendant clones that proliferate from the neural crest (Mintz 1974; McLaren 1976).

If we look more closely at a small part of a tissue, we find that the two cell populations in a chimera or mosaic are normally very finely intermingled. This is probably true for coat pigmentation, where single hairs may contain both populations of melanocytes (McLaren and Bowman 1969), but is most strikingly seen in sections of tissues where the two cell populations can be directly visualized *in situ* (reviewed by McLaren 1976; West 1978).

The pattern in the mouse coat suggests that each descendant clone tends to remain together as a loosely knit unit, whereas the observations on other tissues at the cellular level tell us that considerable cell mingling occurs. It is essential to realise that these two approaches give us different types of information. The first approach tells us about the overall distribution of the two cell populations and may allow us to unravel the arrangement of the lineages of descendant clones. The second approach is more relevant to cell mingling within small regions of a tissue. Thus, cell mingling probably occurs within the large stripes in the mouse coat; and, conversely, the smaller patches seen in other tissues may be part of a larger pattern of zones, equivalent to the stripes of coat melanocytes, that are not apparent by looking at small pieces of tissue.

It is obvious from this discussion that it is essential to define our terms very carefully in order to avoid compounding the confusion.

TERMINOLOGY

The following terms will be used specifically as defined.

A *zone* is an area or volume of tissue in a chimaera or mosaic that is occupied predominantly by one cell population and is bordered by regions predominantly occupied by the other cell population. (A stripe in the coat of a mouse chimaera is an example of a zone.)

A *descendant clone* is any group of clonally-related cells, irrespective of whether or not they remain contiguous throughout

development. Descendant clones can be initiated by any mitotically
active cell, but in this discussion we are only concerned with
descendant clones initiated at the time when cells are *allocated*
to the tissue primordium.

A *patch* has been defined by Nesbitt (1974) as "a group of cells
of like genotype which are contiguous at the time of consideration."

A *coherent clone* is the unit defined by Nesbitt (1974) as "a
group of clonally related cells which have remained contiguous
throughout the history of the embryo."

The time of *allocation* (McLaren 1976) is the time at which cell
mixing between lineages of different tissue primordia becomes minimal.

HYPOTHETICAL PATTERNS OF TISSUE GROWTH

Four hypothetical growth patterns are shown in Fig. 1. In
each, the inner group of six circles represents six cells allocated
to a hypothetical tissue primordium. These cells divide and form a
linear tissue represented by the outer string of circles.

Nesbitt (1974) considered three types of growth: (1) strict
coherent clonal growth, where no cell mingling occurs; (2) non-
clonal growth, where extensive cell mingling randomises the distribution of daughter cells; and (3) limited coherent clonal growth,
where some cell mingling occurs but is insufficient to produce a
completely random cell distribution.

The first two types of growth are represented by Figs. 1a and
1b respectively. In Fig. 1a, the six primordial cells initiate six
descendant clones that can be clearly seen as four zones in the
adult tissue. This type of strict coherent clonal growth may occur
in insects, but almost certainly does not occur in mammals.

The other extreme, non-clonal growth, is shown in Fig. 1b.
Extensive cell mingling has totally disrupted the spatial integrity
of the six descendant clones, and the four zones can no longer be
seen in the adult tissue. The arrangement of cells in the adult
tissue is random, and adjacent cells of the same population form
small patches.

The third category, limited coherent clonal growth, is the
most complex and includes an almost infinite number of possible
growth patterns. The degree of cell mingling may vary with time
and between different parts of the tissue. Figs. 1c and 1d illustrate two possible patterns. The pattern shown in Fig. 1c could

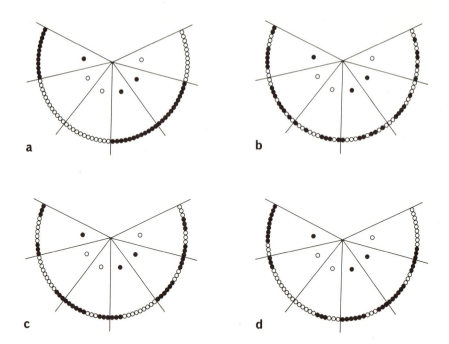

FIGURE 1. Four possible patterns of tissue growth. A hypothetical
    linear tissue (outer circles) may develop from a row of six
    progenitor cells (inner circles) by:

    (a) strict coherent clonal growth;
    (b) non-clonal growth;
    (c) limited coherent clonal growth with extensive cell
         mixing between descendant clones; or
    (d) limited coherent clonal growth with local cell mixing
         between adjacent descendant clones.

arise if cell mingling was very extensive early on, and caused mixing of cells between the six descendant clones; but slowed later in
development and allowed daughter cells to remain adjacent in some
cases. Thus, patches of coherent clones can be seen, but the six
descendant clones, initiated earlier, have been dispersed over the
whole tissue.

    A second type of limited coherent clonal growth is shown in
Fig. 1d. In this case, cell mingling early in development has been
less extensive and some zones of descendant clones can still be
identified. However, local cell mingling occurred and the cells
within a zone have been dispersed into smaller patches. In extreme
cases, the cell mingling may be sufficient to randomise the cells

within a zone, but frequently there would be some tendency for daughter cells to remain together. In this last example, shown in Fig. 1d, two superimposed patterns are apparent: a detailed pattern of patches, made up of coherent clones (or, in extreme cases, individual cells), is superimposed on a broad pattern of zones made up of descendant clones.

BIOLOGICAL PATTERNS OF VARIEGATION

Although either zones or patches have been seen in a number of variegated tissues (Mintz 1974; McLaren 1976; West 1978), the total pattern of variegation has been studied in most detail for the retinal pigment epithelium (RPE) of chimaeric mice. Sanyal and Zeilmaker (1977) combined the two approaches discussed above and analysed the distribution of black and white RPE cells over the whole tissue at the cellular level by reconstructing maps of the cellular distribution from semi-serial sections. Many of these reconstruction maps showed small patches of cells grouped into larger zones that appeared as sectors, radiating from the optic nerve. This type of pattern is best described by the hypothetical pattern shown in Fig. 1d, where limited coherent clonal growth occurs and cell mingling is restricted to mixing between neighbouring descendant clones. In other reconstruction maps (Sanyal and Zeilmaker 1977) the distribution of patches appeared more random over at least part of the eye, suggesting that cell mingling may sometimes be extensive enough to disrupt the sectors, as shown in Fig. 1c.

COMPARATIVE ANALYSIS OF VARIEGATED PATTERNS

In the past, the distinctions between descendant clones and coherent clones and between zones and patches has not been sufficiently emphasised. This has led to some inappropriate comparisons and some misleading interpretations of differences between chimaeras and mosaics. For example, Gartler (1976) compared the small patches of coherent clones seen in human X-inactivation mosaics with the larger zones (stripes) reported for the coats of mouse chimaeras and concluded that there was a significant difference in the "structure of mosaicism" between mouse chimaeras and human X-inactivation mosaics. The same observations prompted Gartler and Andina (1976) to conclude that "clonal development is not found in normal tissues" of humans. In an earlier paper, however, Linder and Gartler (1965) recognised the important difference between zones and patches when they pointed out that "what is considered a patch in the mice coat color cases .... may well represent areas in which there is merely a sufficient predominance of one cell type, such that the area appears to have a hemizygous phenotype."

Unfortunately, it is not even good enough to compare patches with patches, or zones with zones, because the number of clonal units within a patch or zone depends in part on the proportions of the two cell populations (West 1975, 1976). Deol and Whitten (1972) found fewer patches in sections of the RPE from mouse aggregation chimaeras than in equivalent sections from mouse X-inactivation mosaics. However, it is clear from a number of observations (Deol and Whitten 1972; West 1976; Falconer and Avery 1978) that the proportions of the two cell populations tend to be more nearly equal in X-inactivation mosaics than in chimaeras. If the two groups of animals to be compared have different proportions of the two cell populations, the variation in patch size, caused by differences in these proportions, must be taken into account. This can be done algebraically for linear measurements (West 1975, 1976), but for two- or three-dimensional measurements we have to resort to computer simulation. This topic is dealt with in more detail in the paper by Whitten in this volume.

Removal of the variation in patch size that is due to differences in the proportions of the two cell populations also yields a statistical estimate of the mean size of a coherent clone. This type of analysis was performed for the RPE (Tables 1 and 2). Table 1 shows the estimated mean number of cells per coherent clone for a series of mouse aggregation chimaeras and X-inactivation mosaics at different stages of development. Comparison of the estimated coherent clone sizes between X-inactivation mosaics of different ages indicates that coherent clones tend to increase in size during fetal and postnatal development. The four-fold increase suggests a relative decrease in the amount of local cell mingling, although estimates based on the increase in cell number and tissue area suggest that cell mingling does occur and is sufficient to increase the number of coherent clones three-fold between 12½ days *post coitum* and adulthood (West 1976). At 12½ days *post coitum* the estimated mean coherent clone size is close to one cell. This was initially interpreted as evidence for a random mixture of cells in the tissue, as illustrated in Fig. 1b (West 1976). However, in view of Sanyal and Zeilmaker's (1977) convincing evidence for a pattern of sectors, it seems more likely that this small coherent clone size simply reflects extensive local cell mingling within zones.

Tables 1 and 2 indicate that there is a general similarity in the estimated coherent clone sizes in the RPE of X-inactivation mosaics and some groups of aggregation chimaeras. One group of chimaeras, however, tends to have larger coherent clones, and this suggests that there may be a greater tendency for cells of the same population to stay together in chimaeras of certain genotype combinations.

TABLE 1. Estimated number of cells per two-dimensional coherent clone in the retinal pigment epithelium of a series of mouse aggregation chimaeras and X-inactivation mosaics at various stages of development. (From West 1976).

Age (days *post coitum*)	Mean number of cells per coherent clone*	
	X-inactivation mosaics	Aggregation chimaeras**
12½	1.20 ± 0.09 (12)	1.33 ± 0.18 (10)
13½	1.82 ± 0.26 (10)	—
14½	1.56 ± 0.21 (10)	1.83 ± 0.14 (2)
15½	2.24 ± 0.18 (10)	4.72 ± 0.35 (2)
18½	2.18 ± 0.23 (10)	—
Birth		
20½	2.79 ± 0.10 (10)	4.36 ± 0.56 (8)
Adult	4.85 ± 0.27 (20)	6.05 ± 0.44 (11)

* Expressed as mean ± standard error. The number of eyes is shown in parentheses.

** Made with pigmented and non-pigmented Q (random bred) strain mouse embryos.

    The mean coherent clone sizes derived in the tables are imprecise and should be considered only as statistical estimates for the number of cells per clonal group that would produce the observed mean patch size, on the assumption that the coherent clones are of equal size, of regular shape, and distributed at random. In biological actuality, coherent clones are likely to be quite variable in size and shape. Also, if cell mingling is restricted to a relatively local level, the mean number of coherent clones per patch may be more directly influenced by regional proportions of the two cell populations than by the proportions for the whole tissue. Normally, the proportions are estimated from the entire area analysed.

TABLE 2. Estimated number of cells per two-dimensional coherent clone in the retinal pigment epithelium of adult mouse X-inactivation mosaics and three series of aggregation chimaeras. (From West 1976).

Group	Mean number of cells per coherent clone*
X-inactivation mosaics	4.85 ± 0.27 (20)
Aggregation chimaeras:	
Pigmented-Q ↔ Unpigmented-Q	6.05 ± 0.44 (11)
Pigmented-Q ↔ Recessive	5.70 ± 0.76 (16)
(C57BL x C3H)F₁ ↔ Recessive	8.82 ± 0.77 (19)

* Expressed as mean ± standard error (number of eyes).

Despite these shortcomings, the numerical estimates provide a valid method of comparing different groups with respect to the degree of local cell mingling and coherent clonal growth. In principle, similar methods could be used to compare descendant clones, but the boundaries of the zones may be difficult to recognise and, in some cases, a single descendant clone may become divided into two or more separate zones.

SUMMARY

Both "clonal growth" and cell mingling seem to occur to some degree during histogenesis. Studies on mouse chimaeras and mosaics indicate that cell mingling occurs on a local scale but is not normally extensive enough to randomise the distribution of cells within the tissue. Variegation in at least some tissues can be thought of in terms of two superimposed patterns. Most of the cells of a given descendant clone tend to remain in the same zone of the tissue (as stripes or sectors), but local cell mingling occurs within these zones and between neighbouring zones. This local cell mingling disrupts the zones into small patches of cells. The net result is a pattern of small patches superimposed on a larger pattern of zones. It is essential to distinguish between these two component patterns, particularly when comparing different groups of animals. Comparisons between mouse aggregation chimaeras and X-inactivation mosaics suggests that local cell mixing occurs to a similar extent in the retinal pigment epithelium of the two groups. This similarity may be masked by a greater tendency for cells of the same genotype to stay together in chimaeras of some strain combinations.

I am grateful to the Medical Research Council for financial support.

REFERENCES

Deol, M. S. and W. K. Whitten. 1972. Time of X chromosome inactivation in retinal melanocytes of the mouse. Nature New Biol. 238: 159-160.

Falconer, D. S. and P. J. Avery. 1978. Variability of chimaeras and mosaics. J. Embryol. exp. Morph. 43: 195-219.

Gartler, S. M. 1976. Utilization of mosaic systems in the study
of the origin and progression of tumors. In, Chromosomes and Cancer, J. German, Ed., pp. 313-334. Wiley-Interscience, New York.

Gartler, S. M. and R. J. Andina. 1976. Mammalian X-chromosome
inactivation. Adv. Hum. Genet. 7: 99-140.

Linder, D. and S. M. Gartler. 1965. Distribution of glucose-6-
phosphate dehydrogenase electrophoretic variants in different tissues of heterozygotes. Amer. J. Hum. Genet. 17: 212-220.

McLaren, A. 1976. Mammalian Chimaeras. Cambridge University
Press, Cambridge-London.

McLaren, A. and P. Bowman. 1969. Mouse chimaeras derived from
fusion of embryos differing by nine genetic factors. Nature, Lond.
224: 238-240.

Mintz, B. 1974. Gene control of mammalian differentiation. Ann.
Rev. Genetics 8: 411-470.

Nesbitt, M. N. 1974. Chimeras vs. X inactivation mosaicism in
the mouse. Dev. Biol. 26: 252-263.

Sanyal, S. and G. H. Zeilmaker. 1977. Cell lineage in retinal
development of mice studied in experimental chimaeras. Nature,
Lond. 265: 731-733.

Searle, A. G. 1978. Evidence from mutable genes concerning the
origin of the germ line. In, Genetic Mosaics and Chimeras in Mammals, Liane B. Russell, Ed. Plenum Press, New York and London.

West, J. D. 1975. A theoretical approach to the relation between
patch size and clone size in chimaeric tissue. J. theor. Biol.
50: 153-160.

West, J. D. 1976. Clonal development of the retinal epithelium
in mouse chimaeras and X-inactivation mosaics. J. Embryol. exp.
Morph. 35: 445-461.

West, J. D. 1978. Analysis of clonal growth using chimaeras and
mosaics. In, Development in Mammals 3, M. H. Johnson, Ed. North-
Holland, Amsterdam. In press.

Whitten, W. K. 1978. Combinatorial and computer analysis of
random mosaics. In, Genetic Mosaics and Chimeras in Mammals,
Liane B. Russell, Ed. Plenum Press, New York and London.

COMBINATORIAL AND COMPUTER ANALYSIS OF RANDOM MOSAICS

Wesley K. Whitten

The Jackson Laboratory, Bar Harbor, Maine 04609

*Dedicated to the memory of the late Robert S. Rupp whose persever-
ance and keen three-dimensional insight made this study possible.*

INTRODUCTION

Mosaics are arrays of two or more alternatives which may be
in one, two, or three dimensions, and for each of which there are
many biological examples. Before we can discuss the biological
material intelligently, it is essential to determine some of the
parameters of purely random mosaics. The most obvious attributes
of mosaics are patchiness, and the variation in patchiness. I
shall use the terms run, patch, and cluster to describe aggregates
of like cells in one-, two-, and three-dimensional mosaics, respectively.

I have studied patchiness by extending the combinatorial
analysis developed by Stevens (1939) and others for the study of
runs of like cells seen in linear arrays of alternatives, and by
developing computer programs which generate and display random
arrays while at the same time tabulating aggregates of like cells
according to the number of cells they contain.

LINEAR MOSAICS

I shall start with the simplest form, the linear mosaics, because they are the easiest to comprehend and much is already known
about them. In addition, it is from them that two-dimensional
arrays can be assembled, which, in turn, can be used to develop
three-dimensional mosaics.

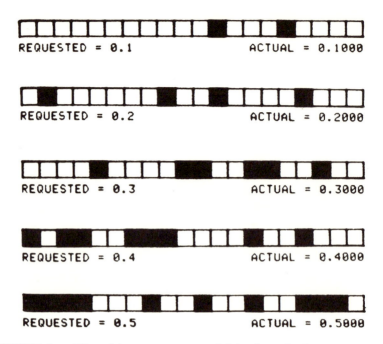

FIGURE 1. Five linear arrays of black and white cells.

Computer displays

Five linear mosaics of black (B) and white (W) cells in which the probability of B ranges from 0.1 to 0.5 are displayed in Figure 1. Within the first four examples are the reciprocal mosaics with white cells of probabilities 0.6—0.9. It is obvious that, as the probability of one cell type increases, the length of the runs of cells of that type tends to increase, whereas, the number of runs of like cells increases to a maximum at p = 0.5 and then decreases.

Included in the program to produce these arrays was a censor component that restricted the samples displayed to those in which the probability did not depart by more than 0.02 from that requested.

Computer analysis

Bob Rupp developed a computer program to generate arrays of 7^6 (117649) B and W cells in which the probability of B varied from 0.1—0.9. At the same time, the runs of B's were tabulated according to length. The number 7^6 was chosen because it was the

largest number with both cube and square roots that could be
accommodated in our computer. This facilitated the production of
straight-sided two- and three-dimensional mosaics, with minimal
surface or volume, the analyses of which could be compared directly
with those of the linear arrays.

A summary of the results obtained is given in column three
of Table 1. This shows that at low probabilities most of the B's
are in single-cell runs, but that even at high probabilities a
significant number of small B runs occur so that the one-cell run
is the mode throughout. At no stage is there a significant percentage of B's in the largest run. The proportion of small runs
decreases as the p increases, but the number of runs increases to
pB = 0.5 and then decreases, confirming the impression given by
the display in Figure 1 and West's (1975) results.

Theoretical validation of computer results

The calculation of the expected number of runs in a procession
of black and white cells is straight forward (Roach 1968). The
number of 1-cell runs of B cells with a probability of p in an
array of N cells is $Np(1-p)^2$, while that of 2-cell runs is
$Np^2(1-p)^2$, and of 3-cell runs $Np^3(1-p)^2$ ... $Np^n(1-p)^2$, whereas the
mean patch size is $\frac{1}{1-p}$.

From the above formulae I calculated the expected number of
runs of each length and the mean run length for arrays of 7^6 cells
(the number used in the computer study) with p = 0.1—0.9. In no
case was there any significant difference between the calculated
and the computer-derived results, thus validating the computer
program.

It is obvious that an infinite patch of B's can only occur
when pB = 1, but then the array is no longer a mosaic. However,
this point is important for comparison with two- and three-dimensional mosaics.

Biological significance

There are many examples of biological linear mosaics: the sex
of a series of offspring, the stained bands on a metaphase chromosome, or the nucleotides on a single strand of DNA. The one most
pertinent to this symposium is the line of cells destined to be the
melanoblasts of the neural crest. These have been discussed by
Lyon (1970), Wolpert and Gingell (1970), Mintz (1971), and others.
They can be represented as two linear mosaics running abreast —
one for each side of the animal. From these cells, two striped
planar mosaics can be developed by simple lateral growth of clones,
as indicated in Figure 2. Similar patterns may be seen in some

TABLE 1. The percentage of B cells in one-, two-, and three-cell patches and in the largest patch in one-, two-, and three-dimensional mosaics of B and W cells in different proportions

Proportion of B cells	Patch size	Dimension(s)		
		one-	two-	three-
0.1	1	80	55	26
	2	18	22	17
	3	1	12	14
	Largest	0	0	0
0.2	1	64	26	5
	2	26	18	4
	3	7	16	3
	Largest	0	0	7
0.3	1	49	12	1
	2	30	10	0
	3	13	11	0
	Largest	0	0	98
0.4	1	36	5	0
	2	29	5	0
	3	17	4	0
	Largest	0	1	100
0.5	1	25	2	0
	2	25	1	0
	3	19	1	0
	Largest	0	10	100
0.6	1	16	0	0
	2	19	0	0
	3	17	0	0
	Largest	0	99	100
0.7	1	9	0	0
	2	13	0	0
	3	13	0	0
	Largest	0	100	100
0.8	1	4	0	0
	2	6	0	0
	3	8	0	0
	Largest	0	100	100
0.9	1	1	0	0
	2	2	0	0
	3	2	0	0
	Largest	0.1	100	100

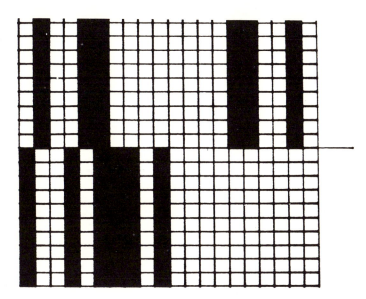

FIGURE 2. Striped planar mosaic simulating lateral clonal growth
from two linear mosaics running abreast.

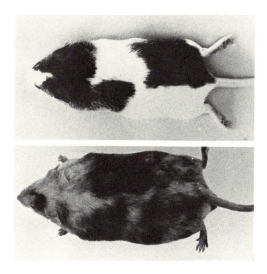

FIGURE 3. Chimeric mice. a. W/W ↔ W/+; b. SJL ↔ C57BL/10.

chimeras, as in Figure 3a, but in this case there may be some non-random clumping characteristic of the $W/W \leftrightarrow W/+$ genotype. The second mouse (Fig. 3b), SJL $\leftrightarrow$ C57BL/10, is much more typical of chimeras and mosaics and indicates there is much more noise in the system than the model in Figure 2 allows.

PLANAR MOSAICS

Cell shape and arrangement

Roach (1968) attempted to analyse two-dimensional mosaics using arrays of square unstaggered cells, but it was difficult to define a patch because such cells have two forms of contact with neighboring cells, side to side and corner to corner (Fig. 4). A more satisfactory approach would have been to study staggered rectangles such as the surfaces of brick walls appear to be. Such

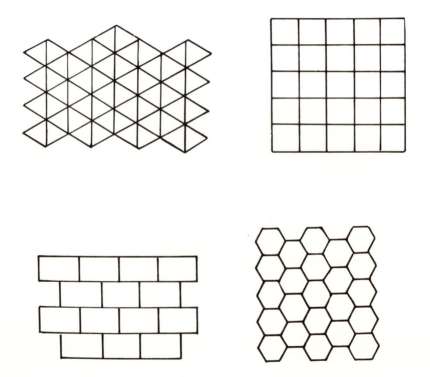

FIGURE 4. Possible shapes of cells packed in two dimensions.

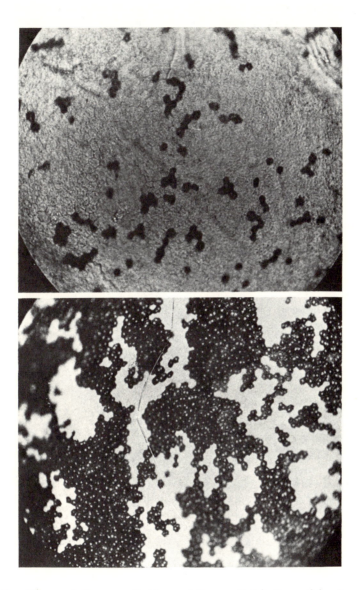

FIGURE 5. Pigment layer of the retinae of 14-day-old mice.
    Top: chimera.
    Bottom: mosaic (Cattanach's translocation). [The mosaic
    is a composite of two photographs because it was not possible
    to keep all of the curved surface in focus.]

rectangles can be considered compressed hexagons that, as Figure 5 indicates, are themselves more realistic representations of sheets of biological cells. A hexagonal cell has 6 equal sides exposed to neighbor contact, so that the simplest patch would be a B cell surrounded by 6 W cells. For models of biological material, it is necessary to assume that all the cells are of equal size. Such an assumption appears more valid for insect material than for mammalian, but Figure 5 indicates that the assumption is not unwarranted even for the latter.

Computer displays

Two-dimensional mosaics of 400 staggered B and W cells are shown in Figs. 6–9. In Figure 6, where pB = 0.1, there are 20 one-cell and 10 two-cell patches. In Figure 7 (pB = 0.2), there are 29 one-cell patches, and the greatest patch contains 5 cells. In Figure 8 (pB = 0.4), there are 17 one- and two-cell patches of B's, and 14 of greater size, but the W cells still form a background lattice with a few of them in islands within the larger black patches. When pB = 0.6, as in Figure 9, the B cells form a background lattice so the picture becomes the "negative" of Fig. 8. Thus mosaics change from "a sea with many islands" to "a land with many lakes" when the probability of one component is between 0.5 and 0.6.

Computer analysis

Bob Rupp developed a program to generate two-dimensional mosaics of 343^2 B and W cells in varying proportions and to tabulate the B patches by size. The summary of this analysis is given in column 4 of Table 1, and it is evident that at low probabilities one-cell patches predominate, but this predominance is not as great as in the linear arrays. Nevertheless, the mode is a one-cell patch from p = 0.1 to p = 0.6. As expected from the display, a dramatic change occurs between p = 0.5 and p = 0.6 so that in the latter almost all of the B cells are part of a background lattice. More refined steps indicate that the changeover takes place near p = 0.52.

Theoretical analysis

Extending the argument used to determine the probability of runs of B cells in linear arrays to two dimensions, it is clear that the probability of a patch composed of one B cell surrounded by 6 W cells is $p(1-p)^6$. When we consider two-cell patches, complications arise because one specific cell may be the partner in 6 different two-cell patches. If we adopt the left to right convention, a specific cell will be the first in only three of these patches — one neighbor to the right above and one below with one on the same level (see Fig. 6). Two-cell patches of B's are surrounded by 8 W cells, so their probability will be $3p^2(1-p)^8$.

Three-cell patches appear in three forms, triangular, straight-linear and bent-linear. The former have 9 neighbors, while the other two have 10 and are more frequent. The probability of the occurrence of three-cell patches is $2p^3(1-p)^9 + 9p^3(1-p)^{10}$. More complicated variations in the shape of larger patches preclude the development of their probability function.

In small arrays, consideration should be given to the effect of the margins on the incidence of patches, because there the number of neighbors is reduced. In our array of 343^2 cells, the margins include about 1% of the cells and can therefore be neglected.

Using the above formulae for the probabilities of small patches, the expected numbers of these were calculated for our standard array of 117649 cells. The results obtained agreed within a few percentage points with those obtained by computer. At pB = 0.56, less than 2% of the B cells occurred as small patches.

Comparison of results

There is remarkable agreement between the results obtained by the visual, computer, and theoretical methods. When the small patches occur in significant numbers, the differences between computer and theoretical values are always less than 10%. No doubt this difference could be reduced by making several determinations and taking the mean. By all three methods, the small patches predominate from p = 0.1 to p = 0.5. Large patches appear at p = 0.5, and at p = 0.6 a background lattice of B-cells contains 99% of all B-cells. Even then, most of the remaining B-cells are in one-, two-, and three-cell patches.

Biological significance

Two-dimensional mosaics are important in development of the derivations of imaginal discs in insects. In mammals, the most obvious planar arrays are in the skin and the pigment layer of the retina.

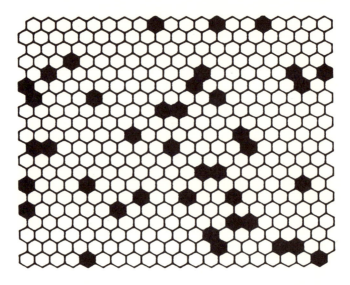

REQUESTED = 0.1   ACTUAL = 0.1000

FIGURE 6

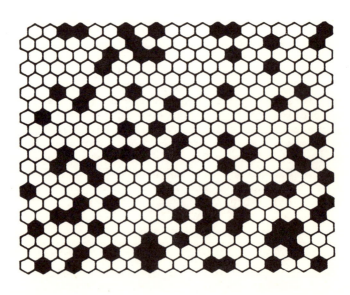

REQUESTED = 0.2   ACTUAL = 0.2000

FIGURE 7

FIGURES 6-9 Two-dimensional mosaic arrays of hexogonal cells,
    with the proportion of black 0.1 and 0.2, 0.4 and 0.6,
    respectively.

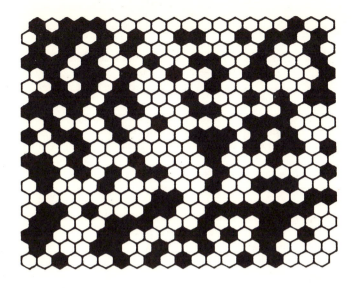

REQUESTED = 0.4   ACTUAL = 0.3900

FIGURE 8

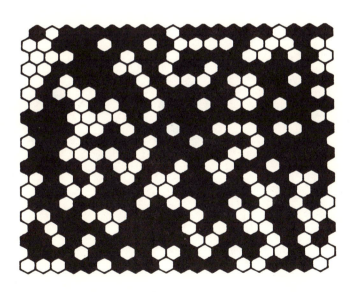

REQUESTED = 0.6   ACTUAL = 0.6075

FIGURE 9

THREE-DIMENSIONAL MOSAICS

Cell shape and arrangement

In order to simulate natural solid mosaics, it is necessary
to make several assumptions about the shape, regularity, and arrangement of the cells concerned. Two potential shapes and organi-
zations are presented in Figure 10. Thompson (1948) has argued
that the 14-sided form meets the requirement for cells packed into
a minimal volume. Such cells have 6 square and 8 larger hexagonal
surfaces, giving a total of 14 to be shared with neighbors, and
there are no edge or corner contacts. It is also possible that in
laminated structures, such as epithelia, a hexagonal cell may sit
directly above or below similar cells. Such a cell would have 6
surface neighbors within its own layer and one in each of the two
adjacent layers, giving a total of 8. In addition, this cell would
have edge contacts with 6 cells in each of the adjacent layers.
Assuming that edge contacts were only half as important as surface
contacts, or that there was some slippage which eliminated half of
them and converted the remaining 6 to minor surfaces, then the
results would also be the equivalent of 14 neighbors, as in the
previous model. Therefore, I have adopted the 14-sided form of
Thompson (1948) in which I assume the sides to be equal and the
cell size to be uniform. The arguments which I develop for arrays
of cells with a minimum of surfaces no doubt will apply to more
complex forms.

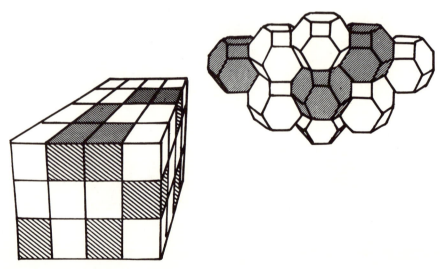

FIGURE 10. Possible shapes and arrangements for cells packed in
three dimensions.

Computer displays

The beginning of a three-dimsnsional mosaic can be represented by overlaying one two-dimensional array with another, as has been done in Figures 11 and 12. The second array was so placed that each cell covered portions of 4 of the first. Thus, each cell in these arrays has 10 neighbors. The addition of a third layer would increase the number of neighbors of cells in the middle array to 14. Thus, this graphical representation portrays the model accurately. In Figure 12 it is obvious that a lattice of B cells is forming, even though the probability of B is only 0.33.

It should be realized that there are twice as many W as B cells in Figure 12, producing a greater, but less obvious, lattice. From this demonstration it is clear that a third dimension greatly facilitates the formation of lattices.

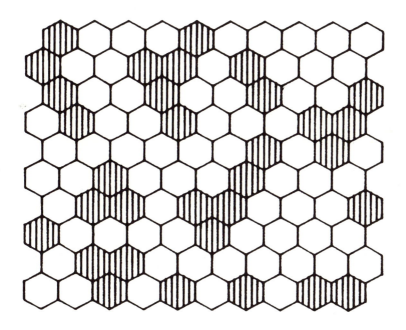

REQUESTED = 0.35   ACTUAL = 0.3300

FIGURE 11. A two-dimensional mosaic of hexagonal cells, some marked with vertical lines.

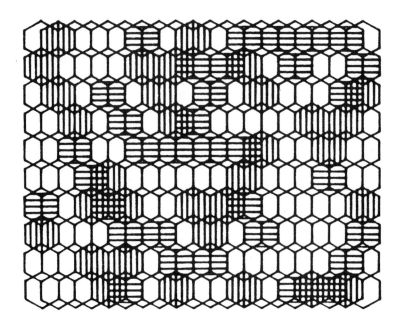

REQUESTED = 0.35   ACTUAL = 0.3300

FIGURE 12. The same array as in Fig. 11, overlaid with a second
   mosaic with some cells marked by horizontal lines. The overlay is placed so that each cell covers part of four cells of
   the original array.

Computer analysis

Bob Rupp developed a difficult program to generate mosaics of
49^3 cells and tabulate the clusters of B cells according to size.
The results of 9 runs, with pB = 0.1—0.9, are summarized in column
5 of Table 1. It is obvious that there are fewer one-cell patches
than in two-dimensional arrays and many fewer than in linear arrays.
This is also portrayed in Figure 13, which graphs the percent of
one-cell clusters in the three forms.

Large clusters develop when pB = 0.2; and by the time pB =
0.3, 98% of B cells are in a background lattice. The critical
change begins at about pB = 0.23 when more than 50% of cells are
found in the lattice.

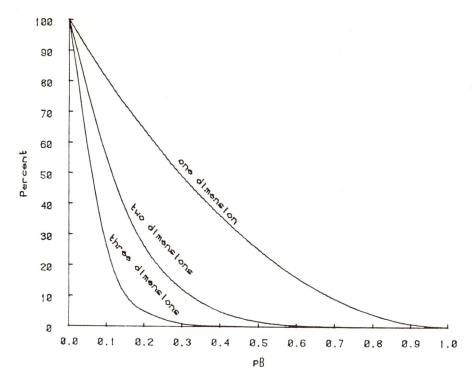

FIGURE 13. Percentage of B cells in one-cell patches in one-, two-, and three-dimensional arrays containing B cells in the proportion of 0.1—0.9.

Theoretical analysis

By the same logic used to analyse two-dimensional mosaics, the probability of one-cell patches in arrays of alternatives in which cells have 14 neighbors is $p(1-p)^{14}$. The probability of two-cell clusters is $7p^2(1-p)^{20}$ and three-cell clusters, $14p^3(1-p)^{25} + 42p^3(1-p)^{28} + 7p^3(1-p)^{30}$. In small arrays, it is essential to make corrections for the reduced number of neighbors of cells on the surfaces which, in this case, make up above 12% of the cells. With these corrections, the results from calculations using the predicted probabilities agree very well with those obtained by computer.

Comparison of results

All methods agree that there are fewer small patches and that background lattices develop rapidly as probability increases. Thus it is clear that both components are present mainly as backgrounds of interlocking lattices for the range of probability of 0.23 to 0.77.

Influence of the number of cells on the appearance of patches in three dimensions

From Table 1, column 5, it is evident that the appearance of patches even of one or two cells is a rare event, except for probabilities less than 0.2. Thus, when p = 0.5, as for a character dependent on inactivation of one X chromosome, 2^{15} cells are required before one can expect a one-cell patch. However, if one allows for the fewer neighbors at the surface so that the mean number of neighbors is 10 then a one-cell patch would be expected once every 2^{11} cells. Such a number of true embryonic cells probably does not appear until after implantation, because two or more sampling events divert many cells to extra-embryonic structures. For a significant number of patches to appear at this stage, as suggested by Nesbitt (1974), it would be necessary to have the cells arranged in very unlikely nonrandom patterns, as in Figure 14.

Biological significance

There is no doubt that most mammalian structures have three dimensions. Even the skin on which mosaic patches occur is several cells thick, which may account for some of the confusing patterns. The method of development of solid tissues and the degree of mixing will determine their final patterns. Analysis of these will be difficult and will have to be built up from sections with only two dimensions. The data presented here will help to visualize the tissue as a whole from such sections. It is clear that parts of interlocking lattices will appear as patches in section.

DISCUSSION

This study has demonstrated that it is possible to quantify random mosaics of one, two, and three dimensions so that, over a wide range, differences of as little as 0.1 in the proportion of cell types produce detectable changes. However, there is one area where this does not hold. In three dimensions, between pB = 0.4 to pB = 0.6, virtually all cells of both components are in one or the other of the background lattices, with almost no one-cell

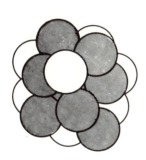 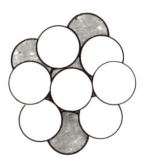

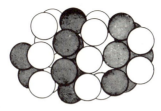

FIGURE 14. Masses of cells comparable to a chimeric embryo at
    aggregation, and to the inner cell mass of a 4½-day embryo.
    Cells arranged to give the maximum number of clusters of like
    cells.

patches. These mosaics are therefore the easiest to characterize
because of the absence of clusters.

The study also indicates that inferences can be made about
more complex arrays from estimates of the proportion of cell types,
and patch size obtained from sections thereof, provided there is
no bias in the method of estimation. For example, it may be easier
to count cells with pigment than those without.

I have considered only random mosaics of *cells*, such as occur
before cell mixing ceases and clonal growth begins. However, it
is obvious from these studies that mosaics of *clones* should develop
in the same proportion and the modal patch will be the single
clone, particularly when it is made up of the minor component.

In Figure 5a one-cell patches predominate and the probability of being pigmented is approximately 0.1. Thus we can conclude that no clonal growth has occurred. In Figure 5b the components are almost equal and there are some one- and two-cell patches. From Table 1 we should expect 2% of each type in this two-dimensional mosaic and could use this tissue from more mature animals to determine the size of clones.

The findings with three-dimensional mosaics make it difficult to comprehend Wegmann's (1970) "intuitive" and much quoted argument that the liver contains about 340 patches. If cell mixing occurred during early development, then two lattices should have formed. The variance found by Wegmann (1970) could have derived from differences in the proportion of each lattice in the samples. More probably, segregation of the genotypes took place in the outgrowths from the primitive gut, but these branched outgrowths coalesced to form the solid liver, and differences in the proportion of the branches were the cause of the variation. The recent finding of 1% one- and two-cell patches by Feder (1976) in chimeric mouse liver is more consistent with our models.

SUMMARY AND CONCLUSIONS

Visual, computer, and combinatorial analyses of mosaics show that patch size varies from single cells to infinite patches or background lattices, depending on the proportion of the components. The proportion of small patches can be calculated for all three dimensions, and the number of such patches decreases rapidly as the number of dimensions of the mosaic increases. Associated with this decrease is the appearance of a background lattice. This cannot occur in a linear mosaic, but begins when $p = 0.52$ for planar mosaics and $p = 0.23$ for cubic mosaics. In the latter case, it follows that both components form interlocking lattices for probabilities ranging from 0.23 to 0.77. No doubt when these mosaics are viewed in section, portions of the lattices appear as patches.

When patches occur, their distribution, according to size, is not normal but hyperbolic, with the one-cell patch being the mode. This indicates that the mean patch size is not a reliable statistic on which to judge mosaics. It would be more realistic to determine the overall proportion of cell types and the distribution of the one-, two-, and three-cell patches.

Because the proportion of small patches is greatest when one component occurs as a distinct minority, such mosaics should be more useful for determining clone size. The blastocyst injection technique (Gardner 1968) could yield a higher proportion of such chimeras than does embryo aggregation.

Finally, two percent of cells of each type occur as one-cell patches in two-dimensional mosaics when the proportion of cell types is equal. This suggests that the clone size for planar tissues, such as the pigment layer of the retina, could be determined in mice with Cattanach's translocation.

Supported by National Institute of Child Health and Human Development Grant HD 04083. The Jackson Laboratory is fully accredited by the American Association for Accreditation of Laboratory Animal Care.

REFERENCES

Feder, N. 1976. Solitary cells and enzyme exchange in tetraparental mice. Nature 263: 67-69.

Gardner, R. L. 1968. Mouse chimaeras obtained by the injection of cells into the blastocyst. Nature 220: 596-597.

Lyon, M. F. 1970. Genetic activity of sex chromosomes in somatic cells of mammals. Phil. Trans. Roy. Soc. London B. 259: 41-52.

Mintz, B. 1971. Clonal basis of mammalian differentiation. Control mechanisms of growth and differentiation. Symp. Soc. Exp. Biol. 25: 345-370.

Nesbitt, M. W. 1974. Chimerics vs. X inactivation mosaics: significance of differences in pigment distribution. Develop. Biol. 58: 202-207.

Roach, S. A. 1968. The Theory of Random Clumping. Methuen, London.

Stevens, W. L. 1939. Distribution of groups in a sequence of alternatives. Ann. Eugenics 9: 10-17.

Thompson, D. W. 1948. On Growth and Form. 2nd ed. McMillan, New York.

Wegmann, T. G. 1970. Enzyme patterns in tetraparental mouse liver. Nature 225: 462-463.

West, J. D. 1975. A theoretical approach to the relation between patch size and clone size in chimeric tissue. J. Theor. Biol. 50: 153-160.

Wolpert, T. G. and D. Gingell. 1970. Striping and the pattern of melanocyte cells in chimaeric mice. J. Theor. Biol. 29: 147-150.

DATA ANALYSIS OF FOUR X-CHROMOSOME INACTIVATION EXPERIMENTS

Victor E. Kane

Mathematics and Statistics Research Department,
Computer Sciences Division, Union Carbide Corporation,
Nuclear Division, Oak Ridge, Tennessee 37830

Some experiments on mosaics result in data that suggest one or more developmental models usually consisting of alternative biological processes having several unknown parameters. If each experimental subject responded in an identical fashion, a mathematical formulation might be appropriate. However, since random fluctuations are often inherent in the developmental system, a statistical model incorporating randomness is necessary. This paper presents the biological assumptions and a developmental model which appear to be used in data analysis of four experiments (Nesbitt 1971; Fialkow 1973; Nance 1964; and Migeon 1971). The simplest statistical estimation scheme is presented here; complete details are given elsewhere (Kane 1975). The emphasis is on the results of the parameter estimates and on hypothesis testing in the four experiments.

BIOLOGICAL ASSUMPTIONS AND DEVELOPMENTAL MODEL

There are two types of cells in most female mammals: cells with the paternal X inactivated and cells with the maternal X inactivated. For simplicity, the two types of cells will be denoted by A and B. Mosaic individuals form a natural statistical framework in that the distribution of A and B cells in various tissues of the adult is dependent on developmental processes. The following assumptions concern the biological processes that give rise to the final observed distribution of A and B cells.

Assumption 1. Each cell undergoes the initial inactivation process independent of every other cell, and all cells have the same probability of being an A cell.

Assumption 2. The process of X inactivation is synchronous.

Assumption 3. After X inactivation has occurred in a cell, this cell cannot alter which X chromosome is inactivated.

Assumption 4. At the time of organ determination, clonal cell growth with respect to A and B cells has not yet occurred in the embryo.

Assumption 5. The rate of growth for A and B cells is identical.

Assumption 6. In the adult, the X chromosome of any given cell is either active or inactive with respect to the quantity being measured.

It is relatively easy to find individual examples in which any one (or more) of the above assumptions is probably not true. Justification and discussion of the assumptions is given in Kane (1978).

Using the above assumptions, Nesbitt (1971) has suggested a scheme of X inactivation in which it is possible to model the between- and within-individual variation that is observed in mosaic populations. The following is a statistical formalization of Nesbitt's biological model. The relevant assumptions are given in parentheses following each step.

Let θ be the probability of an A cell at the time of X inactivation. After inactivation in a cell pool of size n_0, there is a proportion p_0 of A cells (*Assumptions 1 and 2*). This cell pool grows to a size n_0^* with the same proportion p_0 of A cells (*Assumptions 3 and 5*). Then a hypergeometric sampling event occurs. Each of the t tissues to be formed in the adult develops a primordial precursor-cell pool by withdrawing n_{1j} cells $j=1,\ldots,t$ from the large cell pool of size n_0^* (*Assumption 4*). This results in a proportion p_{1j} of A cells in the j-th organ. Then each of the r organs (or tissues) to be experimentally sampled undergoes s-1 stages of growth and hypergeometric sampling. Thus, for the j-th organ the i-th stage consists of withdrawing n_{ij} cells from a large cell pool, $n_{i-1,j}^*$, which has a proportion $p_{i-1,j}$ of A cells. A proportion p_{ij} of A cells is obtained, and this cell pool then grows to a size n_{ij}^* with proportion p_{ij} of A cells (*Assumptions 3 and 5*). The final cell pool then grows into an adult organ of size $n_{s-1,j}^*$ with proportion $p_{s-1,j}$ of A cells (*Assumptions 3 and 5*). In the s-th stage, the experimenter samples r organs, where r is much less than t, and observes n_{sj} cells with a proportion p_{sj} of A cells in the j-th organ (*Assumption 6*). The mathematical developmental model is illustrated in Figure 1. Nesbitt (1971) considers the case s = 2. The motivation for the s stage model stems from the multistage development of organ systems.

A final mathematical assumption is necessary for formulation of the Gaussian and binomial model that enables estimation of θ and n_0, and for the testing of hypotheses arising from the biological model.

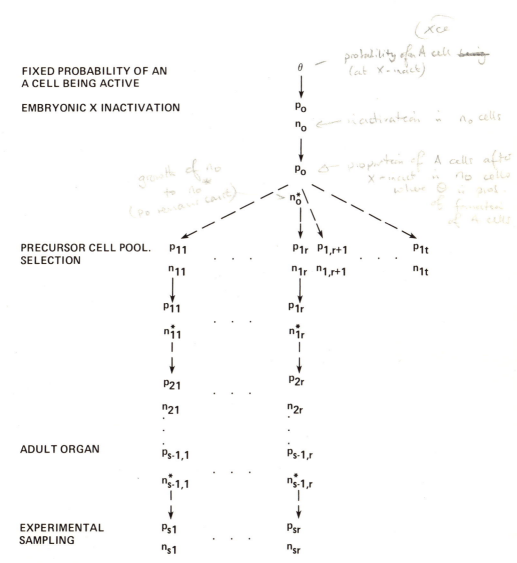

FIXED PROBABILITY OF AN A CELL BEING ACTIVE

EMBRYONIC X INACTIVATION

PRECURSOR CELL POOL. SELECTION

ADULT ORGAN

EXPERIMENTAL SAMPLING

FIGURE 1. Illustration of an s stage model for mammalian development, where r organs are experimentally sampled. Dashed lines represent a sampling event, and continuous lines represent growth.

Assumption 7. The precursor cell pool sizes for an organ (n_{1j}) are small compared to the number of cells in the enlarged cell pool (n_0^*) from which precursor cells are being withdrawn. Also, the cell pool sizes after the (i-1)-th period of growth (n_{ij}^*) are large with respect to the number of cells sampled for the i-th period (n_{ij}).

SELECTED STATISTICAL COMPUTATIONS

The scheme depicted in Figure 1 is a general hypergeometric sampling that may be appropriate for many developmental precursor cell-pool selection experiments. *Assumptions 1–7* enable the hypergeometric sampling to be approximated by binomial sampling which results in

$$E(P_{sj}) = \theta, \tag{1}$$

$$\text{Variance}(P_{sj}) = \theta(1-\theta) \left[1 - (1-n_0^{-1}) \prod_{i=1}^{s} (1-n_{ij}^{-1})\right], \tag{2}$$

$$\text{Covariance}(P_{sj}, P_{sk}) = \theta(1-\theta)/n_0, \tag{3}$$

where $E(P)$ denotes the expected or average observed P. Nesbitt (1971) derived the above moments for s = 2, using a binomial model (Kane 1975).

While the formation of an individual is known to undergo many stages of development, it is not necessary to consider stages other than those for which n_{ij} is small. If n_{ij} is large with respect to n_{kj}, then $(1 - n_{ij}^{-1})$ will be close to 1 and large with respect to $(1 - n_{kj}^{-1})$. Thus, the variance (2) will not change appreciably by neglecting large n_{ij}. This is intuitively appealing, since the experimenter may simply model the major sampling events for an organ to explain the observed variances and covariances. The above argument gives credence to Nesbitt's (1970, 1971) two-stage model, where she in effect postulates that the two major sampling events after inactivation are organ determination and experimental sampling.

The binomial model is useful for estimating θ, n_0, and n_{1j}, but it is difficult statistically to test hypotheses concerning alternative developmental models. However, it is possible to develop a multivariate Gaussian model by using several approximations. The Gaussian model enables statistical testing of many developmental hypotheses. In the Gaussian model, the vector of proportions $(p_{s1}, \ldots, p_{sj})$ has a multivariate Gaussian distribution with mean $\theta \underline{1}$ and covariance matrix $\theta(1-\theta)\Sigma$ where

$$\Sigma = \text{diagonal} \left(\sum_{i=1}^{s} n_{ij} \right) + n_0^{-1} \underline{1} \, \underline{1}' . \tag{4}$$

Considering s=2 and a sample of N individuals, where r tissues are sampled in each individual, the vector of proportions $\underline{P}_{s\alpha} = (P_{s1\alpha},\ldots,P_{sr\alpha})'$ is observed for the α-th individual. The simplest estimators are the moment estimators

$$\hat{\theta} = (Nr)^{-1} \sum_{j=1}^{r} \sum_{\alpha=1}^{N} p_{sj\alpha} = r^{-1} \sum_{j=1}^{r} \overline{P}_{sj} = \overline{P}_s , \tag{5}$$

$$\hat{n}_0^{-1} = [\hat{\theta}(1-\hat{\theta}) \, r(r-1)]^{-1} \sum_{i \neq j} \sum s_{ij} , \tag{6}$$

$$\left(\sum_{i=1}^{s} \hat{n}_{ij}^{-1} \right)^{-1} = [\hat{\theta}(1-\hat{\theta})]^{-1} s_{jj} - \hat{n}_0^{-1} , \tag{7}$$

where

$$s_{ij} = (N-1)^{-1} \sum_{\alpha=1}^{N} (p_{si\alpha} - \overline{P}_{wi})(p_{sj\alpha} - \overline{P}_{sj}) , \tag{8}$$

and for any parameter λ, the quantity $\hat{\lambda}$ denotes an estimate of λ.

Maximum likelihood estimates of θ, n_0, and $\sum_{i=1}^{s} n_{ij}^{-1}$ are statistically superior to the moment estimators, but require computer computations. The moment estimators in (5), (6), and (7) can be altered to account for individuals in which each of the r tissues is not examined, where maximum likelihood estimation techniques are currently not developed for this case.

A consequence of the statistical model is that the moment or maximum likelihood estimates of θ and n_0 do not depend on the number of multistage developmental parameters, i.e., $n_{s1},\ldots,n_{sr}$. For developmental models having an arbitrary number of stages, or a different number of stages for each organ, the estimates of θ and n_0 would not change.

HYPOTHESIS TESTING

It is possible to use the Gaussian model to test many developmental hypotheses of current interest. Letting H_i and A_i, respectively, denote the null and alternative hypotheses, some examples include:

H_1: The experimentally sampled organs are related only by the inactivation event.

A_1: Cell-lineage relationships exist for the experimentally sampled organs.

H_2: Inactivation occurred after tissue differentiation.

A_2: Inactivation occurred before tissue differentiation.

H_3: No change (cell selection) in the relative proportion of A and B cells occurs during organ growth.

A_3: Cell selection exists.

H_4: Random inactivation is present ($\theta = 1/2$).

A_4: Nonrandom inactivation is present ($\theta \neq 1/2$).

H_5: A specified group of experimentally sampled tissues had the same inactivation probability (θ).

A_5: Cell selection exists for the specified group of experimentally sampled tissues.

H_6: There are distinct precursor-cell pools for a specified group of experimentally sampled tissues.

A_6: There is a common precursor-cell pool for the specified group of experimentally sampled tissues.

H_7: The process of inactivation is synchronous throughout the embryo.

A_7: Inactivation is asynchronous.

Another hypothesis-testing problem arises from cell-lineage determinations. The experimentor seeks to determine if various distinct adult cell groups followed the same developmental pathway. Cell pools arising from the same pathway would be more alike in A and B composition than cell pools arising from diverse pathways. Thus, the hypotheses:

H_8: There are distinct precursor cell pools for the first k experimentally sampled tissues.

A_8: There is a common precursor cell pool for the first k experimentally sampled tissues.

Figure 2 depicts the developmental scheme under A_8.

EXPERIMENTAL DATA

Nesbitt's data

Nesbitt (1970, 1971) analyzed approximately 7000 cells of female mice carrying the Cattanach translocation (Cattanach 1961). Females with this translocation have one X chromosome that has a piece of an autosome inserted into it (X^t), while the remaining X chromosome is normal (X^n). Nesbitt and Gartler (1970) demonstrated that it was possible to determine which of the X chromosomes (X^n or X^t) was active in the metaphase cells. These data (Nesbitt 1970, 1972), expressed as proportions, and the total number of cells counted, appear in Table 1.

The results of the statistical analysis appear in Table 2. The estimates of θ and n_0 are relatively stable where the tissue precursor-cell pool sizes are somewhat dependent on the estimation

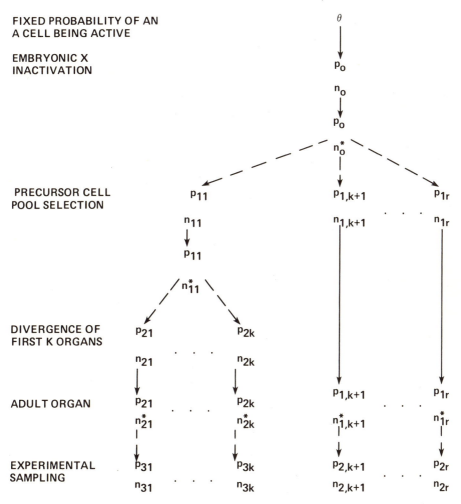

FIXED PROBABILITY OF AN A CELL BEING ACTIVE

EMBRYONIC X INACTIVATION

PRECURSOR CELL POOL SELECTION

DIVERGENCE OF FIRST K ORGANS

ADULT ORGAN

EXPERIMENTAL SAMPLING

FIGURE 2. Illustration of a model for mammalian development for the r organs experimentally sampled, where the first k organs share a common precursor-cell pool. Dashed lines represent sampling, and continuous lines represent growth.

TABLE 1. Proportions of cells with an active X^t and number of cells observed for five tissues (from Nesbitt, 1971).

Animal	Right lung $P_{1\alpha}$	$n_{1\alpha}$	Left lung $P_{2\alpha}$	$n_{2\alpha}$	Abdominal fascia $P_{3\alpha}$	$n_{3\alpha}$	Spleen $P_{4\alpha}$	$n_{4\alpha}$	Thymus $P_{5\alpha}$	$n_{5\alpha}$
1	1.000	82	$-$[†]	$-$	$-$	$-$	$-$	$-$	$-$	$-$
2	.657	35	.361	36	$-$	$-$	$-$	$-$	$-$	$-$
3	.521	48	.717	46	$-$	$-$	$-$	$-$	$-$	$-$
4	.718	47	.553	39	$-$	$-$	$-$	$-$	.590	39
5	.487	39	.370	27	$-$	$-$	$-$	$-$	$-$	$-$
6	.704	54	.553	38	$-$	$-$	.824	34	$-$	$-$
7	.600	45	.658	38	$-$	$-$	$-$	$-$	$-$	$-$
8	.855	62	.849	53	$-$	$-$	$-$	$-$	$-$	$-$
9	.587	45	.349	43	.273	55	$-$	$-$	$-$	$-$
10	.742	98	.673	62	$-$	$-$	$-$	$-$	$-$	$-$
11	.705	44	.889	45	.762	42	$-$	$-$	$-$	$-$
12*	.548	42	.608	46	.375	40	.622	37	.579	38
13	.500	34	.580	43	.300	30	.560	41	$-$	$-$
14*	.217	46	.513	39	.308	39	.571	24	.694	36
15*	.353	51	.457	46	.316	38	.364	33	.686	35
16*	.462	39	.550	40	.538	39	.306	49	.615	26
17*	.552	38	.774	31	.571	42	.634	41	.454	37
18	.488	41	.548	42	.673	52	$-$	$-$	.625	40
19	.625	32	.525	40	.454	33	.538	39	$-$	$-$
20	.573	38	.550	40	.317	41	.467	15	.822	34
21	.629	35	.600	35	$-$	$-$	.342	38	.771	35
22	.690	42	.727	33	.710	31	.788	33	$-$	$-$
23*	.676	37	.480	25	.571	42	.575	40	.639	36
24*	.561	41	.565	46	.611	36	.500	38	.943	35
25*	.410	39	.350	40	.400	40	.189	37	.359	39
26*	.815	38	.703	37	.625	40	.659	44	.667	30
27	.725	98	.730	37	.646	46	$-$	$-$	.688	48
28*	.604	48	.444	45	.615	39	.370	46	.614	44
29	.600	55	.389	36	$-$	$-$	.444	54	.458	48
30	.360	50	.341	44	$-$	$-$	.205	44	.156	45
31*	.489	47	.392	51	.560	50	.477	44	.448	29
32	.500	50	.491	53	$-$	$-$	.590	49	.457	46
33*	.551	49	.574	47	.640	50	.744	43	.642	53
34	.522	46	.250	52	.542	48	.490	51	.400	10

* Denotes animals used in subsequent complete data analyses.

† A "$-$" designates missing data.

TABLE 2. Maximum-likelihood and moment estimates of developmental parameters with asymptotic 90% confidence intervals, using Nesbitt's (1971) data

Estimation procedure*	Probability of an Xt cell being inactivated $\hat{\theta}$	Number of cell at time of X chromosome inactivation $\hat{n}_0$	Precursor cell pool sizes				
			Right lung $\hat{n}_1$	Left lung $\hat{n}_2$	Abdominal fascia $\hat{n}_3$	Spleen $\hat{n}_4$	Thymus $\hat{n}_5$
Maximum likelihood	.526	34	51	158	144	27	12
Confidence intervals	(.480,.572)	(4,64)	(20,∞)	(36,∞)	(34,∞)	(13,∞)	(6,117)
Moment	.536	34	24	144	113	18	31
Confidence intervals	(.484,.587)	(12,∞)	(6,∞)	(12,∞)	(12,∞)	(5,∞)	(7,∞)
Maximum likelihood	$\theta = .5$ assumed	31	57	129	199	28	11
Confidence intervals		(5,57)	(22,∞)	(33,∞)	(39,∞)	(13,∞)	(6,97)
Moment	$\theta = .5$ assumed	33	29	185	338	23	14
Confidence intervals		(11,∞)	(7,∞)	(13,∞)	(14,∞)	(6,∞)	(4,∞)

* Only the 12 animals denoted by a "*" in Table 1 are used in this analysis since the data are complete and is n_{2j}'s are relatively constant.

procedure. Note that the analyses in Table 2 include only the data which closely meet the statistical assumptions; there are no missing data for tissues, and the n_{22}'s are relatively constant within a tissue. Using all the data and assuming s=2 moment estimates are $\hat{\theta}$ = .549, $\hat{n}_0$ = 26, $\hat{n}_1$ = 30, $\hat{n}_2$ = 29, $\hat{n}_3$ = 32, $\hat{n}_4$ = 19, and $\hat{n}_5$ = 17.

Hypothesis-testing results presented by Kane (1975) include:
  (i)   The form of the statistical model is consistent with the observed data.
 (ii)   The five tissues are related by the inactivation event (H_1).
(iii)   Inactivation occurred before tissue differentiation (A_2).
 (iv)   No change occurs during tissue growth in the proportion of X^t inactivated (H_3).

Fialkow's data

Fialkow (1973) analyzed 42 human females heterozygous for G6PD enzyme variants. Six organs were studied (red blood cells, granulocytes, blood lymphocytes, lymph node, skin, and skeletal muscle) with many observations not taken on all the organs for various individuals. Upon graphing, it is uncertain that the data have a Gaussian distribution. The histograms appear to be skewed toward the left of 1/2. The summary statistics for the 6 tissues and precursor-cell pool size estimates appear in Table 3. The hypothesis of random inactivation cannot be rejected; thus, θ is assumed to be 1/2. The estimate of the number of cells at the time of X inactivation is $\hat{n}_0$ = 17.

TABLE 3. Summary statistics from Fialkow's (1973) data

Organ	Red cells	Granu-locytes	Blood lympho-cytes	Lymph node	Skin	Skeletal muscle
Mean proportion	.44	.46	.48	.45	.49	.33
Standard deviation	.15	.13	.11	.16	.12	.22
Number of observations	42	42	20	10	18	5
Estimate of precursor cell pool size (n_2)	31	116	∞	25	427	—

Nance's data

Nance (1964) collected data from the blood of 30 human females
known to be heterozygous for G6PD enzyme variants. The data are
presented graphically in Figure 2 of Nance's paper, and may be
shown in tabular form as follows:

proportion of enzyme A cells	0—.1	.1—.3	.3—.4	.4—.6	.6—.7	.7—.9	.9—1.0
frequency	0	2	4	8	10	5	1

From Nance's Figure 2, it is apparent that a Gaussian approximation
to the distribution of the proportion of A cells would be appropriate. Using the above data, Nance approximated values in an interval by the midpoint of the interval ($\bar{p}$ = .575, s^2 = .03375). Then
assuming that inactivation occurred after organ determination,
Nance estimated the number of blood precursor cells to be 18 by
minimum chi-square methods. Nesbitt (1971) reanalyzed Nance's data
and estimated fewer than 10 precursor cells by her method of moment
estimation. As noted by Nesbitt (1970), it is not possible to estimate the parameters of the two-stage model from a single organ.
However, it may be of interest to study the range of possible values. Using moment estimates for grouped data, $\hat{\theta}$ = .575 and m^{-1} +
n_0^{-1} = .124, where m is assumed to be the precursor-cell pool size
for the G6PD-associated tissue. Figure 3(a) displays values of $\hat{m}$
and $\hat{n}_0$ that are consistent with Nance's data. Using $\hat{n}_0$ = 17 from
Fialkow's data results in $\hat{m}$(G6PD) = 15.

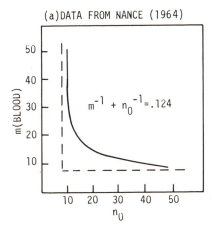
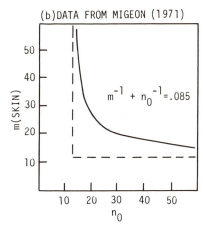

FIGURE 3. Graphic characterization of the two-stage model using
    data from a single organ

Migeon's data

In a study of HGPRT deficiency in humans, Migeon (1971) concluded that there was no selection against HGPRT deficient (HGPRT⁻)
cells. Twenty-one female heterozygotes were sampled. The frequency
distribution is slightly skewed ($\bar{p}$ = .531, s^2 = .0212) toward a
larger proportion of normal cells (HGPRT⁺). However, since the
sample size is small, it is not possible to determine if the skew-
ness is due to sampling variations or to cell selection. A 95%
confidence interval for θ is (.464, .597). Therefore, random inactivation (θ = 1/2) cannot be rejected. (Two subjects were replicated and the weighted average of these observations was taken.)

Migeon shows that due to the larger-than-expected observed
variance, the proportions of HGPRT⁺ cells do not follow a normal
approximation to the binomial sampling scheme. She suggests the
following possible explanations: (1) small size of the cell population at the time of inactivation; (2) tissue and individual variations in the timing of inactivation; (3) discriminant (non-random)
inactivation; (4) post-inactivation selections of one cell type;
and (5) patterns of cell migration. If one considers the variance
of the two-stage model (as well as any higher-stage model), the
variance of the proportions are $\theta(1-\theta)[n_0^{-1} + m^{-1} + n^{-1}]$ as opposed
to the binomial variance, $\theta(1-\theta)n^{-1}$, used by Migeon. Since the n's
were generally very large, n_0 or m could be small and increase the
variance to fit the observed data.

In particular, $\hat{m}^{-1} + \hat{n}_0^{-1}$ = .085 is implied from the data.
Figure 3(b) displays values of $\hat{m}$ and $\hat{n}_0$ that are consistent with
Migeon's data. Using $\hat{n}_0$ = 17 from Fialkow's data results in
$\hat{m}$(skin) = 38.

SUMMARY

A statistical model of embryonic development is presented
which formalizes estimation of the probability that a particular X
chromosome is inactivated. It is possible to estimate the cell-
pool size at the time of both X-chromosome inactivation and organ-
precursor cell-pool selection. Some developmental hypotheses of
interest are also tested statistically. A byproduct of the statistical model is a precise formulation of the biological and statistical assumptions implicitly used in the data analysis of some
mosaic experiments. An analysis of four X-chromosome experiments
is presented to illustrate the application of the statistical
model.

REFERENCES

Cattanach, B. M. 1961. A chemically-induced variegation-type position effect in the mouse. Z. Vererbungslehre $\underline{92}$: 165-182.

Fialkow, P. J. 1973. Primordial cell pool size and lineage relationships of five human cell types. Ann. of Human Genet. $\underline{37}$: 39-48.

Kane, V. E. 1975. Statistical models for X chromosome inactivation. Ph.D. Dissertation, Florida State University.

Kane, V. E. 1978. Stochastic models for X chromosome inactivation. Submitted.

Migeon, B. R. 1971. Studies of skin fibroblasts from 10 families with HGPRT deficiency, with reference to X-chromosome inactivation. Am. J. of Human Genet. $\underline{23}$: 199-210.

Nance, W. E. 1964. Genetic tests with sex-linked marker: glucose-6-phosphate dehydrogenase. Cold Spring Harbor Symp. on Quant. Biol. $\underline{29}$: 415-425.

Nesbitt, M. N. 1970. X chromosome inactivation mosaicism in the mouse. Ph.D. Dissertation, University of Washington.

Nesbitt, M. N. 1971. X chromosome inactivation mosaicism in the mouse. Develop. Biol. $\underline{26}$: 252-263.

Nesbitt, M. N. 1972. Personal communication.

Nesbitt. M. N. and Gartler, S. M. 1970. Replication of the mouse sex chromosome early in the S period. Cytogenet. $\underline{9}$: 212-221.